Thoracic Imaging

A Core Review

Second Edition

Thoracic Imaging

A Core Review

Second Edition

EDITORS

Stephen B. Hobbs, MD, FSCCT

Associate Professor
Departments of Radiology and Medicine
Vice-Chair, Radiology Informatics and Integrated Clinical Operations
Chief, Division of Cardiovascular and Thoracic Radiology
Medical Director, UK HealthCare Imaging Informatics
University of Kentucky
Lexington, Kentucky

Christian W. Cox, MD

Assistant Professor
Division of Thoracic Radiology
Department of Radiology
Mayo Clinic
Rochester, Minnesota

Series Editor
Biren A. Shah, MD, FACR

Clinical Professor of Radiology
Wayne State University School of Medicine
Associate Residency Program Director
Section Chief, Breast Imaging
Detroit Medical Center
Detroit, Michigan

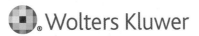

Philadelphia • Baltimore • New York • London
Buenos Aires • Hong Kong • Sydney • Tokyo

Acquisitions Editor: Sharon Zinner
Development Editor: Eric McDermott
Editorial Coordinator: John Larkin
Production Product Manager: Sadie Buckallew
Senior Manufacturing Coordinator: Beth Welsh
Design Coordinator: Stephen Druding
Prepress Vendor: SPi Global

Cataloging-in-Publication Data available on request from the Publisher

ISBN: 978-1-9751-2622-3

Shop.lww.com

To my wife, Fareesh, the love of my life. Your kindness
makes the world a better place.

To my daughters, Ameera and Niya, the prides of my life.
Your spirits brighten every day.

—STEPHEN B. HOBBS

To my mom, Courtney Cox, and my late dad, Robert B. Cox, MD.
To the men who guided and mentored me since the passing of my dad,
particularly Tom Guderian.

—CHRISTIAN W. COX

CONTRIBUTORS

Mohamed Tarek Seleem Ahmed, MBBCh, MSc
Clinical Instructor
Department of Cardiology and Angiology
Alexandria University
Alexandria, Egypt

Tami J. Bang, MD
Assistant Professor
Department of Radiology
University of Colorado–Anschutz Medical Campus
Aurora, Colorado

Michael A. Brooks, MD
Professor
Department of Radiology
University of Kentucky
Lexington, Kentucky

Said Chaaban, MD
Assistant Professor of Medicine
Department of Pulmonary and Critical Care
University of Kentucky
Lexington, Kentucky

Angel O. Coz Yataco, MD, FCCP
Associate Professor of Medicine
College of Medicine
University of Kentucky
Lexington, Kentucky

David W. Grant, Jr., DO
Assistant Professor
Department of Radiology
Uniformed Services University of the Health
    Sciences
Bethesda, Maryland

Christopher Lee, MD
Associate Professor
Department of Radiology
Keck School of Medicine
University of Southern California
Los Angeles, California

James T. Lee, MD
Associate Professor
Department of Radiology
University of Kentucky
Lexington, Kentucky

Conor M. Lowry, MD
Assistant Professor
Department of Radiology
University of Kentucky
Lexington, Kentucky

David A. Lynch, MD
Professor
Department of Radiology
National Jewish Health
Denver, Colorado

Jeremiah T. Martin, MBBch, MSCRD, FRSCI
Clinical Assistant Professor
Ohio University
Athens, Ohio

David Nickels, MD, MBA
Associate Professor
Department of Radiology
University of Kentucky
Lexington, Kentucky

Andrea Oh, MD
Assistant Professor
Department of Radiology
National Jewish Health
Denver, Colorado

Carlos A. Rojas, MD
Associate Professor
Department of Radiology
Mayo Clinic
Jacksonville, Florida

Anne-Marie G. Sykes, MD
Assistant Professor
Department of Radiology
Mayo Clinic Graduate School of Medicine
Rochester, Minnesota

Christopher M. Walker, MD
Associate Professor
Department of Radiology
University of Kansas Medical Center
Kansas City, Kansas

Lara Walkoff, MD
Assistant Professor
Department of Radiology
Mayo Clinic
Rochester, Minnesota

Michael Winkler, MD
Professor
Department of Radiology
Augusta University
Augusta, Georgia

Marianna Zagurovskaya, MD
Associate Professor
Department of Radiology
University of Kentucky
Lexington, Kentucky

The second edition of the *Thoracic Imaging: A Core Review* builds on the success of the first edition by covering the essential aspects of thoracic imaging in a manner that serves as a guide for residents to assess their knowledge and review the material in a format that is similar to the ABR core examination.

The print copy of the *Thoracic Imaging: A Core Review, second edition*, still contains 300 questions. Some questions from the first edition have been kept, while some have been replaced to maximize the relevance to current practice. Approximately 25% to 35% of new questions have been added to the second edition, with the e-book containing an additional 118 questions to the 300 questions in print.

Dr. Hobbs and Dr. Cox have done an excellent job in producing a book that exemplifies the philosophy and goals of the *Core Review Series*. They have done a meticulous job in covering key topics and providing quality images. The questions have been divided logically into chapters so as to make it easy for learners to work on particular topics as needed. There are mostly multiple-choice questions with some extended matching questions. Each question has a corresponding answer with an explanation of not only why a particular option is correct but also why the other options are incorrect. There are also references provided for each question for those who want to delve more deeply into a specific subject.

The intent of the *Core Review Series* is to provide the resident, fellow, or practicing physician a review of the important conceptual, factual, and practical aspects of a subject with multiple choice questions in a format similar to the ABR core examination. The *Core Review Series* is not intended to be exhaustive but to provide material likely to be tested on the ABR core examination and that would be required in clinical practice.

As Series Editor of the *Core Review Series*, it has been rewarding not only to be a coeditor of one of the books in this series but also to work with so many talented individuals in the profession of radiology across the country. This series represents countless hours of work and involvement by many, and it would not have come together without their participation. It has been very gratifying to receive numerous positive comments from residents of the difference they feel the series has made in their board preparation.

I would like to thank Dr. Hobbs and Dr. Cox for their dedication to the series and for doing an exceptional job on the second edition. I believe *Thoracic Imaging: A Core Review, second edition*, will serve as a valuable resource for residents during their board preparation and a useful reference for fellows and practicing radiologists.

Biren A. Shah, MD, FACR
Clinical Professor of Radiology
Wayne State University School of Medicine
Associate Residency Program Director
Section Chief, Breast Imaging
Detroit Medical Center
Detroit, Michigan

PREFACE

We are honored to again be the editors of *Thoracic Imaging: A Core Review*. Current day practice of thoracic imaging requires a robust understanding of not only just imaging but also underlying pathology and management strategies. This book calls upon expert authors in thoracic imaging from across the country to help readers gauge their level of expertise and fill knowledge gaps through evaluation of real cases and scenarios that occur in daily practice. We are grateful for their contributions and assistance in preparing this work.

For residents and practicing radiologists alike, the educational material covered in these pages serves as preparation for both the ABR core board examination and the new Maintenance of Certification Ongoing Longitudinal Assessment (OLA). The questions are divided into different sections directly adapted from the ABR study syllabus to make it easy for readers to work through specific topics. Explanations are concise with key learning points and review references for further exploration if needed.

There are multiple individuals (past fellows, current colleagues, and senior mentors) who contributed to this publication. This work could not have been finished without their efforts. Each of them took time from their lives to research, write, and submit content in a timely manner. Our heartfelt thanks to all of them.

Last, but not least, we are incredibly grateful to our families, who have again endured long hours of work and encouraged us throughout the process.

Stephen B. Hobbs
Christian W. Cox

ACKNOWLEDGMENTS

We would like to acknowledge Peter Sachs, MD, University of Colorado, for contributing to the images found in this work.

CONTENTS

1

Basics of Imaging

Conor M. Lowry, MD

QUESTIONS

1 What is responsible for the following artifact?

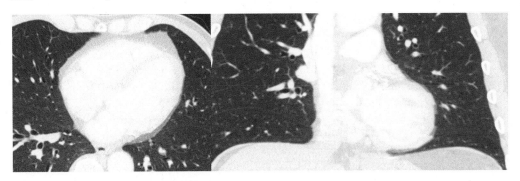

   A. Patient unable to hold breath
   B. Detector malfunction
   C. Patient seizure
   D. Tachycardia

2 Which of the following measurements of CT radiation dose takes into account the anatomic region and tissue being scanned?
   A. CT dose index (CTDI)
   B. Volumetric CT dose index ($CTDI_{vol}$)
   C. Dose–length product (DLP)
   D. Effective dose

3 When protocoling an order for an outpatient chest CT with intravenous contrast, it is discovered that the patient has a stable eGFR of 34 mL/min/ 1.73 mm, and the technologist is concerned about the possible risk of contrast-induced nephropathy (CIN). According to the American College of Radiology, above what eGFR is there very little evidence that IV iodinated contrast is considered an independent risk factor for CIN?
   A. >25 mL/min/1.73 mm^2
   B. >30 mL/min/1.73 mm^2
   C. >35 mL/min/1.73 mm^2
   D. >45 mL/min/1.73 mm^2

4a Explain the appearance of the CT pulmonary angiogram below.

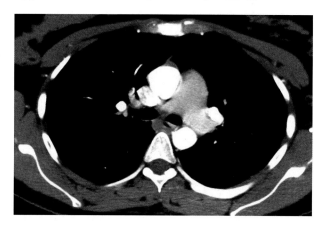

A. Imaging delayed relative to contrast bolus
B. Transient interruption of contrast
C. Imaging early relative to contrast bolus
D. Contrast bolus interrupted by extravasation

4b What physiologic process explains the phenomenon of transient interruption of contrast?

A. Unopacified IVC blood filling atrium due to deep inspiration
B. Flexion in the extremity at the IV site blocking the contrast bolus
C. Cardiac arrhythmia changing flow rates of the bolus
D. Transient decrease in blood pressure slowing bolus progression

5a Apart from red bone marrow, what is the most radiosensitive organ in the chest of a male patient?

A. Lungs
B. Breasts
C. Thyroid
D. Esophagus

5b Apart from red bone marrow, what is the most radiosensitive organ in the chest of a young female patient?

A. Heart
B. Breasts
C. Thyroid
D. Esophagus

6a In addition to chest x-ray, which of the following examinations has the highest rating for initial evaluation of high-energy blunt thoracic trauma according to the ACR Appropriateness Criteria?

A. CTA of the chest
B. CT of the chest without contrast
C. MRI/MRA of the chest with and without contrast
D. Ultrasound of the chest

6b Which of the following examinations has the highest rating for evaluation of suspected cardiac injury after initial radiographs and clinical evaluation?

A. Transthoracic echocardiography
B. CTA coronary arteries
C. Transesophageal echocardiography
D. Cardiac MRI

7a What magnetic resonance artifact is identified by the arrow overlying a known foregut duplication cyst?

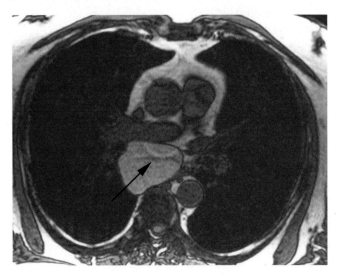

    A. Aliasing
    B. Pulsation
    C. Truncation
    D. Chemical shift

7b In which direction is pulsation artifact?

    A. Anterior to posterior
    B. Parallel to the greatest magnetic field
    C. Z-axis
    D. Phase-encoded axis

8a What is the primary CT finding?

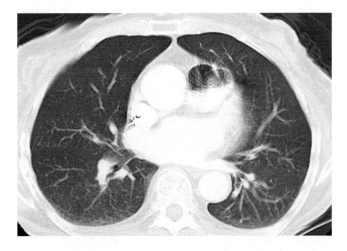

    A. Normal chest CT through pulmonary artery
    B. Pulmonary artery air embolism
    C. Pulmonary artery fat embolism
    D. Pulmonary artery foreign body

8b Give the best recommendation for this asymptomatic patient.
  A. Oblique left lateral decubitus position until resorption.
  B. Emergent surgical consult.
  C. Call code and begin basic life support.
  D. No intervention, patient may leave department.

9 Which of the following would exclude a patient from lung cancer screening with low-dose CT of the chest based on the U.S. Preventive Services Task Force (USPSTF) recommendations?
  A. 50-year-old patient
  B. Greater than 30-pack-year smoking history
  C. Coronary artery disease without angina
  D. Smoking cessation 10 years prior

10 What is the cause of ring artifact on CT?
  A. Volume averaging
  B. Photon starvation
  C. Faulty detector
  D. Beam hardening

11 Which CT imaging parameter change will result in the greatest radiation dose reduction?
  A. Decreasing the mAs by 20%
  B. Decreasing the Z-axis by 20%
  C. Decreasing the kV by 20%
  D. Decreasing the noise index by 20%

12 An incidental 5-mm noncalcified pulmonary nodule is identified in the left lower lobe on a 41-year-old trauma patient with no history of smoking. How should this nodule be followed up?
  A. No routine follow-up
  B. CT at 6 to 12 months, then consider CT at 18 to 24 months
  C. CT at 12 months, then consider CT at 24 months
  D. CT at 3 months, PET/CT, or tissue sampling

13 If a 1.3-cm incidental low attenuation thyroid nodule is identified on a contrast-enhanced chest CT of a 34-year-old female, what is the most appropriate next step?
  A. No further evaluation
  B. PET/CT
  C. Thyroid scintigraphy
  D. Ultrasound of the thyroid

14 A primary care doctor has a patient with a positive PPD, what is the next appropriate test to screen for an active form of tuberculosis?
  A. PA chest radiograph
  B. PA and lateral chest radiograph
  C. Noncontrast chest CT
  D. Chest CT with IV contrast

15 An obese female patient undergoing CT pulmonary angiography experiences pain with injection of 40 mL IV iodinated contrast, which quickly resolves. On physical examination 10 minutes later, the injection site appears as below, and the patient complains of mild increasing pain. What is the best course of action?

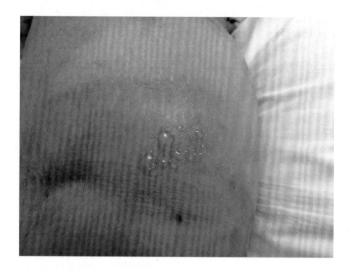

A. No action necessary.

B. Keep the patient for observation.

C. Administer 50 mg IV Benadryl.

D. Surgical consultation.

ANSWERS AND EXPLANATIONS

1 Answer D.   Blurring of the left heart border is noted on the axial image. This is further illustrated on the associated coronal reformation image as a stair step abnormality. This is secondary to cardiac motion, which is accentuated in patients with a faster heart rate. If there were motion artifact along the surface of the diaphragm (best seen on the coronal image), rather than just along the heart, then breathing motion artifact would be a better choice. If the patient was not able to remain still, there would be blurring artifacts to include the chest wall. Motion artifact is not seen with a detector malfunction.

References: Bastos MD, Lee EY, Strauss KJ, et al. Motion artifact on high-resolution CT images of pediatric patients: comparison of volumetric and axial CT methods. *AJR Am J Roentgenol* 2009;193(5):1414–1418.

Kalisz K, Buethe J, Saboo S, et al. Artifacts at cardiac CT: physics and solutions. *Radiographics* 2016;36(7):2064–2083.

2 Answer D.   Both CTDI and DLP are terms related to absorbed dose, which describes the energy from ionizing radiation absorbed per unit mass. The units are expressed in grays (Gy) for absorbed dose. The $CTDI_{vol}$ is simply the most commonly used descriptor for CTDI and is expressed as the average dose over the scanned volume, typically expressed in mGy. Multiplying this $CTDI_{vol}$ value by the scan length results in the DLP (units of mGy $\times$ cm). The effective dose (measured in sieverts, Sv) takes into account the tissue being scanned and its relative radiosensitivity. It takes into account both sex and an age-averaged reference person. Because of the age-averaged reference person, the applicability of effective dose for an individual scan and patient is limited. Effective dose was designed for estimating radiation exposure of entire populations.

Reference: Huda W, Mettler FA. Volume CT dose index and dose–length product displayed during CT: what good are they? *Radiology* 2011;258:236–242.

3 Answer B.   According to the American College of Radiology Contrast manual published in 2018, the eGFR is more accurate in measuring true GFR, and therefore, it is gaining more traction as a risk assessment tool for contrast-induced nephropathy (CIN). In this manual, it mentions that "there is very little evidence that IV iodinated contrast material is an independent risk factor for AKI in patients with eGFR $\geq$ 30 mL/min/1.73 m^2." In practice, any GFR threshold for the use of IV contrast must be determined on an individual patient level with the possible risks and benefits of contrast administration in mind.

References: ACR Manual on Contrast Media (v. 10.3). 2018.

Davenport MS, Khalatbari S, Cohan RH, et al. Contrast material-induced nephrotoxicity and intravenous low-osmolality iodinated contrast material: risk stratification by using estimated glomerular filtration rate. *Radiology* 2013;268(3):719–728.

4a Answer B.

4b Answer A.   As the contrast bolus migrates from the superior vena cava (SVC) to the right atrium during a CT pulmonary angiogram, unopacified blood from the inferior vena cava (IVC) is mixing with the contrast dense blood in the right atrium. If the patient performs deep inspiration during the contrast administration, low thoracic pressure draws an increased volume of unopacified blood from the IVC creating a transient column of low contrast density blood passing through the pulmonary vasculature. Consequently, the CT pulmonary angiogram demonstrates high contrast density in the SVC and aorta while the pulmonary artery appears suboptimally contrast filled. To support the mechanism of the "abdominal–thoracic pump," Wittram and Yoo measured average Hounsfield units (HU) in the right atrium and right ventricle compared to the average HUs in the SVC and IVC to calculate the approximate contributions of the SVC and IVC. Since imaging of the chest takes a variable amount of time, the effect of transient interruption of contrast may not be evenly distributed throughout the lungs as the contrast interruption passes before the imaging is complete. Additionally, these transient breaks in contrast may be mistaken for pulmonary embolism.

Recommendations to minimize transient interruption of contrast focus on limiting deep inspiration immediately prior to imaging. Medical imaging facilities may accomplish this in various ways. For instance, some institutions may perform CT pulmonary angiography at "suspended respiration" rather than full inspiration, while others may work on coaching of patients on proper inspiratory technique with slow gradual deep inspiration.

References: Gosselin MV, Rassner UA, Thieszen SL, et al. Contrast dynamics during CT pulmonary angiogram. *J Thorac Imaging* 2004;19:1–7.

Wittram C, Yoo AJ. Transient interruption of contrast on CT pulmonary angiography: proof of mechanism. *J Thorac Imaging* 2007;22:125–129.

5a **Answer A.**

5b **Answer B.**   The most radiosensitive organs are the red bone marrow, colon, lung, and stomach. In a female patient, the breast is also one of the most radiosensitive (tied with lung). The thyroid is radiosensitive but to a lesser degree than the lung or breast. The esophagus and heart are the least radiosensitive of those listed.

Reference: ICRP. The 2007 recommendations of the International Commission on Radiological Protection. ICRP Publication 103. *Ann ICRP* 2007;37(2–4):1–332.

6a **Answer A.**

6b **Answer A.**   The ACR Appropriateness Criteria designate scores from a range of 1 to 9 for currently available imaging techniques in specific clinical scenarios. These criteria are readily accessible and are useful for guiding clinician imaging requests. A score of 1 to 3 generally corresponds with an exam that is "usually not appropriate." A score of 4 to 6 "may be appropriate," and a score of 7 to 9 is "usually appropriate."

Based on these criteria, chest radiographs and contrast-enhanced chest CT are considered complementary in the setting of blunt trauma and almost always indicated (score of 9). The chest CT should be performed using CTA technique to enhance evaluation for traumatic aortic injury if possible. Noncontrast CT and ultrasound are only sometimes indicated (score of 5). Contrast chest MRI is usually not appropriate (score of 2).

In the setting of suspected cardiac injury after initial evaluation, the highest rating is for transthoracic echocardiography (score of 8). This can exclude cardiac chamber rupture and acute valvular injury. Coronary CTA would only be advised in the setting of suspected coronary injury (score of 5). Transesophageal echo is generally not required unless there is a need to clarify findings on transthoracic echo (score of 5). Cardiac MRI may take 45 minutes to 1 hour and is generally not possible or advisable for patients with significant acute blunt force trauma (score of 4). It may be useful as a problem-solving tool for isolated and specific questions that are not answerable with echocardiography alone.

Reference: Chung JH, Cox CW, Mohammed TL, et al. ACR appropriateness criteria blunt chest trauma. *J Am Coll Radiol* 2014;11(4):345–351.

7a Answer B.

7b Answer D.   Regular or sporadic motion during MR imaging creates motion artifact, which improperly assigns signal to alternative locations greatest in the phase-encoded direction. Regular motion can be macroscopic as in cardiac or respiratory motion or microscopic as in pulsation artifact. In this case, the blood flow within the aorta is sinusoidal creating repetitive artifacts in the phase-encoded axis. The distance between artifacts is proportional to the frequency of the pulsatile flow. Other potential MR artifacts do not create this type of repetitive artifact. In aliasing, the field of view excludes a portion of anatomy that then wraps to the opposite side of the image. Truncation artifact occurs from data lost from fine anatomic detail due to a finite number of spectral components in digital image reconstruction. Finally, chemical shift artifact occurs in well-demarcated borders between fat and water, where the slight difference in proton precession frequency between fat and water creates signal void or overlap at the border in the frequency-encoded direction.

Reference: Arena L, Morehouse HT, Safir J. MR imaging artifacts that simulate disease: how to recognize and eliminate them. *Radiographics* 1995;15:1373–1394.

8a Answer B.

8b Answer A.   Not uncommonly, some small air emboli occur with contrast injection during CT imaging. The small amounts of air are trapped and resorbed in the pulmonary arterioles if not before and the patient remains asymptomatic. These smaller air collections are of greater concern in the setting of a right-to-left shunt where air can transfer to the systemic arterial system and create a vapor lock thereby blocking blood flow in critical small vessels such as the coronary or carotid arteries. In the pulmonary arterial system, a larger amount of air is required before a large enough vessel is blocked to be clinically significant and if large enough, can block cardiac output. In this case, the air injected is greater than average, and if still on the table, the patient may benefit from oblique left lateral decubitus positioning and administration of 100% O_2 until the air collection resorbs.

Reference: ACR Manual on Contrast Media (v. 10.3). 2018.

9 Answer A.   The USPSFT recommends annual screening for lung cancer for those patients (1) who are between 55 and 80 years old, (2) who have at least a 30-pack-year smoking history, (3) who have smoked within the last 15 years, (4) who are willing to undergo treatment if a lesion is discovered, and (5) who do not have a health problem that would otherwise severely limit their life expectancy. Of the choices provided, the 50-year-old patient would be excluded on the basis of age regardless of his or her smoking history. Coronary artery disease without angina would not be expected to severely limit life expectancy to the degree that screening would be unindicated.

References: Donnelly EF, Kazerooni EA, Lee E, et al. ACR appropriateness Criteria Lung Cancer Screening. Available at https://acsearch.acr.org/docs/3102390/Narrative/. Accessed July 29, 2019.

Recommendation Summary. U.S. Preventive Services Task Force. September 2014. Available at http://www.uspreventiveservicestaskforce.org/Page/Topic/recommendation-summary/lung-cancer-screening. Accessed July 29, 2019.

10 **Answer C.** A ring defect on CT is indicative of a miscalibration of one or more CT detectors. Solid-state detectors, which function independently, are at increased risk for ring artifact. While ring artifacts may not be mistaken for pathology, they can degrade image quality. None of the other choices produce discrete ring defects on CT imaging. Volume averaging decreases contrast resolution by averaging the values of two small adjacent objects of differing densities. Photon starvation generally results in streaking artifact manifesting as darkened bands, particularly at the level of the shoulders on chest CT, although can produce round defects in the upper abdomen on reduced dose CT imaging of the chest. Finally, beam-hardening artifacts result from attenuation of low-energy photons causing cupping and streak artifacts.

Reference: Barrett JF, Keat N. Artifacts in CT: recognition and avoidance. *Radiographics* 2004;24:1679–1691.

11 **Answer C.** In the current practice of CT imaging, parameters such as kV are still in the control of the operator, although automation in CT acquisition is increasing. Most current CT scanners employ mA dose modulation, where mAs varies throughout the gantry rotation to account for the natural nonround configuration of the human body. Measures of image quality, such as the noise index, allows for mA modulation while still allowing for some operator control in the trade-off of radiation dose for image quality. Reduced dose chest CT generally employs this method, accepting increased image noise for relative decrease in radiation dose. A decrease in noise index would therefore increase radiation dose.

This question aims primarily at recognizing the relatively linear relationship between reducing the mAs and Z-axis relative to radiation dose reduction versus the nonlinear relationship between kV and radiation dose. By decreasing the kV from 120 to 100 in the setting of coronary CTA, studies have shown a reduction in radiation dose between 47% and 53%. Additionally, in CT contrast studies, the decreased kV also enhances the image contrast from iodinated contrast relative to the surrounding soft tissues due to the k-edge of iodine.

Reference: Kanal KM, Stewart BK, Kolokythas O, et al. Impact of operator-selected image noise index and reconstruction slice thickness on patient radiation dose in 64-MDCT. *AJR Am J Roentgenol* 2007;189;219–225.

12 **Answer A.** Solid incidental pulmonary nodules are encountered on a daily basis when reading chest CT exams. In these clinical scenarios, it is important to be familiar with the most up-to-date Fleischner Society recommendations for follow-up. The most recent update was in 2017 and the recommendation for a patient such as this with no risk factors is "no routine follow-up." This recommendation has been altered from the original 2005 recommendations, which previously did include follow-up for nodules >4 mm. The rationale for this change is that in "high-risk" patients, the average risk of cancer in patients with a nodule <6 mm is <1% and is therefore assumed to be lower in patients considered "low risk." A 6- to 12-month follow-up chest CT is recommended in "low-risk" patients with a nodule measuring 6 to 8 mm. If a nodule is >8 mm, 3-month follow-up, PET/CT, or tissue sampling is recommended.

Reference: MacMahon H, Naidich DP, Goo JM, et al. Guidelines for management of incidental pulmonary nodules detected on CT images: from the Fleischner Society 2017. *Radiology* 2017;284(1):228–243.

13 **Answer D.** Although the thyroid is not usually a clinical concern when chest CT exams are ordered, it is almost always included in the field of view.

Incidental thyroid nodules are prevalent and can create a clinical dilemma for the radiologist of when to recommend further imaging, specifically a thyroid ultrasound. In 2015, the ACR published a white paper providing guidelines for when to follow-up with thyroid ultrasound. If there are no obvious malignant features to the nodule, the guidelines take into account the age of the patient and the size of the incidental nodule. If the patient is <35 years old, a thyroid ultrasound is recommended if the nodule is 1 cm or greater, as in this scenario. If a patient is 35 years or older, an ultrasound is recommended if the nodule is 1.5 cm or greater. PET/CT and thyroid scintigraphy is rarely the first step after incidental identification. An ACR white paper also exists for follow-up recommendation guidelines for "incidentalomas" encountered in the partially imaged upper abdomen.

Reference: Hoang JK, Langer JE, Middleton WD, et al. Managing incidental thyroid nodules detected on imaging: white paper of the ACR Incidental Thyroid Findings Committee. *J Am Coll Radiol* 2015;12:143–150.

14   Answer A.   In the scenario of a person who is at higher risk than the normal population, a PA chest radiograph would be the most appropriate test with a score of 9 with the ACR Appropriateness Criteria. Noncontrast chest CT (score of 4) should be reserved in rare cases where the radiographic findings are considered equivocal. Contrast-enhanced CT (score of 3) is less necessary since lung parenchymal findings are the primary area of concern to evaluate. Lateral radiographs have been shown to not improve the detection of findings related to TB.

Reference: Ravenel JG, Chung JH, Ackman JB. ACR Appropriateness Criteria® imaging of possible tuberculosis. *Am Coll Radiol* 2017;14(5S):S160–S165.

15   Answer D.   In the setting of IV iodinated contrast extravasation, immediate surgical consultation or transfer to emergency care is recommended if the patient demonstrates any of the following: "progressive swelling or pain, altered tissue perfusion as evidenced by decreased capillary refill at any time after the extravasation has occurred, change in sensation in the affected limb, and skin ulceration or blistering." The most common severe complication of IV iodinated contrast extravasation is compartment syndrome, with the likelihood increasing as the quantity of extravasated contrast increases, but small volumes have also been reported to cause compartment syndrome.

If any noticeable amount of extravasation occurs at the injection site, the patient will at least need observation for several hours. Severity and prognosis of IV iodinated contrast extravasation is difficult, and close follow-up is recommended to exclude delayed development of signs and symptoms. Only after the radiologist is comfortable that the patient's signs and symptoms are resolving and no new complaints are arising, can the patient be discharged. Treatment for extravasations not requiring surgical consultation is variable but generally includes elevation of the affected limb and application of a hot or cold compress.

Reference: ACR Manual on Contrast Media (v. 10.3). 2018.

2 Normal Anatomy

David W. Grant, Jr., DO

QUESTIONS

1 Characterize the structure interposed between the aorta and carina.

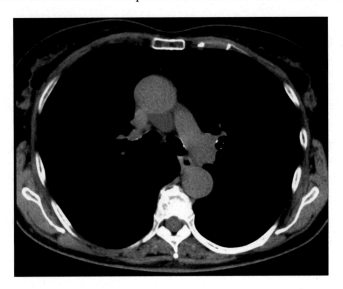

A. Lymphadenopathy
B. Normal anatomic variant
C. Mediastinal cyst
D. Vascular aneurysm

2 Which of the following is responsible for the creation of a juxtaphrenic peak?

A. Superior pulmonary ligament
B. Inferior pulmonary ligament
C. Phrenic nerve
D. Diaphragmatic eventration

3a The provided images were obtained from the same patient at different times. What contrast-enhanced structure is visualized to the left of the aorta on the initial provided image?

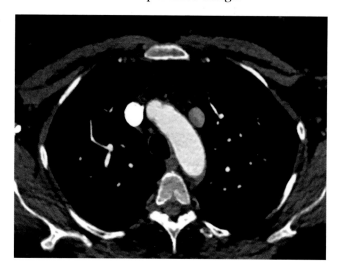 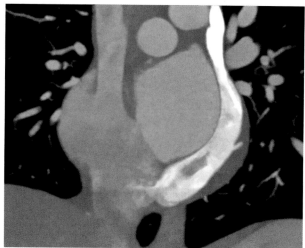

A. Left upper lobe anomalous pulmonary vein
B. Persistent left superior vena cava
C. Aberrant right subclavian artery
D. Hemiazygos vein

3b Which of the following is the typical drainage pathway of this structure (shown in the second provided image above)?

A. Right superior vena cava to right atrium
B. Coronary sinus to right atrium
C. Coronary sinus to left atrium
D. Directly into right atrium

3c In the majority of patients, what type of vascular shunt is associated with this anomaly?

A. Left to right shunt
B. Right to left shunt
C. No associated shunt
D. Bidirectional shunt

4 What forms the medial border of the right paratracheal stripe?

A. Pleura
B. Ascending aorta
C. Trachea
D. Superior vena cava

5 What is the name of the fissure that separates the medial basal bronchopulmonary segment from the other lower lobe segments?

A. Superior accessory fissure
B. Inferior accessory fissure
C. Medial accessory fissure
D. Minor accessory fissure

6   Per the 2009 International Association for the Study of Lung Cancer (IASLC) lymph node map, which lymph node station is associated with the lymph node indicated in the provided image?

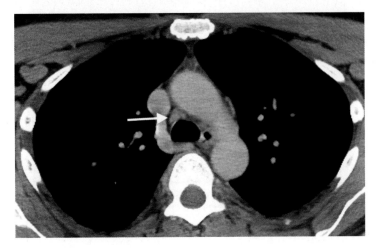

A. Station 2R (Right Upper Paratracheal)
B. Station 4R (Right Lower Paratracheal)
C. Station 4L (Left Lower Paratracheal)
D. Station 6 (Para-aortic)

7   Which segment of lung has been resected?

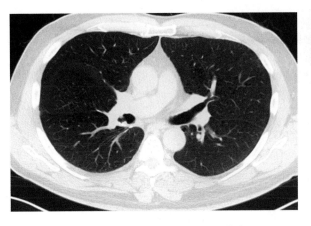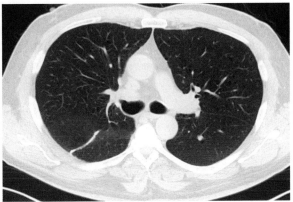

A. Posterior right upper lobe
B. Medial right middle lobe
C. Superior right lower lobe
D. Medial basilar right lower lobe

8   Which of the following is located in the periphery of the secondary pulmonary lobule?

A. Pulmonary vein
B. Pulmonary artery
C. Respiratory bronchiole
D. Terminal bronchiole

9 Which anatomic structure is identified on this CT image by the arrow?

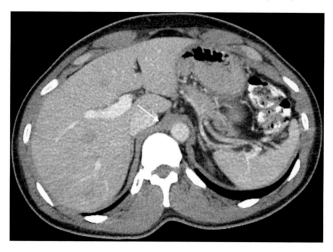

    A. Medial lumbocostal arch
    B. Central tendon of the diaphragm
    C. Psoas muscle
    D. Right diaphragmatic crus

10 Name the normal variant.

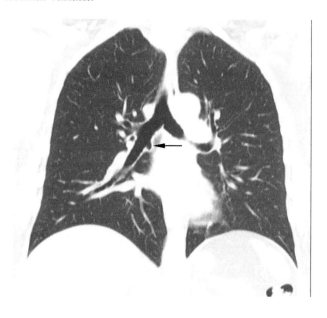

    A. Tracheal bronchus
    B. Bronchial atresia
    C. Bronchus intermedius
    D. Cardiac bronchus

11 Which of the following airways is the first to lack cartilage within its wall?
    A. Terminal bronchiole
    B. Mainstem bronchus
    C. Respiratory bronchiole
    D. Alveolar duct

12a Which window or clear space is demonstrated in this radiograph?

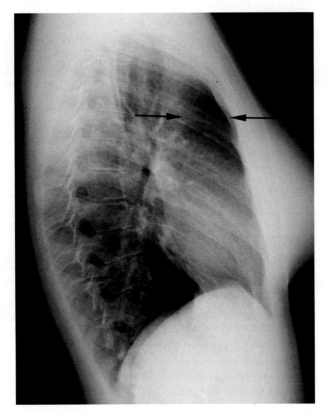

    A. Retrotracheal
    B. Retrocardiac
    C. Retrosternal
    D. Raider triangle

12b The retrosternal window on lateral view correlates with which structure on frontal view?

    A. Anterior junctional line
    B. Posterior superior junctional line
    C. Azygoesophageal recess
    D. Right paratracheal stripe

13a In the intercostal spaces, what is the cranial-to-caudal order of the neurovascular bundle?

    A. Vein → artery → nerve
    B. Nerve → artery → vein
    C. Artery → vein → nerve
    D. Nerve → vein → artery

13b What is the best descriptor for positioning of the neurovascular bundle in the intercostal space?

    A. Cranial (along the undersurface of the superior rib)
    B. Central (midway between the two ribs)
    C. Caudal (along the superior surface of the inferior rib)
    D. Variable (positioning depends on rib level)

14 What is the name for the vascular structure located posterior to bronchus intermedius (annotated by the arrow)?

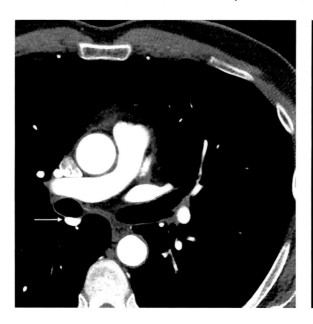 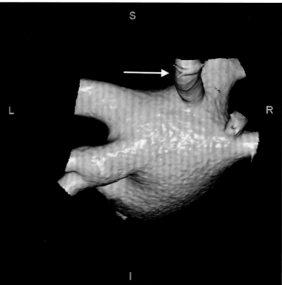

A. Partial anomalous pulmonary venous return
B. Right superior pulmonary vein
C. Right top pulmonary vein
D. Right middle pulmonary vein

15a What is the name of the space denoted by the arrow?

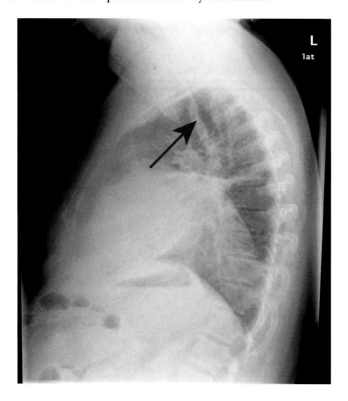

A. Anterior esophageal stripe
B. Tracheoesophageal stripe
C. Anterior junctional line
D. Posterior junctional line

15b What is the upper limit of normal for width of this anatomic space?
  A. 2 mm
  B. 5 mm
  C. 10 mm
  D. 15 mm

16 What vessel is most at risk of injury given the position of the percutaneous pleural catheter?

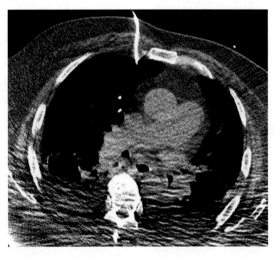

  A. Superior vena cava
  B. Ascending aorta
  C. Right brachiocephalic vein
  D. Right internal thoracic artery

17 What cardiac valve is identified on this lateral chest radiograph by its severe degree of calcification?

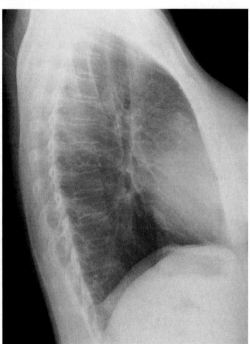

  A. Aortic
  B. Pulmonary
  C. Mitral
  D. Tricuspid

18a What long tubular structure is identified by arrows on these two images?

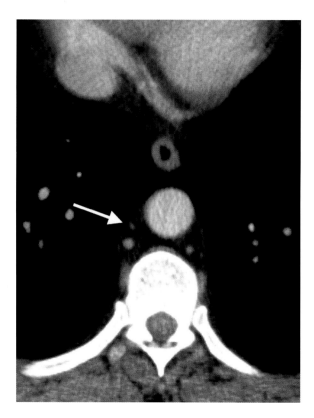 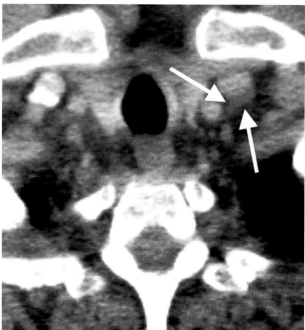

A. Azygos vein
B. Thoracic duct
C. Hemiazygos vein
D. Accessory hemiazygos vein

18b What structure does the thoracic duct typically drain into?

A. Left subclavian vein and internal jugular vein confluence
B. Right subclavian vein and internal jugular vein confluence
C. Superior vena cava
D. Inferior vena cava

18c Which of the following areas is not typically drained (directly or indirectly) via the thoracic duct?

A. Right upper extremity
B. Left upper extremity
C. Right lower extremity
D. Left lower extremity

19 What forms the superior margin of the azygoesophageal recess?

A. Azygos arch
B. Aortic arch
C. Accessory hemiazygos vein
D. Innominate artery

20a What is responsible for the marbled fat appearance in the anterior mediastinum of this adult?

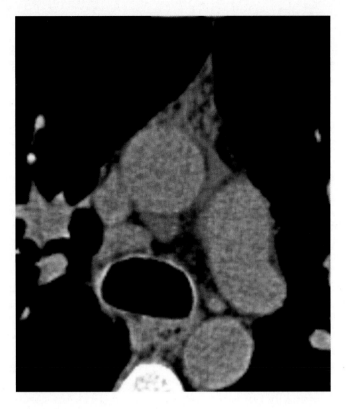

    A. Mediastinal hemorrhage
    B. Infectious mediastinitis
    C. Normal thymus
    D. Thymolipoma

20b In which decade of life should complete fatty replacement of the thymus be expected in all patients?

    A. Second
    B. Fourth
    C. Sixth
    D. Eighth

ANSWERS AND EXPLANATIONS

1 **Answer B.**   Occasionally misinterpreted as lymphadenopathy, a mass, or a mediastinal cyst, a prominent superior pericardial aortic recess is a normal anatomic variant that generally requires no further follow-up. Imaging findings that confirm the presence of the superior pericardial recess include (1) characteristic position of this known pericardial recess, here along the posterior aorta, (2) crescentic shape, (3) fluid density and nonenhancing, and (4) benign appearance relative to adjacent structures. The superior aortic recess can even extend superiorly into the right paratracheal mediastinum. Some benign cystic lesions could overlap with these findings warranting follow-up, but multiplanar reformatted images in the sagittal or coronal plane may better demonstrate extension from the pericardial region. Lymphadenopathy and vascular aneurysm would not have all of these findings.

Reference: Truong MT, et al. Pictorial essay: anatomy of pericardial recesses on multidetector CT: implications for oncologic imaging. *AJR Am J Roentgenol* 2003;181:1109–1113.

2 **Answer B.**   The juxtaphrenic peak is associated with upper lung volume loss of any cause and a resulting appearance of a small triangular opacity at the apex of the diaphragm on a frontal chest radiograph. The peak is formed due to the inferior accessory fissure of an intrapulmonary septum related to the inferior pulmonary ligament. The superior pulmonary ligament would not touch the diaphragm. The phrenic nerve is generally not identifiable on imaging unless pathologic. Diaphragmatic eventration could account for a similar abnormality but is not associated with this term specifically and generally manifests as an additional smooth convexity of the diaphragm.

Reference: Hansell DM, Bankier AA, MacMahon H, et al. Fleischner Society: glossary of terms for thoracic imaging. *Radiology* 2008;246(3).

3a **Answer B.**

3b **Answer B.**

3c **Answer C.**   The superior vena cava (SVC) is the major venous drainage pathway for the head and neck, upper extremities, and thorax to the heart. The SVC lies to the right of midline and forms from the confluence of the left and right brachiocephalic veins. During the 5th week of life, the fetus has anterior and posterior cardinal veins draining its cranial and caudal portions respectively. During development the right anterior cardinal vein, the right common cardinal vein and right horn of sinus venosus join to form the right-sided SVC. The right posterior cardinal vein forms the azygos vein. On the left, a portion of the anterior cardinal vein forms the brachiocephalic vein and left superior intercostal vein with the remainder forming a structure called the ligament of Marshall. The left posterior cardinal vein regresses, and the left horn of the sinus venosus becomes the coronary sinus.

A persistent left SVC is the most common congenital venous variant in the thorax occurring in <0.5% of the general population. The underlying etiology is failure of the left anterior cardinal vein, left common cardinal vein, and left horn of the sinus venosus to regress. The persistent left SVC arises from the confluence of the left subclavian and internal jugular veins and may or may not have communication with a right SVC via a bridging vein. The right SVC can be normal in size, small, or absent. The left SVC drains distally into the right atrium via a dilated coronary sinus. This vein occurs along the course of what would otherwise become the ligament of Marshall in the normal population. In the vast majority of these patients, there is no associated vascular shunt associated with this anomaly. Rarely, there can be an associated abnormal communication with the left atrium such as a levoatrial cardinal vein.

Reference: Sonavane SK, et al. Comprehensive imaging review of the superior vena cava. *Radiographics* 2014;34:1571–1592.

4 **Answer C.** On radiographs, the right paratracheal stripe is formed by the right tracheal wall (medially) and the medial pleura (laterally). It typically measures <4 mm although it can be affected by the degree of inspiration and predominance of mediastinal fat. Pathology that can cause widening of the stripe is frequently best evaluated by CT and includes lymphadenopathy (most common), mediastinal hemorrhage, mediastinal mass, or vessel enlargement.

Reference: Hansell DM, Bankier AA, MacMahon H, et al. Fleischner Society: glossary of terms for thoracic imaging. *Radiology* 2008;246(3).

5 **Answer B.** The inferior accessory fissure separates the medial basal bronchopulmonary segment from the other basilar segments and is typically vertically oriented and frequently complete. It is more common on the right. The superior accessory fissure is in the same plane as the right minor fissure and separates the lower lobe superior segment from the basilar segments. There is no such thing as a medial accessory fissure or minor accessory fissure.

Reference: Godwin JD, Tarver RD. Accessory fissures of the lung. *AJR Am J Roentgenol* 1985;144(1):39–47.

6 **Answer B.** Knowledge of regional lymph nodal stations within the thorax is imperative for the accurate staging of lung cancer. The IASLC lymph node map was developed to create a unified lymph nodal classification and resolve differences in previously described lymph node maps such as the Mountain-Dresler modification of the American Thoracic Society and Naruke lymph node maps.

In this case, the lymph node in question is positioned just anterior to the trachea below the level of the aortic arch consistent with the upper zone, station 4R (right lower paratracheal) per the IASLC lymph node map. In the cranial caudal plane, station 4R is defined as those occurring inferior to the caudal margin of the intersection of the left brachiocephalic vein with the trachea and superior to the lower border of the azygos vein/arch. The anatomic landmark distinguishing the left and right paratracheal stations is the left border of the trachea. As such, all lymph nodes to the right of the left border of the trachea are considered right paratracheal.

Reference: El-Sherief AH, et al. International Association for the Study of Lung Cancer (IASLC) lymph node map: radiologic review with CT illustration. *Radiographics* 2014;34:1680–1691.

7 **Answer C.** Outside of the occasional anatomic variant, the divisions of the tracheobronchial tree into 2 lungs, 5 lobes, and 18 segments are relatively constant as are their relationships on CT imaging. When a segment or lobe has been removed, knowing the expected relationships allows for successful characterizing of the prior resection. The upper and right middle lobar bronchi originate anterior to the lower, and lobectomy of one of these lobes results in surgical clips and bronchial stump anterior to the residual airway. Conversely, resection of a lower lobe results in clips or a stump posterior to the residual airway. A segmentectomy can be more difficult to accurately characterize and requires knowledge of the normal branching. In this case, the suture line courses along the superior right lower lobe and inferior posterior right upper lobe, in the region of the right lower lobe superior segment and posterior right upper lobe segment. The surgical clips and stump are demonstrated along the posterior bronchus intermedius at the expected origin of the right lower lobe superior segmental bronchus.

Reference: Webb WR, Higgins CB. *Thoracic imaging: pulmonary and cardiovascular radiology*, 3rd ed. Philadelphia, PA: Lippincott Williams & Wilkins, 2017:78–104; Chapter 3: The pulmonary hila.

8 Answer A.   The secondary pulmonary lobule serves as the functional unit of the lung and is critical to HRCT evaluation. It is polyhedral in shape measuring approximately 1.5 cm in size with fibrous septa walls (containing pulmonary veins and lymphatics). The center of the lobule is formed by the terminal bronchiole and pulmonary artery (as well as a central set of lymphatics).

Reference: Hansell DM, Lynch DA, McAdams HP, et al. *Imaging of diseases of the chest*, 5th ed. Mosby, 2009:153–204; Chapter 4: Basic HRCT patterns of lung disease.

9 Answer D.   The diaphragm is a skeletal muscle and membranous structure that separates the thorax from the abdomen and aids in respiration. Centrally, the diaphragm is composed of a strong aponeurosis known as the central tendon. Skeletal muscle constitutes the more peripheral aspect of the diaphragm with attachments to the sternum, lower ribs, and upper lumbar region. Posteriorly, the diaphragm is attached to the psoas and quadratus lumborum muscles via ligamentous arches known as the medial and lateral lumbocostal arches (arcuate ligaments), respectively. The posteromedial aspects of the diaphragm form pillars composed of muscular and tendinous components that have been termed the diaphragmatic crura. The tendinous portions of the crura attach to the ventral aspect of L1-L3 on the right and L1 and L2 on the left. Anterior and medially, the muscular portions of the crura form an arch known as the median arcuate ligament. The space between the diaphragmatic crura has been termed the retrocrural space and contains the aorta, lymph nodes, azygos and hemiazygos veins, thoracic duct, and splanchnic nerves.

Reference: Restrepo C, et al. The diaphragmatic crura and retrocrural space: normal imaging appearance, variants, and pathologic conditions. *Radiographics* 2008;28:1289–1305.

10 Answer D.   Congenital variation in the branching of the tracheobronchial tree is not uncommon ranging from 1% to 12% of individuals. In this case, a short segment of bronchus branches from the medial aspect of the bronchus intermedius, opposite the right upper lobe bronchus, and is known as an accessory cardiac bronchus. The bronchus may be blind ending or have some associated aerated cystic or alveolar tissue. Reports of associated infection or hemoptysis have required resection, although the majority are discovered incidentally in asymptomatic individuals. As the name suggests, a tracheal bronchus arises from the trachea and almost invariably provides an accessory bronchus to the right upper lobe. Bronchial atresia refers to an interruption in a normal bronchial branch with noncommunicating peripheral bronchi and associated portions of lung. Finally, the bronchus intermedius is a normal anatomic branch beyond the right upper lobe takeoff, so named as it is the only bronchus beyond a lobar branch, but still peripherally bifurcating into two additional lobar branches.

Reference: Ghaye B, Szapiro D, Fanchamps JM, et al. Congenital bronchial abnormalities revisited. *Radiographics* 2001;21:105–119.

11 Answer A.   There are approximately 23 dichotomous branches that occur from the level of the trachea to the alveolus. These branches are broken into bronchi, which contain cartilage in their wall, and bronchioles, which lack cartilage. The terminal bronchiole is the final airway in the conducting zone and is the first airway to lack cartilage within its wall. The respiratory bronchioles arise from the terminal bronchioles and are therefore the second airway to lack cartilage within their walls. The respiratory bronchioles are the first airways to contain alveoli and the first to participate in gas exchange. The respiratory bronchioles subsequently terminate as alveolar ducts and finally alveoli.

Reference: Webb WR, Higgins CB. *Thoracic imaging: pulmonary and cardiovascular radiology*, 3rd ed. Philadelphia, PA: Lippincott Williams & Wilkins, 2017:602; Chapter 23: Airway disease: bronchiectasis, chronic bronchitis, bronchiolitis.

12a Answer C.

12b Answer A.   The retrosternal window or clear space, also known as the "anterior clear space," represents a narrowing of the mediastinum anterior to the heart and great vessels and posterior to the sternum where the pleurae of the anterior upper lobes come close together or meet. On the lateral chest radiograph, the retrosternal window provides improved visualization of the anterior mediastinum, a potential blind spot on the frontal radiograph as the overlying sternum and mediastinal structures often obscure lesions in the anterior mediastinum. Normal anatomical structures that reside in the anterior mediastinum and retrosternal region include mediastinal fat, lymph nodes, thymic tissue, and internal mammary vessels.

When the pleurae of the anterior upper lobes of the lungs approximate close enough to each other, the anterior junctional line may be seen on frontal chest radiograph. In addition to understanding expected shadows and borders on the normal chest radiograph, recognizing the anterior junctional line can also support the impression of hyperinflation or emphysema, which can accentuate the anterior junctional line.

Reference: Feigin DS. Lateral chest radiograph: a systematic approach. *Acad Radiol* 2010;17:1560–1566.

13a Answer A.

13b Answer A.   The intercostal space neurovascular bundle is ordered vein, artery, and then nerve from superior to inferior (VAN is the acronym to remember). The location of the neurovascular bundle as immediately under the superior rib (cranial in the intercostal space) is critical for those performing interventional procedures to avoid vascular injury. Despite the classic distribution of the intercostal structures, three-dimensional CT angiographic images of the intercostal arteries can demonstrate the potential tortuous route of these arteries. Intercostal vessels can bleed profusely if injured, especially if they bleed into the pleural space.

Reference: Talbot B, Gange C, Chaturvedi A, et al. Traumatic rib injury: patterns, complications, and treatment. *Radiographics*, 2017;37:628–651.

14 Answer C.   A right top pulmonary vein is a relatively uncommon pulmonary vein variant occurring in 10% of patients and has a unique course traversing posterior and medial to the right bronchus intermedius to the superior (or top) aspect of the left atrium. This vein typically drains the superior segment of the right lower lobe, posterior segment of the right upper lobe, and occasionally both. A left "top" pulmonary vein has also been reported. Supernumerary pulmonary veins can be an important preoperative finding in patients undergoing catheter-directed ablation for atrial fibrillation.

Reference: Hassani C, Farhood S. Comprehensive cross-sectional imaging of the pulmonary veins. *Radiographics* 2017;37:1928–1954.

15a **Answer B.**

15b **Answer B.** The tracheoesophageal stripe is identified on lateral chest radiographs as the space between the posterior wall of the air-filled trachea and the anterior wall of the air-filled esophagus. It typically measures up to 5 mm in size. If the posterior trachea does not abut the esophagus, it is generally smaller, up to 2.5 mm, and referred to as the posterior tracheal stripe. Thickening of this stripe (as in this example) generally warrants correlation with CT to evaluate for esophageal lesion, vascular lesion, or other mediastinal pathology.

Reference: Gibbs JM, Chandrasekhar CA, Ferguson EC, et al. Lines and stripes: where did they go?—from conventional radiography to CT. *Radiographics* 2007;27(1):33-48.

16 **Answer D.** The bilateral internal thoracic arteries (internal mammary arteries) serve as blood supply to the anterior chest wall extending from the clavicles to the umbilicus. They most frequently arise directly from the subclavian artery and pass posterior to the subclavian vein with a vertical course between the transversus thoracis muscle posteriorly and the costal cartilages anteriorly. The distal bifurcation results in the musculophrenic artery and superior epigastric artery. Placement of a chest tube via an anteromedial approach (close to the sternum as seen here) places this artery at risk. Injury can be catastrophic with severe chest wall, pleural, and mediastinal hemorrhage. This patient required massive transfusion and artery coil embolization as a result of this placement.

The artery provides an important collateral to the inferior epigastric arteries if there is a coarctation or descending aortic occlusion.

Reference: Glassberg R, Sussman S, Glickstein M. CT anatomy of the internal mammary vessels: importance in planning percutaneous transthoracic procedures. *AJR Am J Roentgenol* 1990;155:397–400.

17 **Answer B.** The lateral radiograph demonstrates severe dystrophic calcification projecting high and anterior relative to the cardiac shadow. The location is that of the pulmonary valve. The other valves would be more posterior and inferior than demonstrated. This patient had long-standing pulmonary stenosis.

Reference: Cressman S, Rheinboldt C, et al. Chest radiographic appearance of minimally invasive cardiac implants and support devices: what the radiologist needs to know. *Curr Probl Diagn Radiol* 2019;48(3):274–288.

18a **Answer B.**

18b **Answer A.**

18c **Answer A.** The thoracic duct serves as the common trunk for a majority of the lymphatic vessels. The duct serves as a continuation of the cisterna chyli (typically located around L1). It courses through the aortic hiatus and ascends in the right posterior mediastinum between the aorta and azygos vein (shown). The hemiazygos and accessory hemiazygos are in the left posterior mediastinum. The thoracic duct is typically identifiable (although small) in patients with a moderate degree of mediastinal fat, but not identifiable on thinner patients. It crosses midline around T5 and continues to the thoracic inlet, anterior to the subclavian artery and anterior scalene, before draining into the angle of the left subclavian and internal jugular veins. Variant drainage includes drainage directly into one of the other neck vessels (internal jugular, external jugular, brachiocephalic of subclavian). Understanding this anatomy is important for cases of chylothorax to guide potential surgical or interventional therapy. The duct drains the lower extremities, abdomen, left chest, left upper extremity, and left neck.

Reference: Liu ME, Branstetter BF, Whetstone J, et al. Normal appearance of the distal thoracic duct. *AJR Am J Roentgenol* 2006;187:1615–1620.

19   **Answer A.**   The azygoesophageal recess is a posterior mediastinal recess located in the right chest. The azygos arch forms the cranial margin. The azygos vein and pleura form the posterior margin. The esophagus generally forms the medial margin.

Reference: Hansell DM, Bankier AA, MacMahon H, et al. Fleischner Society: glossary of terms for thoracic imaging. *Radiology* 2008;246(3).

20a   **Answer C.**

20b   **Answer D.**   The appearance is that of normal thymus. Mediastinal hemorrhage would be expected to demonstrate more areas of mixed high and low attenuation from either direct vessel injury or, more commonly, rupture of the vasa vasorum surrounding the mediastinal vessels. Thymolipoma would demonstrate a combination of fat density and soft tissue; however, there is no actual mass in this case. Similarly, infectious mediastinitis would be much more likely to produce an indurated space-occupying appearance than is demonstrated.

The thymus involutes with age resulting in continual decrease in thymic mass relative to body size. The thymus actually continues to grow in absolute terms until puberty but will start occupying a significantly smaller portion of relative size from infancy. In a study of 309 individuals ranging in age from 6 weeks to 81 years, some remnant thymic tissue was visualized on CT up to the age of 70 years with those in the eighth decade (older than 70) all demonstrating complete fatty replacement of the thymus on CT. The stranded mixed soft tissue and fat appearance shown is typical. Configuration is normally bilobed or triangular. Presence of a significant solid component should raise the possibility of developing thymic neoplasm.

References: Francis IR, Glazer GM, Bookstein FL, et al. The thymus: reexamination of age-related changes in size and shape. *AJR Am J Roentgenol* 1985;145:249–254.

Nishino M, Ashiku SK, Kocher ON, et al. The thymus: a comprehensive review. *Radiographics* 2006;26(2):335–348.

Terms and Signs

Christian W. Cox, MD

QUESTIONS

1a A 57-year-old male presents with recent diagnosis of lung cancer and no interval treatment. The arrow in the CT image is identifying which sign?

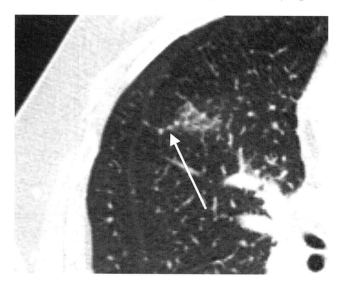

   A. Split pleura
   B. Juxtaphrenic peak
   C. Beaded septum
   D. Bulging fissure

1b In the setting of malignancy, the finding raises concern for which process?

   A. Pulmonary metastases
   B. Pulmonary hemorrhage
   C. Pulmonary embolism
   D. Bacterial pneumonia

2   A 35-year-old male presents with uveitis and mild shortness of breath. Chest radiograph is obtained. What sign best describes the radiograph image provided?

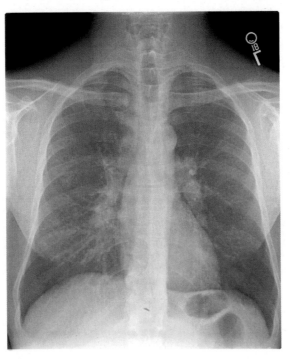

A. Galaxy sign
B. Fleischner sign
C. 1-2-3 sign
D. Golden S sign

3a   A 32-year-old female presents with refractory asthma and chronic sinusitis. Prior bronchoscopy had revealed eosinophilia on bronchoscopic alveolar lavage (BAL). What sign is present on this patient's radiograph?

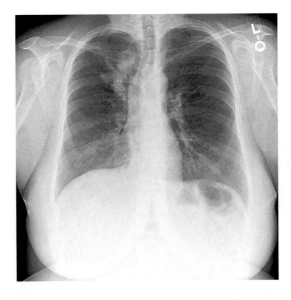

A. Tree-in-bud
B. Hilum overlay
C. Air crescent
D. Finger-in-glove

3b Based on the imaging findings and clinical history, what is the most likely diagnosis?

    A. Allergic bronchopulmonary aspergillosis
    B. Aspergilloma
    C. Semi-invasive aspergillosis
    D. Angioinvasive aspergillosis

3c A follow-up CT of the chest was obtained on the patient and provided below. Do the imaging findings support your prior diagnosis?

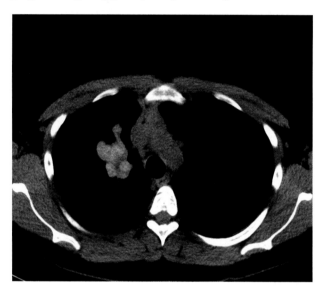

    A. Yes, contrast enhancement of bronchial impaction is common in ABPA.
    B. Yes, high density of bronchial impaction is common in ABPA.
    C. No, a vasculitis such as Churg-Strauss disease should be considered.
    D. No, high density of bronchial impaction suggests a diagnosis other than ABPA.

4a On these inspiratory images, what is the primary radiologic finding?

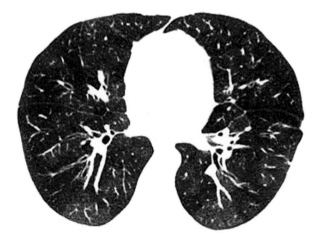

    A. Mosaic attenuation
    B. Consolidation
    C. Bronchiectasis
    D. Architectural distortion

4b Expiratory images of the same patient demonstrate that the previously noted mosaic attenuation is due to which of the following?

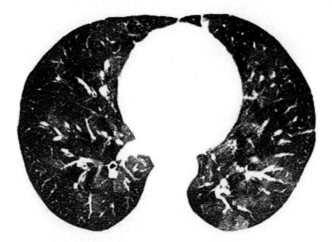

   A. Air trapping
   B. Pulmonary vascular disease
   C. Ground-glass opacity
   D. Photon starvation artifact

4c If this patient had a history of prior toxic fume inhalation injury, which of the following etiologies is most likely?

   A. Hypersensitivity pneumonitis
   B. Asthma
   C. Obliterative bronchiolitis
   D. Follicular bronchiolitis

4d Which of the following connective tissue diseases is most highly associated with obliterative bronchiolitis?

   A. Scleroderma
   B. Rheumatoid arthritis
   C. Lupus
   D. Sjögren syndrome

5 What structure forms the superior border of the aortopulmonary window?

   A. Left pulmonary artery
   B. Aortic arch
   C. Ligamentum arteriosum
   D. Parietal pleura

6 Which of the following causes the "deep sulcus" sign on supine chest radiograph?

   A. Lobar collapse
   B. Pleural effusion
   C. Pneumothorax
   D. Emphysema

7 Pulmonary infarction most commonly involves which of the following vessels?

   A. Bronchial arteries
   B. Pulmonary arteries
   C. Pulmonary veins
   D. Intercostal arteries

8a Which term best describes the finding?

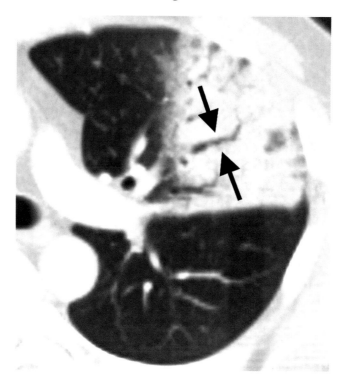

A. Air bronchogram
B. Beaded septum
C. Ring around the artery
D. Air crescent

8b This finding is characteristic of which pulmonary opacity?
A. Mass
B. Consolidation
C. Endobronchial plug
D. Pseudomass

8c Which consolidation correlates highest with an absence of air bronchograms?
A. Streptococcal pneumonia
B. Organizing pneumonia
C. Pulmonary edema
D. Pulmonary infarct

9 Tree-in-bud nodules is a combination of branching opacities and what nodule type?
A. Centrilobular
B. Perilymphatic
C. Random
D. Subpleural

10 The Monod sign indicates what underlying pathology?

   A. Mycetoma
   B. Angioinvasive fungal infection
   C. Cavitary neoplasm
   D. Granulomatosis with polyangiitis

11a A 60-year-old male presented 1 week ago with cough, shortness of breath, and negative chest radiographs. Patient is prescribed antibiotics for presumed pneumonia but returns with continued shortness of breath and the chest radiograph below. Which sign best characterizes the radiographic finding?

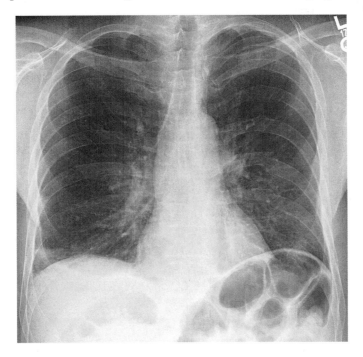

   A. Spine sign
   B. Flat waist sign
   C. Hampton hump
   D. Scimitar

11b Which process is most suggested by this finding?

   A. Pulmonary edema
   B. Bacterial pneumonia
   C. Pleural neoplasm
   D. Pulmonary embolism

12a What term best describes the pattern in the CT image provided?

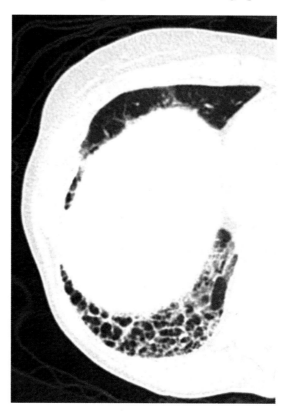

A. Emphysema
B. Honeycombing
C. Mosaic attenuation
D. Air trapping

12b An additional CT image from the same study is provided below. What is the most likely diagnosis?

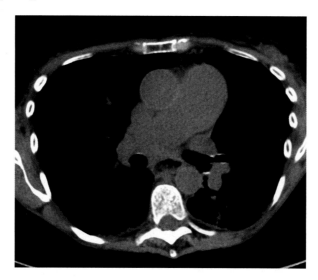

A. Idiopathic pulmonary fibrosis
B. Hypersensitivity pneumonitis
C. Scleroderma
D. Asbestosis

13a What is the best descriptor of the pattern of nodule distribution shown?

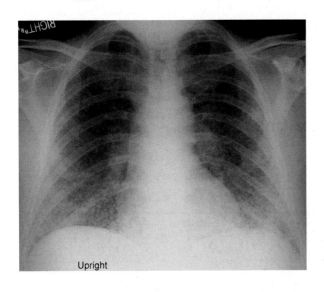
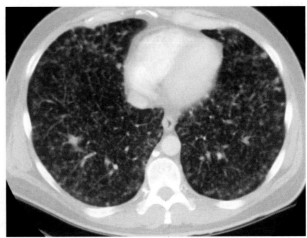

A. Centrilobular
B. Peribronchovascular
C. Miliary
D. Perilymphatic

13b What is the diagnosis for a miliary distribution of nodules?

A. Sarcoidosis
B. Disseminated fungal infection
C. Disseminated mycobacterial infection
D. Metastasis

14a The nodule is best described by which term?

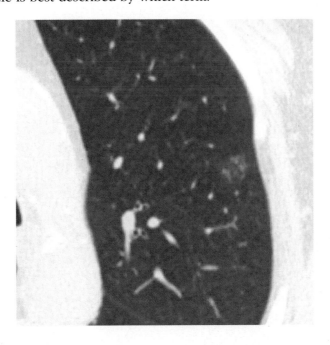

A. Solid
B. Halo lesion
C. Multicystic
D. Ground glass

14b Which characteristic of the nodule best defines it as ground glass?

A. Association with pleural tail
B. Visible vessels within the nodule
C. Presence of air bronchograms
D. Visible on soft tissue windows

15 Which of these radiologic signs is demonstrated?

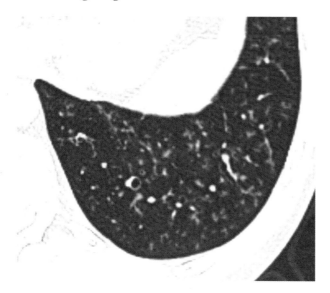

A. Silhouette sign
B. Signet ring sign
C. Reversed halo sign
D. Halo sign

ANSWERS AND EXPLANATIONS

1a **Answer C.**

1b **Answer A.** The beaded septum sign is associated with perilymphatic nodularity where disease is spreading along the lymphatics causing irregular and nodular thickened interlobular septa. First described in the setting of malignancy, the CT evidence of a beaded septum was highly correlative with pulmonary metastases. Histopathologic correlation in the same study confirmed involvement of pulmonary capillaries and lymphatics.

Primarily, this finding assists in characterizing a nodular pattern as perilymphatic, or characterizing a septal thickening pattern as nodular. The beaded septum sign can also be seen in other diseases with perilymphatic distribution, particularly sarcoidosis. Other provided options to include pulmonary hemorrhage, pulmonary embolism, and bacterial pneumonia can produce septal thickening and/or poorly defined nodularity but do not manifest with nodular septal thickening like the beaded septum sign.

References: Hansell DM, Bankier AA, MacMahon H, et al. Fleischner Society: glossary of terms for thoracic imaging. *Radiology* 2008;246(3):697–722.

Ren H, et al. Computed tomography of inflation-fixed lungs: the beaded septum sign of pulmonary metastases. *J Comput Assist Tomogr* 1989;13(3):411–416.

2 **Answer C.** In the radiograph provided, the bilateral hila demonstrate symmetric fullness with thickening of the right paratracheal stripe, accounting for the 1 (right hilum), 2 (left hilum), 3 (right paratracheal stripe) sign of lymphadenopathy in the setting of sarcoidosis. While this sign is highly suggestive of sarcoidosis, the differential would include other granulomatous diseases such as silicosis, coal worker's pneumoconiosis, or granulomatous infection. Less likely, but not excluded, would be a neoplastic process such as lymphoma or small cell carcinoma.

Reference: Webb WR, Higgins CB. Chapter 15: The pulmonary hila. In: *Thoracic imaging: pulmonary and cardiovascular radiology*, 2nd ed. Philadelphia, PA: Lippincott Williams & Wilkins, 2011:466.

3a **Answer D.**

3b **Answer A.**

3c **Answer B.** Finger-in-glove is a characteristic finding in allergic bronchopulmonary aspergillosis (ABPA), which often presents as refractory asthma. Bronchial atresia or other chronic bronchial obstruction would be alternative considerations, although the clinical history to include bronchial eosinophilia correlates better with ABPA. High density of the bronchial impaction is also characteristic of ABPA caused by the dense collection of *Aspergillus* in the secretions. In a recent study of 155 patients with diagnosed ABPA, hyperattenuation of the mucoid impaction on CT correlated with greater serologic severity and increased frequency of relapses. Additional imaging findings seen on CT for ABPA would include upper lobe predominant bronchiectasis, bronchial wall thickening, and tree-in-bud opacities.

References: Agarwal R, Gupta D, Aggarwal AN, et al. Clinical significance of hyperattenuating mucoid impaction in allergic bronchopulmonary aspergillosis: an analysis of 155 patients. *Chest* 2007;132:1183–1190.

Marshall GB, Farnquist BA, MacGregor JH, et al. Signs in thoracic imaging. *J Thorac Imaging* 2006;21:76–90.

4a **Answer A.**

4b **Answer A.**

4c **Answer C.**

4d **Answer B.** The inspiratory CT demonstrates geographic areas of mosaic attenuation, defined as patchwork regions of differing attenuation by the Fleischner Society Glossary. Differential considerations include (1) interstitial lung disease, (2) air trapping, and (3) occlusive pulmonary vascular disease. Of these causes, air trapping is accentuated by expiration (as demonstrated on the expiratory images of this patient). This air trapping is characteristic of small airways disease such as hypersensitivity pneumonitis, obliterative (constrictive) bronchiolitis, or asthma. Causes of obliterative bronchiolitis include prior infection (especially adenovirus or respiratory syncytial virus), collagen vascular disease (especially rheumatoid arthritis), drug toxicity, industrial toxic inhalation injury, and chronic transplant rejection (both heart/ lung and graft versus host disease in bone marrow transplant).

Reference: Hansell DM, Bankier AA, MacMahon H, et al. Fleischner Society: glossary of terms for thoracic imaging. *Radiology* 2008;246(3):697–722.

5 **Answer B.** The aortic arch forms the superior border. The other choices form the inferior (left pulmonary artery), medial (ligamentum arteriosum), and lateral borders (parietal pleura of the left lung). The anterior border is formed by the ascending aorta, and the posterior border is formed by the descending aorta.

Reference: Hansell DM, Bankier AA, MacMahon H, et al. Fleischner Society: glossary of terms for thoracic imaging. *Radiology* 2008;246(3):697–722.

6 **Answer C.** Supine positioning of the patient on chest radiograph redistributes a pneumothorax from the typical location along the lung apex inferiorly along the lower lung. Therefore, the deep sulcus sign represents a lucent distention of the sulcus by redistributed pleural air. Pleural effusion increases basilar opacity with layering fluid and may obscure the costophrenic angle. Collapse of a lower pulmonary lobe also increases basilar opacity with nonaerated lung and decreases lung volume. Finally, emphysema hyperinflates the lung and may flatten the diaphragm, but would not accentuate the costophrenic angle on supine imaging.

Reference: Kong A. The deep sulcus sign. *Radiology* 2003;228:415–416.

7 **Answer B.** Infarction is the result of pulmonary artery occlusion in almost all cases. Pulmonary vein–related infarction is recognized but extremely uncommon. Ischemic necrosis may or may not be present due to the bronchial arteries remaining patent and serving as a secondary vascular supply. Pulmonary embolism and pulmonary involvement of vasculitis are the most frequent causes.

Reference: Hansell DM, Bankier AA, MacMahon H, et al. Fleischner Society: glossary of terms for thoracic imaging. *Radiology* 2008;246(3):697–722.

8a **Answer A.**

8b **Answer B.**

8c **Answer D.** Air bronchograms are air-filled bronchi contrasted by surrounding alveoli filled with blood, pus, cells, water, or other debris. On chest radiograph and computed tomography, this produces a branching black structure with surrounding white lung. In contrast, the beaded septum is a sign describing white nodules tracking along an interlobular septum indicating a perilymphatic pattern. The ring around the artery sign appears as black air tracking around the artery on lateral radiograph related to pneumomediastinum. Finally, an air crescent develops as a crescent-shaped lucency within an early cavitary lesion suggestive of improving immune status in the setting of neutropenic invasive fungal infection.

The air bronchogram is a characteristic finding in the setting of consolidation and assists in differentiating this pulmonary opacity from others. Mass, by definition, is a 3-cm rounded pulmonary opacity without air bronchograms. An endobronchial plug, usually caused by mucus, will produce an inverted appearance of a white bronchus outlined by black lung. Fluid trapped within a fissure may appear as a pseudomass and does not contain air bronchograms.

Pulmonary infarct generally occurs without air bronchograms as the associated hemorrhage fills the bronchi in the area of the infarct. Streptococcal pneumonia, organizing pneumonia, and pulmonary edema are all classic examples of consolidations with produce air bronchograms on radiograph and CT. So the presence of air bronchograms on noncontrast CT can be helpful in decreasing the likelihood of infarct when evaluating peripheral consolidation.

References: Hansell DM, Bankier AA, MacMahon H, et al. Fleischner Society: glossary of terms for thoracic imaging. *Radiology* 2008;246(3):697–722.

Revel MP, Triki R, Chatellier G, et al. Is it possible to recognize pulmonary infarction on multisection CT images? *Radiology* 2007;244(3):875–882.

9 **Answer A.** The tree-in-bud pattern reflects endobronchial filling of the branching distal airways and as such is a type of centrilobular nodule pattern. The differential diagnosis includes a variety of infectious and inflammatory bronchiolar conditions but most common causes include endobronchial spread of infection and aspiration. In the past, the term tree-in-bud was synonymous with endobronchial spread of tuberculosis, but this is now recognized as a finding present in multiple other diseases.

Reference: Nupur V, Jonathan HC, Tan-Lucien HM. Tree-in-bud sign. *J Thorac Imaging* 2012;27(2):W27.

10 **Answer A.** The Monod sign reflects a mycetoma mass within a preexisting cavity. Frequently, the mass is gravity dependent and can move with prone or decubitus imaging. The mycetoma itself forms from conglomerate hyphae, mucin, fibrin, and debris. Overlapping appearance with cavitary masses and nodules can sometimes occur, and some use the "air crescent sign" (originally reserved for angioinvasive fungal disease with immune reconstitution) to also refer to a mycetoma. Intracavitary hematoma can present similarly as well.

References: Ashley N, Peter S, Thomas SL. et al. Monod sign. *J Thorac Imaging* 2013;28(6):W120.

Palla A, Desideri M, Rossi G, et al. Elective surgery for giant bullous emphysema: a 5-year clinical and functional follow-up. *Chest* 2005;128:2043.

11a **Answer C.**

11b **Answer D.** The peripheral wedge-shaped opacity in the right lower lung is already suspicious for pulmonary infarct, and considering the classic history of shortness of breath with an initial negative chest radiograph, Hampton hump is the primary consideration to be excluded. While a pulmonary infarct could produce a positive spine sign, this sign is a **lateral** radiograph finding where the radio-opacity of the spine increases from cranial to caudal direction; the opposite of the expected decrease in opacity at the lung base seen on a normal lateral chest radiograph. Atelectasis in the left lower lobe produces the flat waist sign along the left heart border, and a thick curvilinear anomalous pulmonary venous drainage in the medial lower lobe produces the scimitar finding of scimitar (or hypogenetic lung) syndrome, neither of which have the appearance as shown on this chest radiograph.

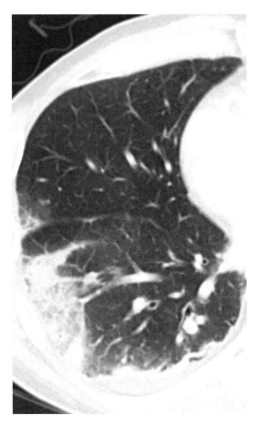 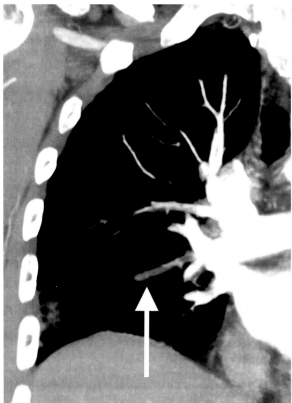

Hampton hump is a radiographic finding, which raises concern for pulmonary embolism resulting in a peripheral consolidation from an infarct, and CT angiogram of the pulmonary arteries is next imaging study favored by the ACR Appropriateness Criteria. The subsequent CTA images provided confirm the presence of central pulmonary embolism (white arrow) associated with the peripheral pulmonary infarct. While neoplasm and atypical infection could have this appearance, the short interval development and clinical presentation makes these considerations only after pulmonary embolism has been excluded. The focal nature of the finding nearly excludes the consideration of pulmonary edema.

References: ACR Appropriateness Criteria. Cardiac Section, Topic "Suspected Pulmonary Embolism". Available at https://acsearch.acr.org/docs/69404/Narrative/

Pipavath SN, Godwin DJ. Acute pulmonary thromboembolism: a historical perspective. *AJR Am J Roentgenol* 2008;191:639–641.

12a Answer B.

12b Answer C.   According to the Fleischner Society "Glossary of Terms for Thoracic Imaging," pulmonary fibrotic cystic airspaces with thick walls define honeycombing, and therefore, honeycombing represents fibrotic changes of the lung. Generally peripheral in distribution, honeycombing is a useful finding for consideration of fibrosing interstitial pneumonias. Emphysema can have some overlap in appearance, particularly in the setting of combined pulmonary fibrosis and emphysema (CPFE), although the thicker walls and basilar peripheral distribution are not characteristic of emphysema. Mosaic attenuation and air trapping do not produce well-defined walls but rather distinct areas of variable lung density on inspiratory and expiratory CT imaging, respectively.

While any of the diagnoses provided could cause honeycombing at the lung bases, the significant enlargement of the pulmonary artery and the dilated debris-filled esophagus best correlate with scleroderma, also called systemic sclerosis.

References: Bhalla M, Silver RM, Shepard JO, et al. Chest CT in patients with scleroderma: prevalence of asymptomatic esophageal dilatation and mediastinal lymphadenopathy. *AJR Am J Roentgenol* 1993;161:269–272.

Hansell DM, Bankier AA, MacMahon H, et al. Fleischner Society: glossary of terms for thoracic imaging. *Radiology* 2008;246(3):697–722.

Solomon JJ, Olson AL, Fischer A, et al. Scleroderma lung disease. *Eur Respir Rev* 2013;22(127):6–19.

13a Answer C.

13b Answer A.   The nodule distribution is miliary. The miliary pattern is characterized by innumerable tiny nodules <3 mm in size diffusely throughout the lungs. It is technically a subclass of randomly distributed nodules, but the random descriptor is generally reserved for larger and less profuse nodules. This distribution implies hematogenous spread of infection or malignancy with common pathogens being tuberculosis, fungal infection (such as histoplasmosis), and thyroid cancer. Sarcoid can present with miliary pattern but is quite unusual by comparison. Centrilobular nodules are generally airway-centered processes such as endobronchial infection, respiratory bronchiolitis, or subacute hypersensitivity pneumonitis. Perilymphatic nodules are a more common presentation for sarcoidosis or pneumoconiosis. This was a case of disseminated histoplasmosis.

Reference: Hansell DM, Bankier AA, MacMahon H, et al. Fleischner Society: glossary of terms for thoracic imaging. *Radiology* 2008;246(3):697–722.

14a Answer D.

14b Answer B.   Accurately characterizing the density of a pulmonary opacity on CT is critical to considering the correct differential for the finding. In this case, several surrounding pulmonary vessels as well as vessels internal to the nodule are visually denser that the nodule itself, confirming that it is ground glass in density. A solid nodule will obscure the internal vessels on noncontrast CT and be as dense if not denser than the adjacent vessels. A "halo" lesion or nodule is a specific type of part solid nodule defined by a central solid density with surrounding ground-glass opacity, which is not evident here. Nodules with multicystic components are often seen in the setting of solid, part solid, and ground-glass nodules with internal well-defined round lucencies that are the density of air.

In addition to visualization of vessels internal to the nodule, ground-glass components of a nodule can be evaluated by switching from lung window to a soft tissue window. Ground-glass portions will disappear, where solid portions will remain visible on the soft tissue window, keeping in mind that vessels can also be visible on soft tissue window. Association of a pleural tail may raise suspicion for malignancy but plays no part in determining the density of the nodule. Air bronchograms are best visualized when a bronchus passes through a solid density such as a solid nodule or consolidation. A transiting airway may or may not be visible in a ground-glass nodule but does not assist in characterizing the lesion as ground glass.

Reference: Hansell DM, Bankier AA, MacMahon, et al. Fleischner Society: glossary of terms for thoracic imaging. *Radiology* 2008;246(3):697–722.

15 **Answer B.**   The signet ring sign represents a dilated bronchus (the ring) with a smaller adjacent pulmonary artery (the signet). The bronchus should be similar in size to the adjacent artery and when dilated represents bronchiectasis. By definition, bronchiectasis is irreversible, and it should be noted that occasionally bronchial dilatation can resolve. More rarely, some causes of pulmonary arterial vasoconstriction can result in a similar appearance such as chronic thromboembolic disease.

Note that this signet ring sign has no relation to the musculoskeletal sign reflecting scapholunate dissociation or the presence of renal papillary necrosis in genitourinary imaging.

References: Hansell DM, Bankier AA, MacMahon H, et al. Fleischner Society: glossary of terms for thoracic imaging. *Radiology* 2008;246(3):697–722.

Ouellette H. The signet ring sign. *Radiology* 1999;212(1):67–68.

Intensive Care Unit Radiographs

Tami J. Bang, MD

QUESTIONS

1a A 56-year-old man with acute respiratory distress syndrome has been in the ICU for 10 days and presents with the chest radiograph shown. What is the most acute finding?

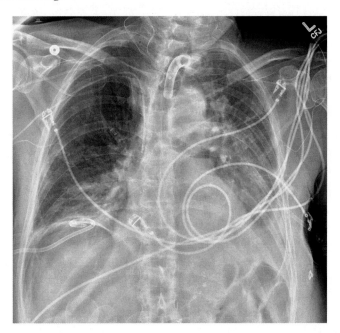

A. Pleural effusion
B. Esophageal intubation
C. Pneumoperitoneum
D. Pneumonia

1b What accounts for the well-demarcated bowel loops?

A. Oral contrast
B. Air on both sides of the bowel wall
C. Ascites surrounding bowel loops
D. Bowel wall thickening

2a   What is the optimum position of an endotracheal tube in an adult patient?

A. Midthoracic trachea
B. At the level of the clavicles
C. Right mainstem bronchus
D. Greater than 6 cm above the carina

2b   How does an endotracheal tube (ETT) tip move relative to head positioning?

A. ETT moves down when head is elevated.
B. ETT moves down when head is lowered.
C. ETT moves up when head is lowered.
D. ETT doesn't move with head positioning.

3a   What support device is labeled by the arrow?

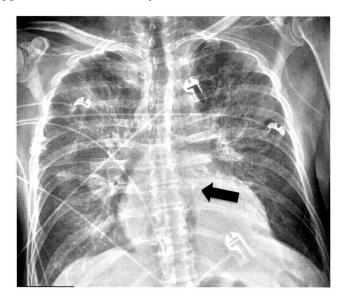

A. Peripherally inserted central catheter
B. Impella device
C. Intra-aortic balloon pump
D. ECMO cannula

3b   What complication is the primary concern for the malpositioned device (arrow) as shown?

A. Stroke
B. Arrhythmia
C. Pulmonary embolism
D. Renal or mesenteric ischemia

4   On a chest radiograph, what is the approximate location of the superior vena cava and the right atrial junction (superior cavoatrial junction)?

A. Midthoracic trachea
B. Carina
C. T9/T10 disc space
D. Two vertebral body heights below the carina

5a This is a chest radiograph for left central line placement. If no prior imaging is available, what is the next best step in the management of the patient?

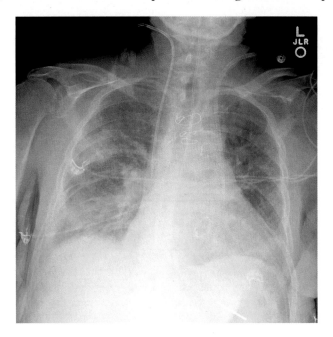

    A. Follow-up chest radiograph in 6 hours.
    B. Evaluate flow return and obtain blood gas.
    C. Pull and replace the left central line.
    D. Place a left thoracostomy tube.

5b A prior CT scan was reviewed on the same patient. What is the most likely explanation for the course of the left central line?

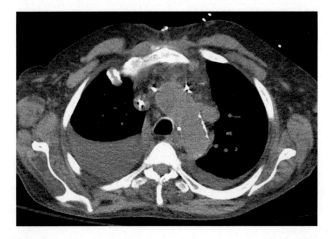

    A. Placement in the left subclavian artery
    B. Placement in the left common carotid artery
    C. Extravascular placement
    D. Placement in a left superior vena cava

6 An intubated patient in the ICU had morning chest radiographs taken 6 hours apart. What is the most likely cause for the left lung findings?

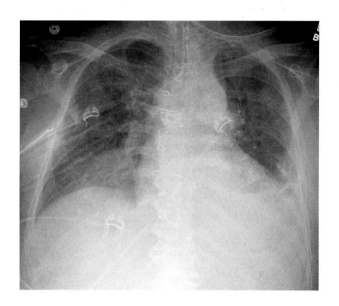
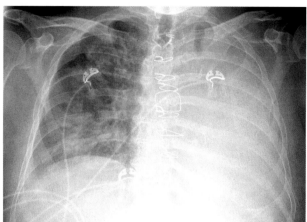

A. Pneumonia
B. Hematoma
C. Pleural effusion
D. Mucous plug

7a A left ventricular assist device (LVAD) is shown. What part of the device is indicated by the arrow?

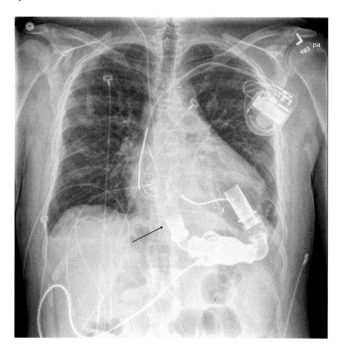

A. Reservoir
B. Outflow cannula
C. Drive line
D. Pump

7b Where is blood flow directed after leaving the outflow cannula?

    A. Aorta
    B. Left ventricle
    C. Left atrium
    D. Pulmonary artery

7c This device is considered:

    A. MR safe at all fields
    B. MR conditional at 1.5 T
    C. MR conditional at 3.0 T
    D. MR unsafe

8a Where is the indicated lead positioned?

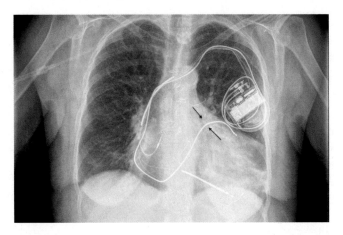

    A. Pulmonary artery
    B. Left atrium
    C. Coronary sinus
    D. Right ventricle

8b What is the primary indication for placement of biventricular pacemaker?

    A. Bradycardia
    B. Heart failure
    C. History of ventricular fibrillation
    D. Supraventricular tachycardia

9 What is the best way to differentiate extrapleural hematoma from hemothorax?

    A. Free layering configuration
    B. Increased density
    C. Blood return in chest tube
    D. Displacement of extrapleural fat

10 What is a long-term consequence of endotracheal tube balloon overinflation?

    A. Chronic infection
    B. Tracheal stenosis
    C. Reactive airways disease
    D. Hemorrhage

11a What device tip is denoted by the arrow?

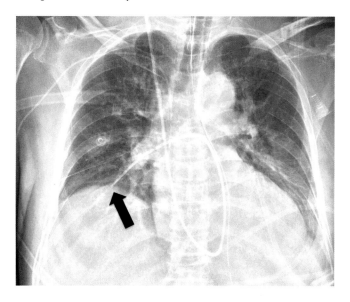

A. Pulmonary artery catheter
B. Peripherally inserted central catheter
C. Left ventricular assist device
D. ECMO cannula

11b What is the primary concern for the positioning of the device (arrow) in this case?

A. Falsely elevated pressure reading
B. Pulmonary artery pseudoaneurysm
C. Infection
D. Air embolism

12 What is the likely location of this catheter (arrow)?

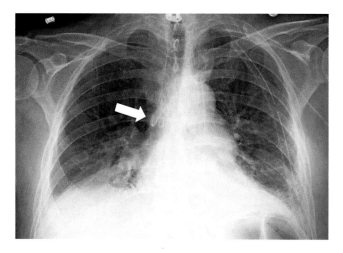

A. Superior vena cava
B. Inferior vena cava
C. Azygos vein
D. Right pulmonary artery

13a What is the primary abnormality?

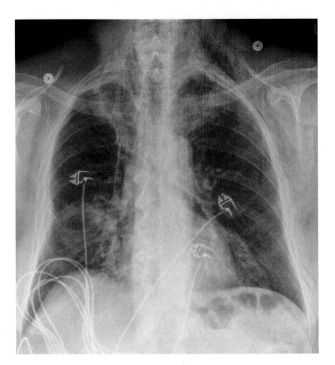

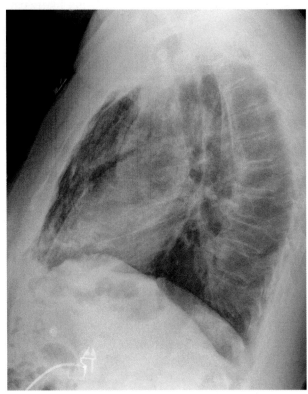

A. Pneumothorax
B. Pneumopericardium
C. Pneumoperitoneum
D. Pneumomediastinum

13b In a different patient, what accounts for the lucency inferior to the heart?

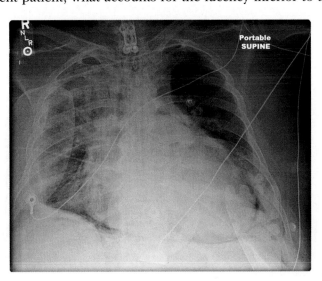

A. Pneumothorax
B. Pneumopericardium
C. Pneumoperitoneum
D. Pneumomediastinum

14 A chest radiograph is obtained for increased postoperative oxygen requirement. What is the likely cause?

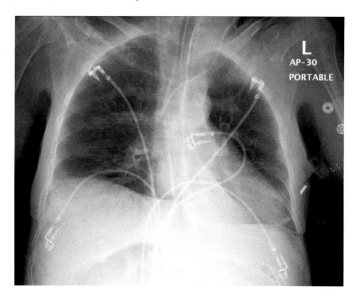

A. Mucous plugging
B. Pleural effusion
C. Pneumonia
D. Pulmonary embolus

15 Compare the preoperative image of a patient (image left) and the postoperative image taken on postoperative day 1. What accounts for the new density at the apex of the left hemithorax (arrowhead)?

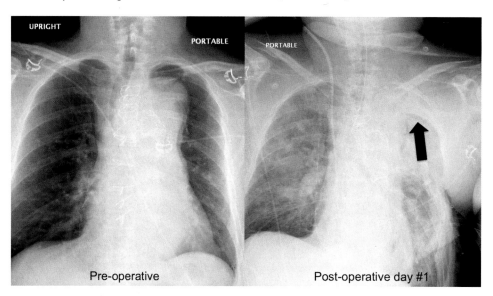

A. Mediastinal hemorrhage
B. Tension pneumothorax
C. Pericardial tamponade
D. Left upper lobe atelectasis

16a What is the most common location for lead fracture of a transvenous pacer?

    A. At the pacemaker attachment
    B. Terminal lead tip
    C. Venous access site
    D. Cavoatrial junction

16b What is a common cause of pacemaker lead fracture?

    A. Metal fatigue
    B. Friction motion between leads
    C. Electrical short circuit
    D. Compression between the clavicle and first rib

17 What is generally the most appropriate initial management of vascular catheter fracture and dislodgement?

    A. No treatment
    B. Snare
    C. Vascular surgery
    D. Suction aspiration

18 What is the role of a Sengstaken-Blakemore tube?

    A. Direct drainage of bleeding gastric ulcer
    B. Enteric feeding following gastrectomy
    C. Balloon tamponade of bleeding esophageal varices
    D. Temporary plombage treatment of mycobacterial pneumonia

19a What is this imaging sign commonly called?

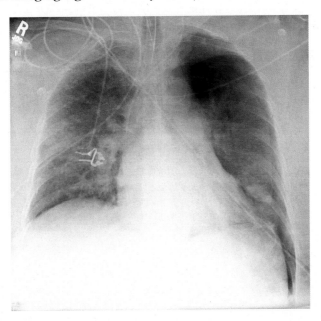

    A. Deep sulcus sign
    B. Silhouette sign
    C. Air crescent sign
    D. Scimitar sign

19b   Where is the air located associated with the deep sulcus sign?

    A. Posterior lateral pleural space
    B. Anterior lateral pleural space
    C. Left upper quadrant
    D. Lateral chest wall

20   A chest x-ray was obtained for evaluation of feeding tube placement. What best describes the location of the feeding tube tip?

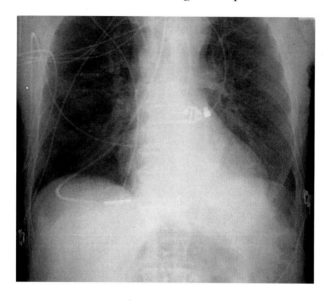

    A. In the right lower lobe bronchus
    B. In the right middle lobe bronchus
    C. In the right pleural space
    D. In a large hiatal hernia

ANSWERS AND EXPLANATIONS

1a   Answer C.

1b   Answer B.   Pneumoperitoneum can result from a variety of benign and emergent conditions and can be a harbinger of a serious underlying condition. Common causes include surgery, peritoneal dialysis, or recent instrumentation. Toxic causes include bowel ischemia, infectious or inflammatory gastrointestinal conditions, or penetrating trauma. Steroids can cause asymptomatic benign pneumoperitoneum. "Free air" rises to a nondependent location in a body cavity. In the upright position, pneumoperitoneum will be seen as curvilinear lucencies outlining the abdominal surface of the diaphragm. In the ICU, supine radiography is employed in intubated nonambulatory patients. Right upper quadrant air can be seen in the subdiaphragmatic space distinct from the liver. Normal bowel gas only outlines the intraluminal surface. The serosal surfaces have similar radiographic soft tissue attenuation as the surrounding mesenteric fat and are not as well delineated. When gas is on the extraluminal surface of the bowel wall, this creates a radiodense line known as the Rigler sign.

Reference: Ly JQ. The Rigler sign. *Radiology* 2003;228(3):706–707.

2a   Answer A.

2b   Answer B.   Endotracheal tubes provide ventilatory support to critically ill patients to aid with oxygenation. Malposition can occur in up to 15% of patients. Postplacement chest radiography of intubated patients can detect malposition prior to complications. Optimal position is in the midthoracic trachea approximately 5 cm above the carina with the head in the neutral position where the mandible overlies the lower cervical spine on frontal view. Head flexion causes the tube to move caudally while head extension causes it to move cranially ("the hose follows the nose"). High placement of an ETT can lead to extubation, hypopharyngeal intubation, gastric distension, and poor ventilation as well as lead to vocal cord injury. Low placement can result in mainstem bronchus intubation, ipsilateral lung overinflation, and increased risk of pneumothorax and atelectasis of the opposite lung. Bronchial intubation usually occurs on the right due to the more vertical course of the right mainstem bronchus. Esophageal intubation can be fatal and may present as an ETT lateral to the trachea, an esophageal air column parallel to the trachea, or gastric distension. Obtaining a right posterior oblique radiograph can aid in diagnosis by separating the trachea and the inadvertently intubated esophagus.

Reference: Godoy MC, Leitman BS, de Groot PM, et al. Chest radiography in the ICU: part I, evaluation of airway, enteric, and pleural tubes. *AJR Am J Roentgenol* 2012;198(3):563–571.

3a   Answer C.

3b   Answer D.   Intra-aortic balloon pump (IABP) is a long tubular balloon that is inserted from a femoral artery approach into the descending thoracic aorta. It inflates during diastole and deflates during systole, providing circulatory support in patients with cardiogenic shock. If inserted too deep (high termination), this can result in occlusion of left subclavian, vertebral, or carotid arteries—consequences include limb ischemia or stroke. However, if IABP positioning is too low, the balloon may be inflated across the renal or mesenteric arteries, resulting in ischemia. Additionally, distal position results in less effective circulatory support. The ideal position of the IABP is just caudal to the aortic arch—approximately 2 cm distal to the left subclavian artery origin. Other complication of IABP placement include aortic dissection or very rarely balloon rupture with gas embolization.

References: Godoy MC, Leitman BS, de Groot PM, et al. Chest radiography in the ICU: part 2, evaluation of cardiovascular lines and other devices. *AJR Am J Roentgenol* 2012;198(3): 572–581.

Winer-Muram HT. Abnormally positioned tubes and catheters. In: Rosado-de-Christenson, ML (ed.). *Diagnostic imaging: chest*, 2nd ed. Altona, Manitoba: Amirsys, 2012:10–13.

4 **Answer D.** The superior cavoatrial junction (CAJ) is the point between the superior vena cava (SVC) and the true right atrium. The CAJ is the midpoint on an oblique line between the crista terminalis anteriorly and the crista dividens posteriorly. Because the SVC has a most posterior insertion on the right atrium, the CAJ is located more inferior than usually anticipated on chest radiography. Various techniques have been described to confirm adequate positioning of central venous catheters, to include two vertebral body heights below the carina, within 4 cm of the carina, and alignment with the inferior bronchus intermedius.

References: Baskin KM, Jimenez RM, Cahill AM, et al. Cavoatrial junction and central venous anatomy: implications for central venous access tip position. *J Vasc Interv Radiol* 2008;19(3):359–365.

Ridge CA, Litmanovich D, Molinari F, et al. Radiographic evaluation of central venous catheter position: anatomic correlation using gated coronary computed tomographic angiography. *J Thorac Imaging* 2013;28(2):129–133.

Webb, WR. Pulmonary edema, the acute respiratory distress syndrome, and radiology in the ICU. In: Webb WR, Higgins CB (eds.). *Thoracic imaging: pulmonary and cardiovascular radiology*, 2nd ed. Philadelphia, PA: Lippincott Williams & Wilkins, 2011:348–374.

5a **Answer B.**

5b **Answer D.** Central venous lines provide venous access to administer fluids, medications, and pressure monitoring. Common types of central lines include internal jugular and subclavian lines and peripherally inserted central catheters (PICC). Optimal position of a central line tip is in the downstream superior vena cava at the cavoatrial junction. Intracardiac placement risks cardiac injury or rhythm disturbances, while high positioning could lead to thrombus formation or intravenous introduction of potentially toxic drugs that are meant to be diluted. Malpositioned catheters may lie in the internal jugular, contralateral subclavian, or azygos veins. Inadvertent arterial positioning can lead to thromboembolic events and stroke.

Variant anatomy can cause unexpected positioning on radiography and can be confirmed by review of cross-sectional imaging. A persistent left SVC is not an infrequent anomaly, which can cause an aberrant course of a left central line projecting along the left upper mediastinum. A diligent search for a vascular anomaly should be undertaken with available images. If no cause is found, communication with the care team should raise the possibility of arterial catheterization. Intravenous fluids should be maintained to prevent thrombus formation. Confirmation of arterial catheterization includes evaluation of blood color, arterial blood gas measurements, catheter transduction, and assessment of pulsatile waveform. A CT scan or contrast injection under fluoroscopy can confirm the diagnosis. The line should remain in place and consultation obtained for endovascular or surgical management.

References: Godoy MC, Leitman BS, de Groot PM, et al. Chest radiography in the ICU: part 2, evaluation of cardiovascular lines and other devices. *AJR Am J Roentgenol* 2012;198(3):572–581.

Pikwer A, Acosta S, Kölbel T, et al. Management of inadvertent arterial catheterisation associated with central venous access procedures. *Eur J Vasc Endovasc Surg* 2009;38(6):707–714.

6 **Answer D.** Central endobronchial obstruction can cause obstructive atelectasis following reabsorption of gas from the alveoli. A central mucous plug can cause relatively rapid and impressive whole lung atelectasis. By knowing the intubation status of the patient and recognizing the ipsilateral volume loss, one can make a confident diagnosis of a mucous plug and not mistake the "white out" appearance for a large pleural effusion. Bronchoscopy can confirm the diagnosis and clear the mucoid impaction.

Reference: Collins J, Stern EJ, eds. *Chest radiology: the essentials*. Philadelphia, PA: Lippincott Williams & Wilkins, 2008.

7a **Answer B.**

7b **Answer A.**

7c **Answer D.** Left ventricular assist devices (LVADs) are implantable devices used for patients in end-stage heart failure prior to heart transplantation, during cardiac recovery, or for those patients ineligible for transplant. Several different types of LVADs are in use (HeartMate II shown, Thoratec, Inc.). All devices currently approved (including HeartMate II, the HeartMate 3, and HeartWare) are considered MR UNSAFE. Basic design features usually include an inflow cannula attached to the left ventricle, a pump, and an outflow cannula attached to the aorta. The connection between the outflow cannula and the ascending aorta is normally radiolucent, and the position must be inferred by radiography. Potential complications include postoperative hemorrhage, pericardial tamponade, thrombus formation, aortic valve stenosis, aortic valve insufficiency, right-sided heart failure, and infection. These complications are generally best evaluated by chest CT.

References: Carr CM, Jacob J, Park SJ, et al. CT of left ventricular assist devices 1. *Radiographics* 2010;30(2):429–444.

Sigakis CJG, Mathai SK, Suby-Long TD, et al. Radiographic review of current therapeutic and monitoring devices in the chest. *Radiographics* 2018;38(2):1027–1045.

8a **Answer C.**

8b **Answer B.** On a frontal chest radiograph, the approximate position of the coronary sinus runs at an oblique angle from the inferior right heart border to the superior left heart border. A pacer lead in the coronary sinus allows for pacing of the left ventricle and in this patient indicates placement of a dual-chamber biventricular pacer. Heart failure is the primary indication for biventricular pacing, as they have shown improved cardiac function in refractory heart failure patients.

References: Costelloe CM, et al. Radiography of pacemakers and implantable cardioverter defibrillators. *AJR Am J Roentgenol* 2012;199(6):1252–1258.

Singh JP, Gras D. Biventricular pacing: current trends and future strategies. *Eur Heart J* 2012;33(3):305–313.

9 **Answer D.** The pleura is surrounded by a thin layer of fat external to the parietal layer of the pleura. An extrapleural hematoma occurs outside the fat layer causing inward medial displacement of the extrapleural fat. Other indications of an extrapleural hematoma, as may be seen due to thoracentesis, include a focal lobular contour and fixed position despite repositioning of the patient.

Reference: Godoy MC, Leitman BS, de Groot PM, et al. Chest radiography in the ICU: part I, evaluation of airway, enteric, and pleural tubes. *AJR Am J Roentgenol* 2012;198(3): 563–571.

10 **Answer B.** The endotracheal tube balloon should not expand normal tracheal contours. Overinflation of the balloon is associated with tracheal injury. Acutely, this can cause tracheal rupture, most frequently of the posterior membranous wall within 7 cm of the carina. Quick onset of subcutaneous emphysema, pneumomediastinum, and pneumothorax are frequently seen as a result of such a tracheal injury. In the long term, this can result in chronic damage including tracheal stenosis or tracheobronchomalacia. Subglottic tracheal stenosis as a result of endotracheal tube overinflation is increasingly recognized with prolonged intubation >7 days being an additional risk factor. Such tracheal stenosis usually takes weeks to months to develop after the associated injury.

Reference: Godoy MC, Leitman BS, de Groot PM, et al. Chest radiography in the ICU: part I, evaluation of airway, enteric, and pleural tubes. *AJR Am J Roentgenol* 2012;198(3):563–571.

11a **Answer A.**

11b **Answer B.** The pulmonary artery catheter (Swan-Ganz catheter) is a catheter with a specially designed tip placed in the pulmonary artery for hemodynamic monitoring of critically ill patients. It is inserted into the central venous system, through the right heart, and into the proximal pulmonary arterial system. Ideal position is in the proximal right or left pulmonary arteries within 2 cm of the hilum. Potential complications of distal placement such as in this case include pulmonary artery occlusion (and potentially pulmonary infarction) or more rarely, pulmonary artery injury such as pseudoaneurysm, dissection, or rupture.

References: Godoy MC, Leitman BS, de Groot PM, et al. Chest radiography in the ICU: part 2, evaluation of cardiovascular lines and other devices. *AJR Am J Roentgenol* 2012;198(3): 572–581.

Winer-Muram HT. Abnormally positioned tubes and catheters. In: Rosado-de-Christenson, ML (ed.). *Diagnostic imaging: chest*, 2nd ed. Altona, Manitoba: Amirsys, 2012:10–13

12 **Answer C.** The azygos vein is usually oriented in the anterior–posterior direction as it empties into the superior vena cava. It is located at the junction of the trachea and the right mainstem bronchus. On chest radiography, a catheter directed into the azygos vein appears to loop or turn in the SVC at the level of the right mainstem bronchus origin. A lateral radiograph may show the posterior direction of the catheter.

References: Godoy MC, Leitman BS, de Groot PM, et al. Chest radiography in the ICU: part 2, evaluation of cardiovascular lines and other devices. *AJR Am J Roentgenol* 2012;198(3):572–581.

Winer-Muram HT. Abnormally positioned tubes and catheters. In: Rosado-de-Christenson, ML (ed.). *Diagnostic imaging: chest*, 2nd ed. Altona, Manitoba: Amirsys, 2012:10–13.

13a **Answer D.**

13b **Answer D.** Pneumomediastinum can result from a variety of causes including alveolar rupture, tracheobronchial tree laceration, gastrointestinal tract injury (especially the esophagus), or extraluminal gas tracking into the thorax from other sites. Mechanically ventilated patients are at increased risk for pneumomediastinum. The first case shown was related to recent bronchoscopy. The streaky lucencies overlying the mediastinum on the frontal and lateral projections are typical.

Mediastinal gas collecting along the inferior margin of the heart can sometimes outline the superior diaphragmatic surface. Usually, the anterior medial left hemidiaphragm is not distinguishable due to the isodense soft tissue interface between the diaphragm and the heart. A pneumomediastinum air gap separates these two surfaces allowing visibility of the left side of the diaphragm, which creates a continuous diaphragm sign as seen in the second case shown.

References: Bejvan SM, Godwin JD. Pneumomediastinum: old signs and new signs. *AJR Am J Roentgenol* 1996;166(5):1041–1048.

Schmitt ER, Burg MD. Continuous diaphragm sign. *West J Emerg Med* 2011;12(4):526–527.

14 Answer A.   There is a triangular opacity in the medial left lung base, obscuring the descending aorta and the left hemidiaphragm. This is associated with downward and medial retraction of the fissure. These findings are compatible with left lower lobe atelectasis. Intubated patients are at high risk for mucous plugging—this should be a primary consideration when new lobar atelectasis is encountered in the setting of intubation.

References: Abbott GF, Carter BW. Left lower lobe atelectasis. In: Rosado-de-Christenson ML (ed.). *Diagnostic imaging: chest*, 2nd ed. Altona, Manitoba: Amirsys, 2012:1–64.

Kazerooni EA, Gross BH. Thoracic imaging in the critically Ill. In: Kazerooni EA, Gross BH (eds.). *Cardiopulmonary imaging*. Philadephia, PA: Lippincott Williams & Wilkins, 2004:217–254.

15 Answer A.   The follow-up radiograph performed on postoperative day 1 shows increasing mediastinal widening and development of a cap-like opacity at the apex of the left hemithorax (left apical cap).

In the setting of mediastinal hemorrhage, the hematoma results in widening of mediastinal contours and extends into the potential space at the left apical extrapleural space. Presence of a new left apical cap suggests acute mediastinal hematoma, which may be postoperative or traumatic.

Reference: Harris JH, Harris WH, Jain S, et al. To reduce routine computed tomographic angiography for thoracic aortic injury assessment in level II blunt trauma patients using three mediastinal signs on the initial chest radiograph: a preliminary report. *Emergency Radiology* 2018;25:387–391.

16a Answer C.

16b Answer D.   Pacemakers are used to treat a variety of cardiac conduction disturbances and can be either temporary or permanent. Permanent pacers have a pulse generator with a battery pack and control unit that is implanted into the anterior chest wall. One or more leads are positioned endovascularly as needed. Biventricular pacing can treat congestive heart failure, and an automatic implantable cardioverter–defibrillator (AICD) may be added to reduce the risk of ventricular tachyarrhythmias. Complications can include pneumothorax, vascular injury, myocardial perforation, and lead fracture. Lead fractures can occur at the venous access site, from compression between the clavicle and first rib; at the battery pack; or at the lead tip. Patients who rotate the generator in the subcutaneous skin pocket ("twiddler's syndrome") can cause lead traction and dislodgement.

Reference: Godoy MC, Leitman BS, de Groot PM, et al. Chest radiography in the ICU: part 2, evaluation of cardiovascular lines and other devices. *AJR Am J Roentgenol* 2012;198(3):572–581.

17 Answer B.   When an intravascular foreign body is discovered, careful evaluation can determine the necessity of removing the object, best approach, safety concerns, and technique. A snare loop is the simplest and most commonly found device that can retrieve a variety of foreign bodies. A snare consists of an adjustable loop that works similar to a "lasso" to tighten around intravascular catheters for extraction.

Reference: Kaufman JA, Lee MJ. *Vascular and interventional radiology*. Philadelphia, PA: Elsevier Health Sciences, 2013.

18 Answer C.   Bleeding esophageal varices can be a life-threatening condition, and prompt treatment is necessary for patient stabilization. Volume repletion, with pharmacologic and surgical interventions, is a mainstay of treatment. Mechanical balloon tamponade can be accomplished with a Sengstaken-Blakemore tube. It is inserted through the mouth or nose and the balloon tip is inflated for compression of bleeding varices. Tubes that have an opening near the top are called Minnesota tubes. Complications include esophageal perforation, rupture, ulceration, and necrosis. Due to modern endoscopic advances, Sengstaken-Blakemore tubes are much less frequently employed than in the past.

Reference: Shen TC, Tu CY. Common procedure-related complications in the ICU: a pictorial review. *J Intern Med Taiwan* 2013;24(6):453–460.

19a Answer A.

19b Answer B.   Pneumothorax in a supine patient collects anteriorly and basally in the nondependent portion of the chest. When it accumulates laterally, the lateral costophrenic angle is accentuated producing the deep sulcus sign. Other signs of pneumothorax include diaphragmatic depression, increased sharpness of the cardiac borders and pericardial fat pads, inferior pleural line, or double diaphragmatic contour. Lateral decubitus views may be helpful for future evaluation.

Reference: Kong A. The deep sulcus sign. *Radiology* 2003;228(2):415–416.

20 Answer C.   A feeding tube is identified overlying the right lung. The course of the tube extends into the right bronchial tree but makes an L-shaped curve that is not compatible with being inside the lung parenchyma. This tube has pierced the visceral pleura and resides within the pleural space. This should be considered an emergent finding, and the caregivers should be prepared for a high likelihood that this patient will require a chest tube after removal of the feeding tube. There is no identifiable hiatal hernia, although feeding tubes can loop inside hernias on occasion.

Reference: Godoy MC, Leitman BS, de Groot PM, et al. Chest radiography in the ICU: part I, evaluation of airway, enteric, and pleural tubes. *AJR Am J Roentgenol* 2012;198(3):563–571.

5 Infectious Pneumonia

Christopher Lee, MD

QUESTIONS

1a In the CT image, an imaging feature that reliably differentiates between cytomegalovirus pneumonia and *Pneumocystis jiroveci* pneumonia is:

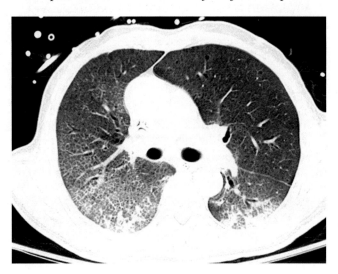

    A. Ground-glass opacities
    B. Consolidations
    C. Crazy-paving pattern
    D. Not present

1b At what CD4+ cell count does PJP infection generally begin to occur?
    A. 400 cells/mm³
    B. 200 cells/mm³
    C. 100 cells/mm³
    D. 50 cells/mm³

2   This 66-year-old nursing home patient with pneumonia has a past medical history of diabetes, chronic respiratory insufficiency requiring tracheostomy, and chronic renal insufficiency. Considering the CT appearance, the most likely etiologic agent of pneumonia is:

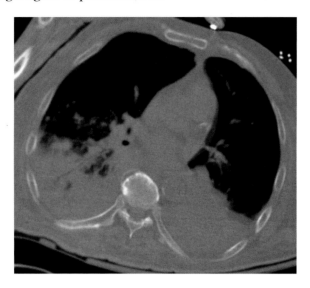

A. *Pseudomonas aeruginosa*
B. Cytomegalovirus
C. *Pneumocystis jiroveci*
D. Histoplasmosis

3a Two weeks after significant head injury, this 74-year-old patient developed overnight respiratory decline in the ICU. CT pulmonary angiogram was obtained, which is shown below. After obtaining a protected bronchial washing for culture, the best intervention is to commence therapy with:

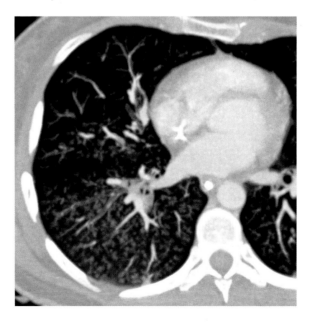

A. Sulfamethoxazole and trimethoprim
B. Isoniazid and rifampin
C. Levofloxacin
D. Ceftazidime and vancomycin

3b Which of the following is a risk factor for community-acquired methicillin-resistant *Staphylococcus aureus* (MRSA) infection?

A. Female gender
B. Incarceration
C. High socioeconomic status
D. Silica exposure

4 This 37-year-old patient was referred to the outpatient imaging center with complaints of a nonproductive cough for 5 months. The most appropriate subsequent intervention is:

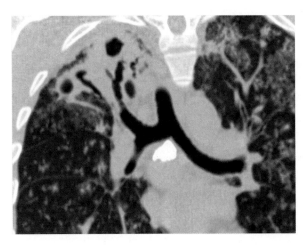

A. Left mainstem bronchial intubation
B. Bronchoscopy with bronchoalveolar lavage
C. Initiation of antimicrobial therapy
D. Contrast esophagram

5 A 26-year-old patient with known HIV/AIDS presents with respiratory distress. The most likely etiologic agent responsible for the findings present on the image provided is:

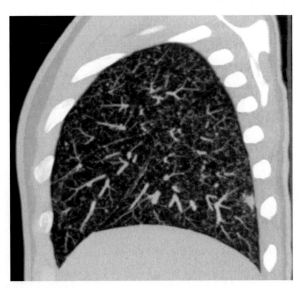

A. *Coccidioides immitis*
B. Cytomegalovirus
C. *Pneumocystis jiroveci*
D. *Nocardia asteroides*

6a In the setting of pulmonary septic emboli, what is the most common cardiac source of infection?

    A. Tricuspid valve
    B. Mitral valve
    C. Pulmonic valve
    D. Aortic valve

6b What is the most common infectious agent to cause septic emboli?

    A. *Streptococcus pneumoniae*
    B. *Enterobacter aerogenes*
    C. *Haemophilus influenzae*
    D. *Staphylococcus aureus*

7 In an immunocompromised patient with dyspnea and fever and a chest radiograph showing diffuse pulmonary parenchymal opacities, what is the next most appropriate imaging examination for further evaluation?

    A. Chest CT without IV contrast
    B. Chest CT with IV contrast
    C. FDG-PET/CT
    D. No further imaging

8 What is the typical patient demographic of nonclassic pulmonary MAC infection?

    A. Middle-aged men with HIV/AIDS
    B. Elderly men with COPD
    C. Young women with cystic fibrosis
    D. Elderly women without underlying lung disease

9 This patient underwent orthotopic heart transplant 3 months prior. Based on the image provided, what is the most likely cause of the nodule?

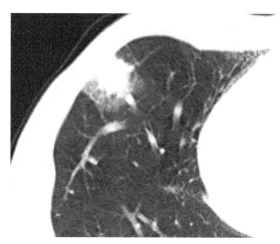

    A. *Aspergillus*
    B. Cytomegalovirus
    C. Posttransplant lymphoproliferative disease
    D. Rounded atelectasis

10 A 61-year-old male presents with declining pulmonary function tests. The etiology of the process evident on the image provided is most likely to be:

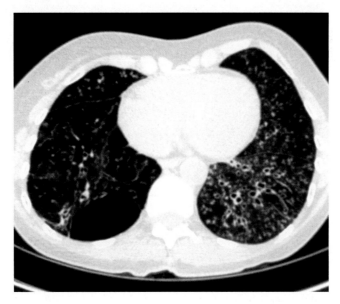

A. Allergic bronchopulmonary aspergillosis
B. Cystic fibrosis
C. Sarcoidosis
D. Recurrent infection

11 Chest radiographs were obtained 6 days apart in this 19-year-old male with positive H1N1 viral culture. What is the most likely cause of progression in the second chest radiograph?

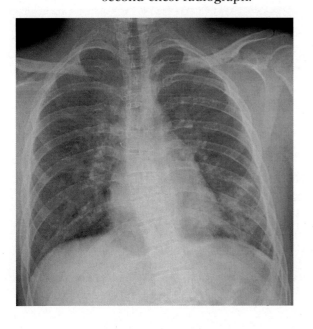 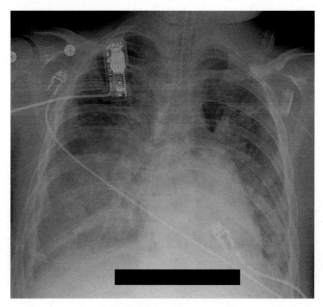

A. Pulmonary hemorrhage
B. Cardiogenic pulmonary edema
C. Alveolar proteinosis
D. Diffuse alveolar damage

12 In this patient with acute myeloid leukemia is diagnosed with invasive aspergillosis, what does the imaging sign demonstrated indicate?

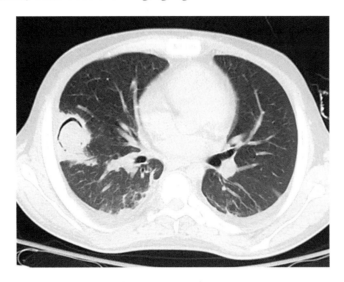

A. Neutropenia
B. Acute infection
C. Healing infection
D. Superinfection

13a What is the most likely pathogen in the setting of a community-acquired pneumonia in an immunocompetent patient?

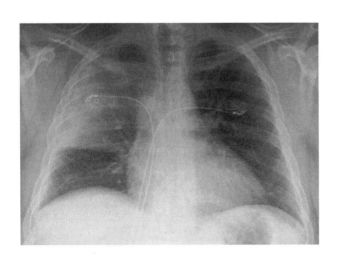
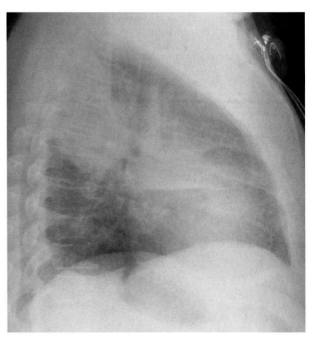

A. *Streptococcus pneumonia*
B. *Legionella pneumophila*
C. Influenza A
D. *Mycoplasma pneumoniae*

13b What lung segment is largely spared by the pathologic process demonstrated in the right upper lobe?

A. Apical segment
B. Posterior segment
C. Anterior segment
D. Apicoposterior segment

14 A HIV/AIDS patient noncompliant with his HAART medications presents with a rash and the accompanying CT image. What is the most likely diagnosis?

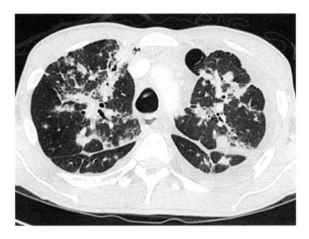

A. CMV pneumonia
B. MAC infection
C. Cryptococcal pneumonia
D. Kaposi sarcoma

15a What complication of airspace disease is identified in the right upper lobe?

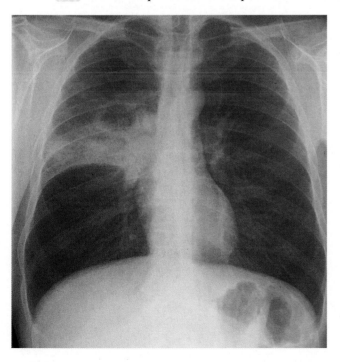
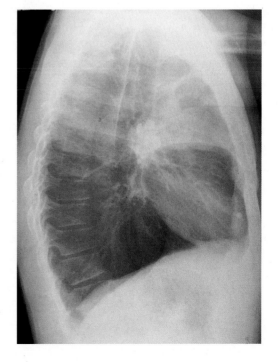

A. Pleural effusion
B. Pneumothorax
C. Cavitation
D. Pulmonary hemorrhage

15b What is the likely pathogen given the complication, presuming this is an infectious process?

A. Mixed anaerobic infection
B. *Staphylococcus aureus*
C. *Pseudomonas aeruginosa*
D. *Mycobacterium tuberculosis*

16 A patient presents with a history of tuberculosis and new-onset hemoptysis. In addition to the accompanying CT image, what imaging can be performed to confirm the diagnosis?

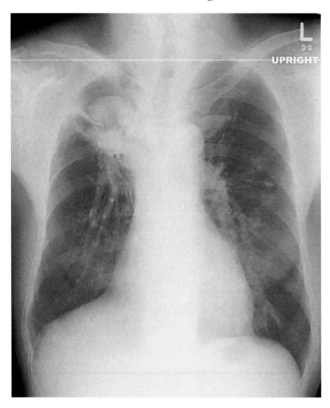
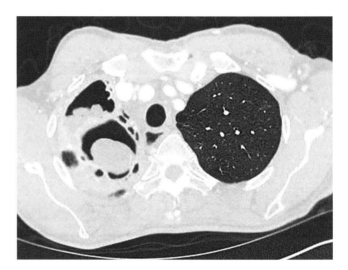

A. PET/CT
B. Prone chest CT
C. Pre- and postcontrast chest CT
D. Inspiratory and expiratory chest CT

17 What is the most common cause of lobar consolidation in an HIV patient?

A. Bacterial pneumonia
B. Viral pneumonia
C. Fungal pneumonia
D. Tuberculosis

18 Given a history of HIV infection and slowly progressive symptoms, what is the most likely diagnosis?

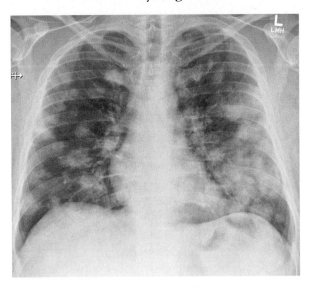
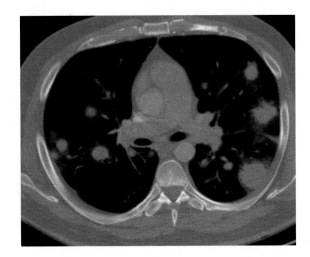

    A. Septic emboli
    B. Angioinvasive fungal infection
    C. Lymphoma
    D. Organizing pneumonia

19a A patient presents with the following imaging, with a concurrent diffuse rash progressing from macules to blisters and finally scabbing. What is the likely cause of the pulmonary parenchymal abnormality?

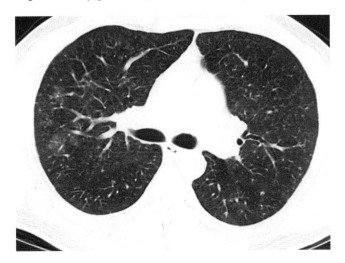

    A. Varicella pneumonia
    B. Kaposi sarcoma
    C. Pulmonary hemorrhage
    D. Sarcoidosis

19b What is the most common residual appearance of healed varicella pneumonia?
    A. Linear scar formation
    B. Rounded atelectasis
    C. Diffuse, tiny, calcified pulmonary nodules
    D. Pulmonary cysts

ANSWERS AND EXPLANATIONS

1a   Answer D.

1b   Answer B.   The image provided is of a patient with an acute presentation of AIDS and respiratory failure due to a coinfection with cytomegalovirus (CMV) and *P. jiroveci* (PJ).

However, differentiation between CMV and PJ pneumonia is challenging, as both can manifest with ground-glass opacities, a crazy-paving pattern, and consolidations. For this reason, cultures, serum markers, and CD4 lymphocyte counts are important adjuncts to CT in the diagnosis of CMV and PJ pneumonia.

Different pulmonary infections/diseases have typical CD4+ cell count levels in which they appear in HIV patients. At CD4 counts below 500 cells/mm^3, tuberculosis, bacterial infections, and Kaposi sarcoma may occur. PJ pneumonia is an AIDS-defining infection and appears at CD4+ counts below 200 cells/mm^3. CD4+ counts below 50 cells/mm^3 are necessary for other infections such as CMV pneumonia, invasive aspergillosis, nontuberculous mycobacterial infection, cryptococcosis, and disseminated histoplasmosis.

References: Kunihiro Y, Tanaka N, Matsumoto T, et al. The usefulness of a diagnostic method combining high-resolution CT findings and serum markers for cytomegalovirus pneumonia and pneumocystis pneumonia in non-AIDS patients. *Acta Radiol* 2015;56:806–813.

Tanaka N, Kunihiro Y, Yanagawa N. Infection in immunocompromised hosts: imaging. *J Thorac Imaging* 2018;33:306–321.

2   Answer A.   *P. aeruginosa* pneumonia is a common cause of nosocomial pneumonia with a high mortality rate in critically ill patients. Bronchial wall thickening and pleural effusion are signs more common with *P. aeruginosa* than with CMV or *P. jiroveci*. Additionally, the dependent lung distribution makes aspiration-related pneumonia a distinct possibility in this setting. This patient is chronically ill, ventilated, and immunocompromised; this is a common context for *P. aeruginosa* pneumonia.

References: Okada F, Ono A, Ando Y, et al. Thin-section CT findings in Pseudomonas aeruginosa pulmonary infection. *Br J Radiol* 2012;85:1533–1538.

Omeri AK, Okada F, Takata S, et al. Comparison of high-resolution computed tomography findings between Pseudomonas aeruginosa pneumonia and Cytomegalovirus pneumonia. *Eur Radiol* 2014;24:3251–3259.

3a   Answer D.

3b   Answer B.   The CT image in this hospitalized patient demonstrates extensive tree-in-bud nodular opacities, most prominent within the right lower lobe, compatible with infectious bronchiolitis. The tree-in-bud pattern represents impaction of centrilobular bronchioles with mucus, fluid, and/or pus with associated peribronchiolar inflammation. The tree-in-bud pattern is highly specific for infection, though it may occur with a wide variety of organisms.

Late-onset (>5 days after admission) hospital-acquired pneumonia should be treated initially with broad-spectrum antibiotics, including those with efficacy treating methicillin-resistant *S. aureus* (MRSA) and *Pseudomonas*. Sulfamethoxazole and trimethoprim covers community-acquired MRSA but would not be used empirically for hospital-acquired MRSA.

More recently, MRSA is increasing as a cause of community-acquired pneumonia in otherwise healthy children and adults. Some subsets of the population, such as those of low socioeconomic status, intravenous drug abusers, or incarcerated individuals, are at greater risk for community-acquired MRSA infections.

References: American Thoracic Society; Infectious Diseases Society of America. Guidelines for the management of adults with hospital-acquired, ventilator-associated, and healthcare-associated pneumonia. *Am J Respir Crit Care Med* 2005;171:388–416.

Nguyen ET, Kanne JP, Hoang LM, et al. Community-acquired methicillin-resistant *Staphylococcus aureus* pneumonia: radiographic and computed tomography findings. *J Thorac Imaging* 2008;23:13–19.

Rossi SE, Franquet T, Volpacchio M, et al. Tree-in-bud pattern at thin-section CT of the lungs: radiologic-pathologic overview. *Radiographics* 2005;25:789–801.

4 **Answer B.** A patient with the provided history and CT findings of an apical cavitary lesion and bilateral tree-in-bud opacities should be assumed to have *Mycobacterium tuberculosis* infection until proven otherwise. However, initiation of antimicrobial therapy before obtaining a good sputum sample might prevent effective culture of the organism and subsequent tailoring of therapy based on drug sensitivities of the organism. A left mainstem bronchial intubation would not prevent infection of the right lung; infection is already present. This pattern is bilateral and upper lung zone predominant, which is not typical of aspiration. A bronchoscopy, which was performed in this case, can provide a good sample for cultures. The sputum culture was positive for a strain of *M. tuberculosis* without significant drug resistance.

Reference: Nachiappan AC, Rahbar K, Shi X, et al. Pulmonary tuberculosis: role of radiology in diagnosis and management. *Radiographics* 2017;37:52–72.

5 **Answer A.** Present on the image is a pattern of uniform, randomly distributed micronodules, with some nodules contiguous with the fissural and pleural surfaces. On chest radiographs, this distribution creates a miliary pattern. Although *C. immitis*, CMV, *P. jiroveci*, and *N. asteroides* can manifest as pulmonary parenchymal nodules, the random micronodular pattern present on the image is typical of disseminated fungal or mycobacterial infection. The differential diagnosis would also include hematogenous miliary metastases, but the clinical history can often assist in distinguishing between the two. Also, a study of multiple pulmonary nodules in AIDS patients demonstrated that size <1 cm generally correlated with infection.

References: Edinburgh KJ, Jasmer RM, Huang L, et al. Multiple pulmonary nodules in AIDS: usefulness of CT in distinguishing among potential causes. *Radiology* 2000;214:427–432.

Lichtenberger JP, Sharma A, Zachary KC, et al. What a differential a virus makes: a practical approach to thoracic imaging findings in the context of HIV infection—part I, pulmonary findings. *AJR Am J Roentgenol* 2012;198:1295–1304.

6a **Answer A.**

6b **Answer D.** The tricuspid valve is the most commonly affected cardiac structure resulting in pulmonary septic emboli. This is related to the inflow from the systemic venous system in the setting of sepsis, long-term indwelling catheter use, and IV drug abuse. The pattern of pulmonary septic emboli is most frequently characterized by peripheral predominant, randomly distributed, nodular areas of consolidation. They may be wedge-shaped and cavitate. A "feeding vessel" sign has been described, which refers to a vessel supplying the infarcted parenchyma, but this is only occasionally helpful in clinical practice. *S. aureus* is the most commonly implicated organism.

References: Dodd JD, Souza CA, Müller NL. High-resolution MDCT of pulmonary septic embolism: evaluation of the feeding vessel sign. *AJR Am J Roentgenol* 2006;187:623–629.

Engelke C, Schaefer-Prokop C, Schirg E, et al. High-resolution CT and CT angiography of peripheral pulmonary vascular disorders. *Radiographics* 2002;22:739–764.

7 Answer A. In an immunocompromised patient with an acute respiratory illness and an abnormal chest radiograph with multiple, diffuse, or confluent opacities, CT chest without IV contrast receives a rating of "usually appropriate" according to the ACR Appropriateness Criteria. CT chest with IV contrast receives a rating of "may be appropriate," and FDG-PET/CT receives a rating of "usually not appropriate."

Reference: Lee C, Colletti PM, Chung JH, et al. ACR Appropriateness Criteria acute respiratory illness in immunocompromised patients. *J Am Coll Radiol* 2019;16:S331–S339.

8 Answer D. The nonclassic form of nontuberculous mycobacterial infection typically affects elderly women without underlying lung disease, termed the Lady Windermere syndrome. CT characteristics of nonclassic nontuberculous mycobacterial infection consist of tree-in-bud pattern, centrilobular nodules, and bronchiectasis, most severely affecting the right middle lobe and lingula. The classic form of nontuberculous mycobacterial infection typically affects elderly men with COPD. MAC is a common opportunistic infection in AIDS patients with CD4 counts <50 cells/mm^3; CT findings include small nodules, consolidations, and lymphadenopathy. MAC, along with other bacterial and fungal organisms, is frequently detected in patients with cystic fibrosis.

References: Reich JM, Johnson RE. Mycobacterium avium complex pulmonary disease presenting as an isolated lingular or middle lobe pattern. The Lady Windermere syndrome. *Chest* 1992;101:1605–1609.

Rossi SE, Franquet T, Volpacchio M, et al. Tree-in-bud pattern at thin-section CT of the lungs: radiologic-pathologic overview. *Radiographics* 2005;25:789–801.

9 Answer A. In the setting of heart transplant, new pulmonary parenchymal nodules are more likely infectious than neoplastic, though both should be considered depending on the clinical context. In this case, there is a solid nodule with surrounding ground-glass opacity, known as the halo sign. This sign is associated with invasive fungal infection, especially angioinvasive aspergillosis, which is a common opportunistic infection following transplant. CMV pneumonia much more commonly presents with diffuse ground-glass opacities than an isolated discrete nodule. There are no features to suggest rounded atelectasis in this case.

Posttransplant lymphoproliferative disease (PTLD) should be considered for nodules/masses in a posttransplant patient; however, it typically occurs at least 1 year after transplantation. Nodular disease prior to that time frame is much more likely to be infectious. PTLD is also commonly accompanied by intrathoracic lymphadenopathy.

Reference: Smith JD, Stowell JT, Martinez-Jimenez S, et al. Evaluation after orthotopic heart transplant: what the radiologist should know. *Radiographics* 2019;39:321–343.

10 Answer D. Predominant findings on the image provided are cylindrical bronchiectasis in the lower lobes with centrilobular micronodules. Given the lower lobe distribution, the most likely etiologies of bronchiectasis are prior infections and/or chronic aspiration. Cystic fibrosis, sarcoidosis, and allergic bronchopulmonary aspergillosis demonstrate upper lobe predominant bronchiectasis. There are no reticulations or architectural distortion to suggest traction bronchiectasis secondary to fibrotic lung disease. Follicular bronchiolitis and diffuse panbronchiolitis may present with diffuse centrilobular micronodules but are extremely rare by comparison. Given the degree of bronchiectasis in this case, underlying immunodeficiency should be considered.

References: Milliron B, Henry TS, Veeraraghavan S, et al. Bronchiectasis: mechanisms and imaging clues of associated common and uncommon diseases. *Radiographics* 2015;35:1011–1030.

Winningham PJ, Martinez-Jimenez S, Rosado-de-Christenson ML, et al. Bronchiolitis. *Radiographics* 2017;37:777–794.

11 **Answer D.**   Commonly known as swine flu, H1N1 influenza A virus spread across the world in 2009, causing variable degrees of respiratory tract infection. While generally self-limited, a small subset of patients with H1N1 pneumonia progressed to more severe or fulminant disease, especially in those with underlying chronic lung disease. In these cases, pathology most commonly showed diffuse alveolar damage. H1N1 virus also tended to affect a younger population relative to common seasonal influenza pneumonia. According to the final estimate of burden published by the Centers for Disease Control and Prevention, 87% of deaths occurred in those <65 years old, with children and working adults having risks of hospitalization and death 4 to 7 times and 8 to 12 times greater, respectively, than estimates of impact due to seasonal influenza.

References: Marchiori E, Zanetti G, D'Ippolito G, et al. Swine-origin influenza A (H1N1) viral infection: thoracic findings on CT. *AJR Am J Roentgenol* 2011;196:W723–W728.

Shrestha SS, Swerdlow DL, Borse RH, et al. Estimating the burden of 2009 pandemic influenza A (H1N1) in the United States (April 2009–April 2010). *Clin Infect Dis* 2011;52:S75–S82.

12 **Answer C.**   Angioinvasive aspergillosis occurs in severely immunosuppressed patients and is particularly common in leukemic patients with neutropenia. Early in the disease course, invasion of the pulmonary vasculature by the fungal hyphae results in vascular thrombosis, pulmonary infarction, and hemorrhage. The hemorrhage creates ground-glass opacity surrounding the nodule on CT, known as the halo sign. After recovery of a neutropenic patient's granulocyte count—typically 2 weeks after disease onset—the devitalized necrotic center separates from the surrounding rim of hemorrhagic tissue. On CT, this appears as a peripheral crescentic collection of air surrounding the nodule, known as the "air crescent sign." The presence of the air crescent sign portends a favorable prognosis, as it is associated with relatively improved survival.

References: Fan K, Lee C. Imaging evolution of an invasive fungal infection in a neutropenic patient. *Ann Am Thorac Soc* 2019;16:271–274.

Franquet T, Müller NL, Giménez A, et al. Spectrum of pulmonary aspergillosis: histologic, clinical, and radiologic findings. *Radiographics* 2001;21:825–837.

13a **Answer A.**

13b **Answer A.**   *Streptococcus pneumoniae* is the most common pathogen in the immunocompetent patient to present as a lobar pneumonia. Note that the term lobar is somewhat misleading, as currently many patients do not fully progress to lobar pneumonia if treated appropriately early in the course of disease. Air bronchograms are common in lobar pneumonias but not specific for infection. Of note, a "bulging fissure" sign is classically associated with *Klebsiella pneumoniae* (more frequent in alcoholics and nursing home residents) but may be present in other bacterial pneumonias, including *Streptococcus* given the higher prevalence. *Proteus*, *Morganella*, and *Legionella* are other pathogens that may present with a lobar pattern. *Legionella* may rapidly progress to complete lobar consolidation.

The right upper lobe has three segments: anterior, posterior, and apical segments. The anterior and posterior segments abut the minor fissure, and either could be involved based on the frontal view. However, the lateral view confirms that a majority of the consolidation is located in the anterior and posterior segments with sparing of the apical segment. The apicoposterior segment is a segment of the left upper lobe, unless variant anatomy is present.

References: Franquet T. Imaging of community-acquired pneumonia. *J Thorac Imaging* 2018;33:282–294.

Washington L, Palacio D. Imaging of bacterial pulmonary infection in the immunocompetent patient. *Semin Roentgenol* 2007;42:122–145.

14   Answer D.   Kaposi sarcoma is a low-grade mesenchymal tumor caused by human herpes virus 8. Most HIV patients with the disease have CD4 counts <200 cells/mm³. Kaposi sarcoma primarily affects the skin but can disseminate with multi-organ involvement. Pulmonary involvement occurs in 18%-47% of cases but is usually preceded by cutaneous or visceral involvement. Thoracic imaging manifestations of Kaposi sarcoma include ill-defined ("flame-shaped") nodular opacities with perihilar and peribronchovascular predominance, peribronchovascular interstitial thickening, small peripheral nodules, hilar and mediastinal lymphadenopathy, and pleural effusions.

References: Lichtenberger JP, Sharma A, Zachary KC, et al. What a differential a virus makes: a practical approach to thoracic imaging findings in the context of HIV infection—part I, pulmonary findings. *AJR Am J Roentgenol* 2012;198:1295–1304.

Restrepo CS, Martinez S, Lemos JA. Imaging manifestations of Kaposi sarcoma. *Radiographics* 2006;26:1169–1185.

15a   Answer C.

15b   Answer A.   Multiorganism anaerobic infection is considered the most frequent cause of cavitation and lung abscess development. This is followed in frequency by *S. aureus* and *Pseudomonas*. Aspiration is a frequent cause of multiorganism infection in the hospital and ICU setting, which includes an increased risk of anaerobic infection. Although postprimary tuberculosis often cavitates with a predilection for the upper lobes, the lateral view shows that the cavity is within the anterior segment of the right upper lobe, while postprimary tuberculosis has a predilection for the apical and posterior segments.

Depending on the clinical scenario, follow-up radiographs may be warranted to exclude an underlying neoplasm.

References: Franquet T. Imaging of community-acquired pneumonia. *J Thorac Imaging* 2018;33:282–294.

Washington L, Palacio D. Imaging of bacterial pulmonary infection in the immunocompetent patient. *Semin Roentgenol* 2007;42:122–145.

16   Answer B.   An aspergilloma, or mycetoma, is a saprophytic infection that occurs in patients with underlying structural lung disease. Patients generally have normal immunity. Pathologically, an aspergilloma presents as a mobile mass of fungal mycelia, tissue debris, and inflammatory cells within a preexisting cavity or other airspace; tissue invasion is characteristically absent. The most common causes of structural lung disease are prior tuberculosis and fibrotic sarcoidosis. On imaging, the Monod sign, which refers to the air surrounding the fungal ball, is often confused with the air crescent sign in invasive aspergillosis. In a simple aspergilloma, the fungal ball is mobile within the cavity and gravitates to dependent areas, which can be confirmed with prone CT imaging. Patients are often asymptomatic, but massive hemoptysis may occur, which may require emergent embolization or surgery.

References: Fan K, Lee C. Imaging evolution of an invasive fungal infection in a neutropenic patient. *Ann Am Thorac Soc* 2019;16:271–274.

Franquet T, Müller NL, Giménez A, et al. Spectrum of pulmonary aspergillosis: histologic, clinical, and radiologic findings. *Radiographics* 2001;21:825–837.

17   Answer A.   Community-acquired bacterial pneumonia remains the most common cause of infectious pneumonia, even in the immunosuppressed. This typically manifests as bronchopneumonia or lobar pneumonia depending on the pathogen, and recurrent pneumonias are considered an AIDS-defining illness. Tuberculosis is possible and should be a consideration, especially if significant lymphadenopathy is present. Viral pneumonias are much more likely to present with an interstitial pattern than lobar consolidation.

Reference: Lichtenberger JP, Sharma A, Zachary KC, et al. What a differential a virus makes: a practical approach to thoracic imaging findings in the context of HIV infection—part I, pulmonary findings. *AJR Am J Roentgenol* 2012;198:1295–1304.

18 **Answer C.** This is a case of B-cell lymphoma in the setting of HIV/AIDS. Extranodal lymphoma is more common in HIV than in nonimmunosuppressed patients. Additionally, doubling time can be quite rapid, which limits the use of doubling time for distinguishing this from infection. Both septic emboli and angioinvasive fungal disease would present much more acutely with dyspnea and pulmonary symptoms than this patient. Note that several nodules demonstrate a halo sign, which is a nonspecific finding but may be seen in angioinvasive aspergillosis. Kaposi sarcoma is the most common AIDS-related neoplasm and classically presents with a peribronchovascular distribution. In the past, gallium scans were used to help distinguish the two (gallium uptake is positive in lymphoma), but this is typically accomplished with biopsy today. Organizing pneumonia is more likely to present with peripheral airspace disease that is less nodular than shown here. Of note, organizing pneumonia may demonstrate a reversed halo sign, which represents ground-glass opacity surrounded by consolidation—essentially the reverse of the halo sign.

References: Bligh MP, Borgaonkar JN, Burrell SC, et al. Spectrum of CT findings in thoracic extranodal non-Hodgkin lymphoma. *Radiographics* 2017;37:439–461.

Lichtenberger JP, Sharma A, Zachary KC, et al. What a differential a virus makes: a practical approach to thoracic imaging findings in the context of HIV infection—part I, pulmonary findings. *AJR Am J Roentgenol* 2012;198:1295–1304.

19a **Answer A.**

19b **Answer C.** The appearance shown is typical of acute varicella pneumonia, which frequently presents as ill-defined pulmonary nodules and ground-glass opacities. This diagnosis should be considered when the imaging features are present within the context of skin lesions characteristic of the chickenpox rash. Varicella-zoster virus infection may result in pneumonia 10 % to 20% of the time (more common than pneumonia associated with zoster/shingles). The risk of pneumonia increases with immunodeficiency, pregnancy, and lymphoma/leukemia. Onset is generally 2 to 3 days after appearance of the rash. The morbidity and mortality of adult-onset chickenpox are considerably higher than childhood chickenpox. Healed varicella pneumonia frequently manifests as diffuse, tiny (2 to 3 mm), calcified pulmonary nodules.

References: Kim JS, Ryu CW, Lee SI, et al. High-resolution CT findings of varicella-zoster pneumonia. *AJR Am J Roentgenol* 1999;172:113–116.

Koo HJ, Lim S, Choe J, et al. Radiographic and CT features of viral pneumonia. *Radiographics* 2018;38:718–738.

Diffuse Lung Disease

Marianna Zagurovskaya, MD

QUESTIONS

1a A 26-year-old black man presents with chronic dry cough and tender nodules on shins. What is the most likely diagnosis?

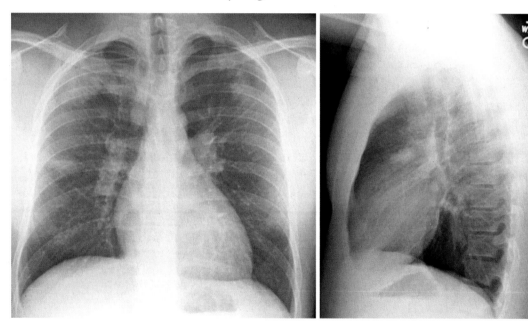

A. Tuberculosis
B. Sarcoidosis
C. Lymphoma
D. Pneumoconiosis

1b What radiologic study is used for staging of sarcoidosis?

    A. CT chest

    B. Virtual bronchoscopy

    C. Chest x-ray

    D. PET/CT

1c What typical sarcoidosis findings are present here?

    A. Subcarinal lymphadenopathy

    B. Paratracheal and bilateral hilar lymphadenopathy

    C. Scattered pulmonary cysts

    D. Macronodular lung opacities with mid and lower lung predominance

1d What is the classic distribution of perilymphatic nodularity in sarcoidosis?

    A. Diffuse symmetric

    B. Bilateral asymmetric without lobe sparing

    C. Upper lung–predominant bilateral

    D. Lower lung–predominant bilateral

2a What are the key lung findings in this 40-year old woman with chronic cough?

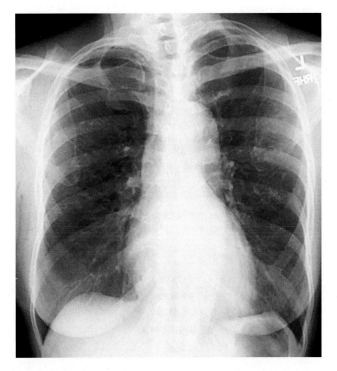

    A. Reticulonodular opacities

    B. Calcified micronodules

    C. Diffuse honeycombing

    D. Diffuse ground-glass opacities

2b Axial and coronal CT images of the same patient are shown. What would be the most important positive information to conclude on the diagnosis?

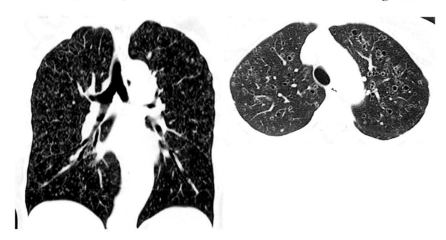

    A. Smoking history
    B. History of illicit drug use
    C. Recent viral upper respiratory infection
    D. Exposure to environmental inhaled antigens

2c What is the pathologic hallmark in pulmonary Langerhans cell histiocytosis (PLCH)?

    A. Bronchiolocentric fibroblast-rich interstitial infiltration late in the disease
    B. Bronchiolocentric smooth muscle proliferation regardless of the phase of the disease
    C. Occlusion of arterioles with dislodged infected material
    D. Sloughing off the alveolar epithelium with airway sparing

3a This 36-year-old female presents with an acute exacerbation of chronic shortness of breath. What is the next best step?

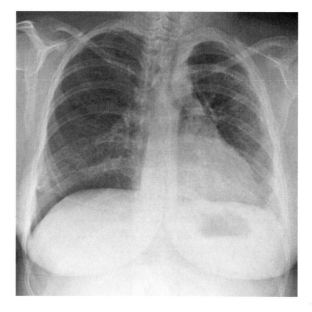

    A. Antibiotics trial
    B. Referral to pulmonologist
    C. CT chest
    D. Urgent call to the referring clinician

3b Coronal and axial images are obtained from the same patient. What is the most likely diagnosis?

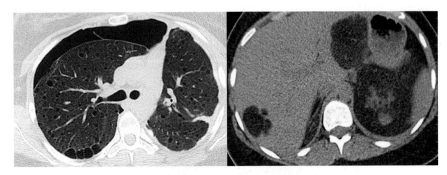

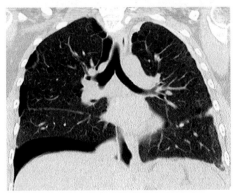

A. Lymphangioleiomyomatosis (LAM)
B. Pulmonary Langerhans cell histiocytosis (PLCH)
C. Lymphocytic interstitial pneumonia (LIP)
D. Chronic pneumocystis pneumonia

3c Which patient population is most frequently affected by an isolated lymphangioleiomyomatosis?

A. Young females
B. Elderly females
C. Young males
D. Elderly males

4a A 29-year-old nonsmoking man presents with laryngeal lesions and recurrent pneumonia. What are the key findings?

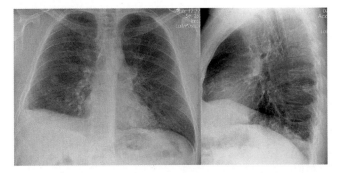

A. Hydrostatic edema with right-sided pleural effusion
B. Bilateral hilar lymphadenopathy with right lung base consolidation
C. Partially cavitating lung nodules and elevated right hemidiaphragm
D. Bilateral honeycombing and right pleural calcifications

4b These CT images are obtained from the same patient. What is the most likely diagnosis?

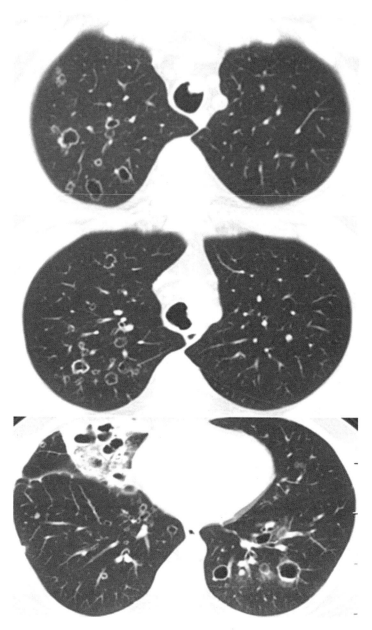

    A. *Mycobacterium avium* infection
    B. Relapsing polychondritis
    C. Wegener granulomatosis
    D. Respiratory papillomatosis

4c What is the best imaging modality to detect large airway intraluminal lesion?

    A. Two-view chest radiography
    B. Chest CT
    C. F-18 PET/CT
    D. Thoracic MRI

5a A 36-year-old woman presents with xerostomia and dry eyes. What is the best next radiologic study for evaluation of her progressive dry cough?

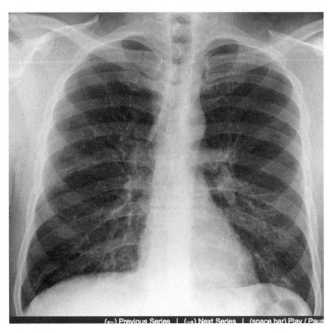

A. High Resolution Chest CT
B. Cardiac MRI
C. Dynamic airway CT chest
D. Echocardiography

5b Axial CT images are obtained from the same patient. What is the most likely diagnosis?

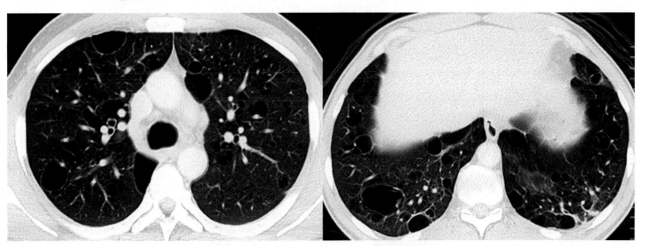

A. Pulmonary Langerhans cell histiocytosis
B. Lymphocytic interstitial pneumonia
C. Lymphangioleiomyomatosis
D. Idiopathic pulmonary fibrosis

5c The images are obtained from a middle-aged woman with dysproteinemia and a history of Sjögren syndrome. What is the correct statement in regard to the lung changes?

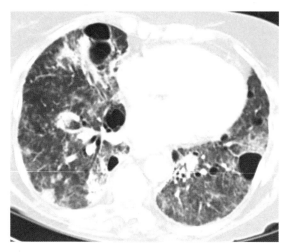 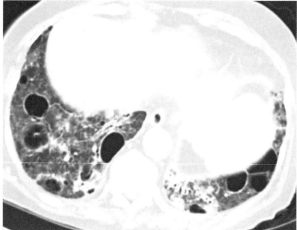

A. At least 25% of patients with Sjögren syndrome have these lung manifestations.
B. A majority of the patients present with acute illness.
C. The course of the disease is unpredictable.
D. Half of patients with this lung disease progress into lymphoma.

6 Given the radiograph and the corresponding chest CT findings, what is the likely cause of interlobular septal thickening in this patient?

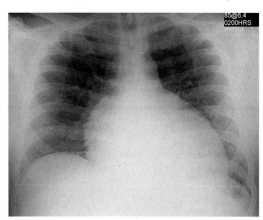 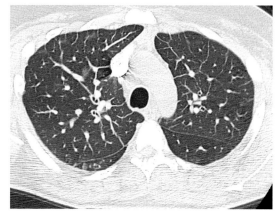

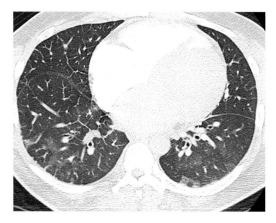

A. Cardiogenic pulmonary edema
B. Fibrotic interstitial lung disease
C. Lymphangitic carcinomatosis
D. Lymphangiectasia

7a   A 45-year-old man with new diagnosis of HIV presents with chronic cough. What is the most likely pathophysiology of imaging abnormalities?

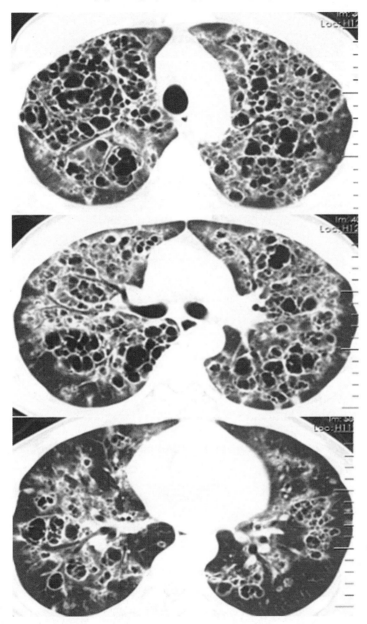

A. Chronic atypical infection
B. Recurrent aspiration
C. Smoking-induced lung injury
D. Drug-induced alveolitis

7b   What is the most likely diagnosis?

A. *Pneumocystis jiroveci* infection
B. Pulmonary Langerhans cell histiocytosis (PLCH)
C. Septic emboli
D. Lymphangioleiomyomatosis (LAM)

8a This 60-year-old man has previously worked in a foundry. What are the main radiographic abnormalities?

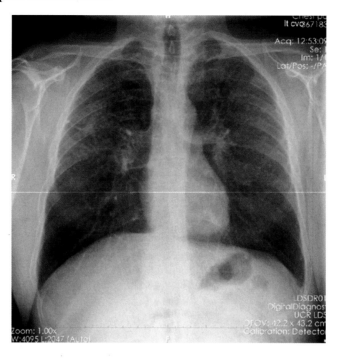

A. Multifocal ill-defined consolidation
B. Bilateral small lung nodules
C. Bilateral diffuse interstitial thickening
D. Subtle bilateral lung cysts

8b These images are obtained from the same patient. What is the most likely diagnosis?

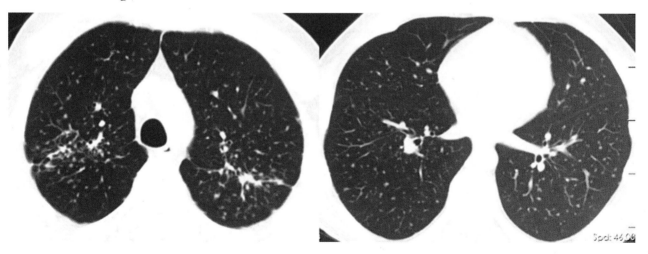

A. Pneumoconiosis
B. Granulomatosis with polyangiitis
C. Healed varicella
D. Miliary fungal infection

8c What are the classic imaging findings in simple chronic silicosis?

    A. Geographic ground-glass opacities with interlobular septal thickening
    B. Calcified pleural plaques
    C. Perilymphatic nodules
    D. Upper lobe confluent airspace opacities with cephalad hilar retraction

9a What is the most likely diagnosis?

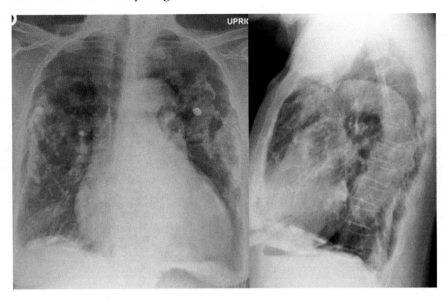

    A. Asbestos exposure
    B. Bilateral mesothelioma
    C. Multifocal round atelectasis
    D. Squamous cell carcinoma

9b A different patient with prior work on a shipyard is evaluated for abnormal pulmonary function test. What is the most likely diagnosis?

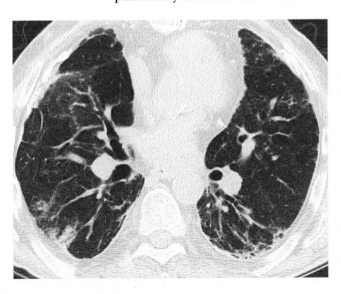
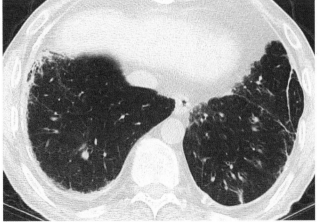

    A. Sarcoidosis
    B. Silicosis
    C. Asbestosis
    D. Berylliosis

9c What is the relationship between incidence of bronchogenic lung cancer and asbestos exposure?

A. The same as in those without exposure

B. Decreased in comparison to those without exposure

C. Increased in comparison to those without exposure

D. Controversial

10a Compare initial (left) and 1-month follow-up (right) CT images. What is the most likely cause of recurrent pneumothorax in this 87-year-old man with PET-positive scalp lesions?

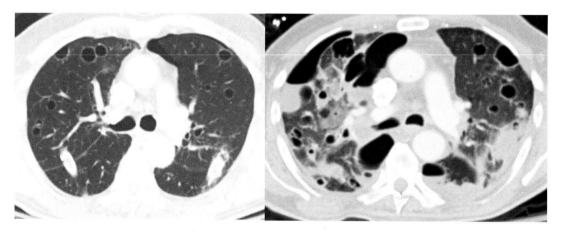

A. Lymphangioleiomyomatosis

B. Pulmonary Langerhans cell histiocytosis

C. Pulmonary metastatic disease

D. Birt-Hogg-Dube syndrome

10b A 45-year old smoker presents with unintentional weight loss. What is the most likely cause of the non-calcified pulmonary nodules?

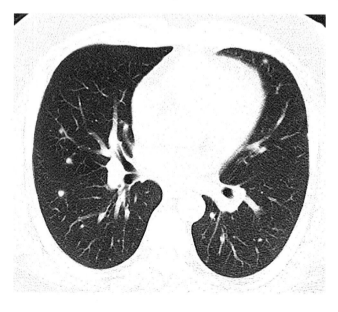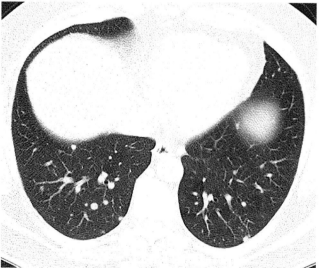

A. Hematogenous metastases

B. Granulomatous disease

C. Pulmonary papillomatosis

D. Septic emboli

11a This 61-year-old man has worked in the aerospace industry. What is the most likely diagnosis?

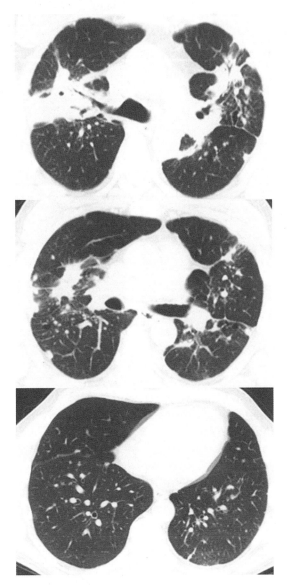

    A. Sarcoidosis
    B. Chronic beryllium disease
    C. Usual interstitial pneumonia
    D. Silicosis

11b What is the pathologic hallmark of pulmonary chronic beryllium disease?
    A. Caseating granulomas indistinguishable from those in tuberculosis
    B. Noncaseating granulomas indistinguishable from those in sarcoidosis
    C. Caseating granulomas indistinguishable from those in granulomatosis with polyangiitis
    D. Noncaseating granulomas indistinguishable from those in Langerhans cell histiocytosis

12a What is the main radiographic pattern here?

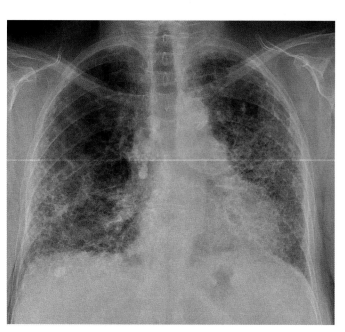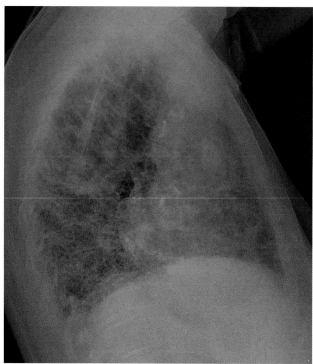

    A. Reticular opacities
    B. Multifocal peribronchial airspace disease
    C. Upper lung–predominant fibrosis
    D. Emphysematous changes

12b CT axial image from a 37-year-old female with mixed connective tissue disease. What type of interstitial pneumonia is the most likely present here?

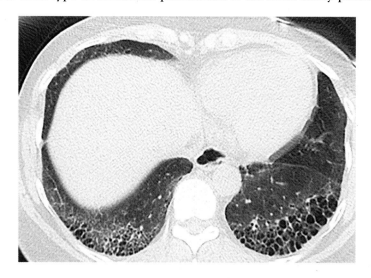

    A. Nonspecific interstitial pneumonia (NSIP)
    B. Usual interstitial pneumonia (UIP)
    C. Lymphocytic interstitial pneumonia (LIP)
    D. Organizing pneumonia (OP)

12c Based on the current ATS guidelines for IPF, what is the correct statement regarding the UIP pattern in this patient?

A. Definite UIP
B. Probable UIP
C. Indeterminate for UIP
D. Suggestive of an alternative diagnosis to UIP

12d This patient is evaluated for idiopathic pulmonary fibrosis. According to the 2018 ATS guidelines, the imaging findings would be consistent with which of the following definitions?

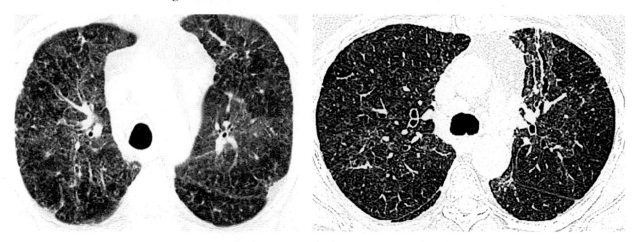

A. Definite UIP
B. Probable UIP
C. Indeterminate for UIP
D. Suggestive of an alternative diagnosis to UIP

13a A 26-year-old woman presents with rapidly progressing severe respiratory failure. What is the most likely diagnosis?

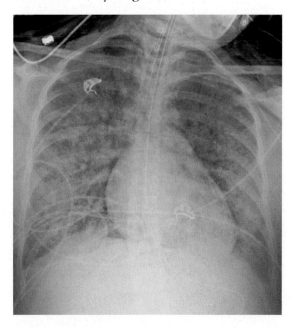

A. Cardiogenic pulmonary edema
B. Noncardiogenic pulmonary edema
C. Infectious pneumonia
D. Aspiration

13b CT axial images obtained later from the same patient. What is the most likely pathomorphologic mechanism responsible for imaging abnormalities?

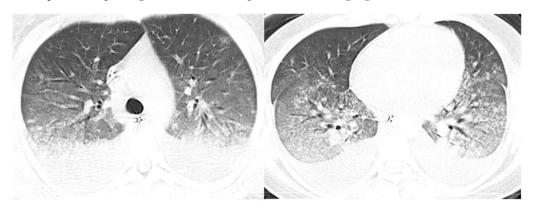

    A. Accumulation of lipoproteinaceous material in the alveoli
    B. Replacement of alveoli and interstitium by fibroblasts
    C. Diffuse alveolar damage
    D. Increased oncotic pressure

13c CT axial images are obtained from the same patient several months later. What is the most likely diagnosis?

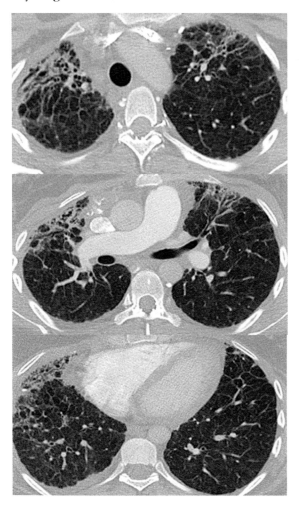

    A. Nonspecific interstitial pneumonia
    B. Fibroproliferative ARDS
    C. End-stage sarcoidosis
    D. Idiopathic pulmonary fibrosis

13d What is the correct statement regarding diffuse alveolar damage (DAD)?
   A. Similar survival in acute and organizing phases.
   B. Unlikely to be present in accelerated idiopathic pulmonary fibrosis.
   C. Has clear clinical demarcation between acute and chronic lung parenchymal changes.
   D. Recovery correlates with the degree of basement membrane damage and reparative processes.

14a These CT axial images were obtained from a 58-year-old woman with scleroderma. What is the most likely diagnosis?

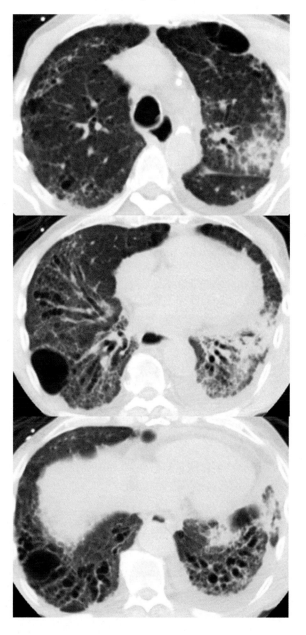

   A. Nonspecific interstitial pneumonia
   B. Usual interstitial pneumonia
   C. Hypersensitivity pneumonitis
   D. Pulmonary fibroelastosis

14b Based on these images, what is the most likely imaging pattern of ILD in this patient with CREST syndrome?

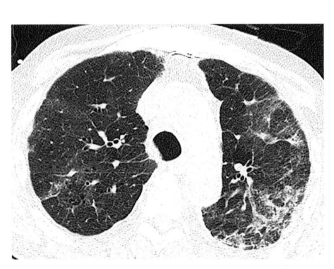 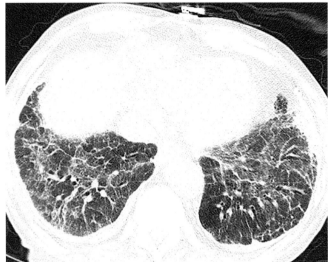

    A. NSIP

    B. Probable UIP

    C. Definite UIP

    D. Desquamative interstitial pneumonia (DIP)

14c Which of the following is a well-recognized etiology of nonspecific interstitial pneumonia?

    A. Bacterial pneumonia

    B. Connective tissue disease

    C. Emphysema

    D. Tuberculosis

14d What is the correct statement regarding nonspecific interstitial pneumonia (NSIP)?

    A. Five-year survival in fibrotic NSIP is similar to that in IPF.

    B. If honeycombing is a predominant feature, biopsy should be performed.

    C. Histologic evidence of NSIP is enough for the final diagnosis of idiopathic form.

    D. Response to corticosteroids is variable depending on NSIP type.

15a A 72-year-old woman presents with fatigue. What is the most likely diagnosis?

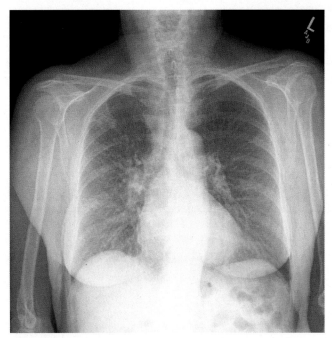

    A. Emphysema
    B. Pulmonary edema
    C. Lymphangitic carcinomatosis
    D. Silicosis

15b What is the key imaging finding?

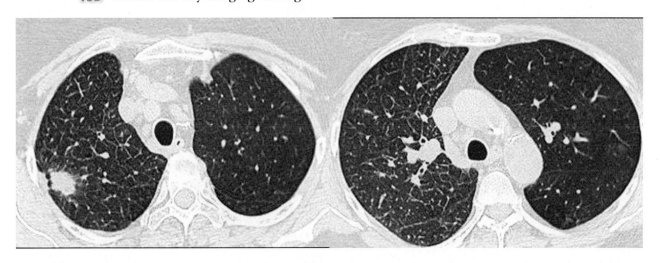

    A. Pleural thickening and fibrosis
    B. Lung volume loss
    C. Ground-glass opacities
    D. Nodular interstitial thickening

15c What is the best next step?
    A. Trial of antibiotics
    B. Trial of corticosteroids
    C. Oncology consult
    D. Percutaneous biopsy

15d What is the most common adenocarcinoma associated with lymphangitic carcinomatosis?

A. Bronchogenic
B. Breast
C. Gastric
D. Colonic

16a Please review initial (left) CT images of 48-year-old man dyspnea on exertion and a strong smoking history. Three-month follow-up images (right) are obtained after smoking cessation and steroids trial. What is the most likely diagnosis?

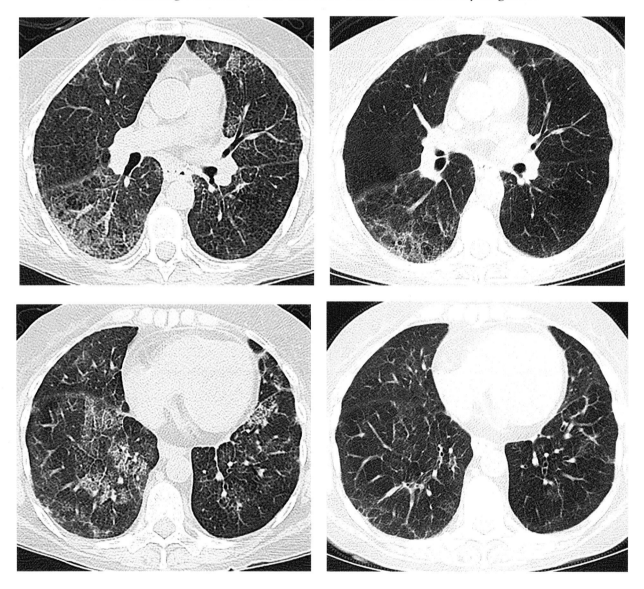

A. Usual interstitial pneumonia
B. Desquamative interstitial pneumonia
C. Pulmonary edema
D. Hypersensitivity pneumonitis

16b What are the similarities between desquamative and nonspecific interstitial pneumonia?

A. Both have strong association with smoking history
B. Both have similar to respiratory bronchiolitis distribution of findings
C. Both present with ground-glass opacities
D. Both have high incidence of subpleural cysts

ANSWERS AND EXPLANATIONS

1a **Answer B.**

1b **Answer C.**

1c **Answer B.**

1d **Answer C.** The clinical scenario along with Garland triad (right upper paratracheal and bilateral hilar lymphadenopathy with preserved cardiac borders) and upper/mid lung–predominant opacities on radiographs favors thoracic sarcoidosis.

Clinical staging is based on chest radiograph pattern. Five-part "Scadding" classification system exists: 0—normal chest x-ray (5% to 15%); I—lymphadenopathy (LN) with clear lungs (50%); II—LN and pulmonary disease, 25% to 30%; III—isolated pulmonary disease (15%); and IV—lung fibrosis (10% to 15%). Definite diagnosis requires presence of noncaseating epithelioid cell granulomas in more than 1 organ or positive Kveim-Siltzbach skin test.

High-resolution CT is helpful in distinguishing active interstitial inflammation from irreversible fibrosis, assessment of atypical features, and differential diagnosis. Typical manifestations are seen in 60% to 70% of cases and include bilateral hilar and right paratracheal lymphadenopathy, perilymphatic micronodularity along bronchovascular bundles and fissures (patchy; upper and mid lung predominant), perihilar opacities, and fibrotic changes. Other pulmonary parenchymal findings, isolated mediastinal lymphadenopathy, pleural/airway involvement, honeycombing, and mycetoma are considered atypical. Perilymphatic nodularity may improve, stabilize, or progress into fibrosis. FDG uptake in thoracic sarcoidosis is nonspecific, variable in intensity, and most predominant in involved lymph nodes, parenchymal nodules, and opacities.

Half of sarcoidosis patients are asymptomatic in stages I to II. Pulmonary function worsens with an increasing stage, but radiologic staging does not correlate well with severity of pulmonary function abnormalities. Often, radiographic abnormalities appear worse than the degree of functional impairment. Spontaneous remission occurs in 60% to 90% in stage I, 40% to 70% in stage II, 10% to 20% in stage III, and 0% in stage IV disease.

Treatment may not be indicated in stage I alone. Oral steroids are used as first-line therapy beyond stage I and before end-stage fibrosis with associated improved radiologic findings during the treatment. Cytotoxic drugs and immunomodulators may be considered for complicated or severe refractory sarcoidosis. Lofgren syndrome (fever, polyarthritis, erythema nodosum, and bilateral hilar lymphadenopathy) has spontaneous remission rate more than 85%. Steroids are not usually required. Recurrence of disease in a pulmonary allograft after lung transplantation is 47% to 67%, but frequently not clinically significant.

References: Criado E, Sanchez M, Ramirez J, et al. Pulmonary sarcoidosis: typical and atypical manifestations at high-resolution CT with pathologic correlation. *Radiographics* 2010;30(6):1567–1586.

Prabhakar HB, Rabinowitz CB, Gibbons FK, et al. Imaging features of sarcoidosis on MDCT, FDG PET, and PET/CT. *AJR Am J Roentgenol* 2008;190(Suppl):S1–S6.

Wu JJ, Shiff KR. Sarcoidosis. *Am Fam Physician* 2004;70(2):312–322.

2a **Answer A.**

2b **Answer A.**

2c **Answer A.** Frontal chest radiograph shows upper and mid lung–predominant bilateral reticulonodular opacities and increased lung volumes. These features could be seen in pulmonary Langerhans cell histiocytosis (PLCH), lymphangioleiomyomatosis, and emphysema. There is no evidence of honeycombing or decreased lung volumes. Ground-glass opacities are reserved for CT abnormalities, and not present here. No calcified micronodules are present.

Upper and mid lung–predominant centrilobular micronodules and thin-walled, bizarre-shaped cavitary lesions sparing the costophrenic angles are hallmarks of smoking-related PLCH. Upper and mid lung–predominant micronodules could be seen in upper respiratory viral infection or respiratory bronchiolitis related to smoking but have no association with cystic lesions. Vegetations on cardiac valves (usually tricuspid) with history of illicit drug use could lead to septic emboli but show a predilection to the lower lungs, migratory character, and foci of peripheral consolidation with frequent cavitation. Hypersensitivity pneumonitis (HP) caused by exposure to inhaled antigens presents with centrilobular micronodules and ground-glass opacities, but cysts seen in HP are distinct from the thin-walled cavitary lesions of PLCH.

PLCH lesions evolve from early bronchiolocentric multicellular dense infiltrates with Langerhans cells (with characteristic Birbeck granules) into a predominantly fibroblast-containing lesion with bronchiole dilatation (mid to late phase) followed by end-stage fibrotic stellate scars with paracicatricial airspace enlargement.

Presence of Langerhans cells within bronchial mucosa or alveolar parenchyma is not specific for PLCH and could be seen in COPD, lung cancer, and other interstitial lung diseases. More definite diagnosis of PLCH requires correlation of smoking history, radiologic features, and combination of nodular and cystic lesions on light microscopy containing aggregates of Langerhans cells. TGF-beta is an essential factor in the development of Langerhans cells, sustained chronic inflammation, and airway-centered fibrosis.

Pneumothorax is seen in approximately 15% of PLCH cases (predominantly unilateral), is associated with worse outcome, and does not seem to benefit from steroid use but may require surgical management or mechanical pleurodesis. Steroids may be beneficial in selected cases for parenchymal stabilization or complicating pulmonary hypertension, but smoking cessation is the most important factor in disease stabilization (up to 50%), or even regression in early stages (25% of cases).

References: Abbott GF, Rosado-de-Christenson ML, Franks TF. From the archives of the AFIP pulmonary Langerhans cell histiocytosis. *Radiographics* 2004;24:821–841.

Caminati A, Harari S. Smoking-related interstitial pneumonias and pulmonary Langerhans cell histiocytosis. *Proc Am Thorac Soc* 2006;3(4):299–306.

Kim HJ, Lee KS, Johkoh T, et al. Pulmonary Langerhans cell histiocytosis in adults: high-resolution CT—pathology comparisons and evolutional changes at CT. *Eur Radiol* 2011;21:1406–1415.

3a **Answer D.**

3b **Answer A.**

3c **Answer A.** Frontal chest radiograph demonstrates a moderate right pneumothorax (best seen overlying the diaphragm as a thin linear opacity), reticular opacities, and subtle bilateral scattered cystic lesions. The presence of pneumothorax in a symptomatic patient requires an emergent notification of a referring physician for a possible chest tube placement. After stabilization, CT of the chest would aid in the evaluation for additional findings and cause of the pneumothorax.

Bilateral scattered thin-walled small cystic lesions without zonal predilection in a female patient with hepatic and renal fat-containing masses are most suggestive of LAM in a patient with tuberous sclerosis (TS)—LAM–TS complex.

In LAM, thin-walled uniform round or oval cysts result from air trapping due to smooth muscle–like cell proliferation along the bronchioles, blood vessels, and lymphatics. Cysts frequently enlarge as the disease progresses. Pneumothorax is seen up to 50% of the patients, sometimes with associated chylous effusion (10% to 20%). Lungs are hyperinflated due to air trapping in half of the patients. Reticular pattern is common on CXR (up to 90%) and results from summation of thin-walled cystic lesions. Hilar and abdominal lymphadenopathy is frequent, caused by proliferation of abnormal smooth muscle cells along lymphatic vessels.

The disease is seen in symptomatic females of childbearing age that present with dyspnea (70%), pneumothorax (50%), or chylous pleural effusion (28%). Chyloptysis and hemoptysis are also seen due to obstruction of pulmonary blood and lymphatic vessels by LAM cells.

Characteristic LAM findings in females with tuberous sclerosis (TS) are seen only in 30% of the cases with overall gender-free occurrence of LAM in TS not exceeding 1%. Interestingly, a greater number of cystic lesions and likelihood of pneumothorax and chylous effusions are seen in sporadic LAM as opposed to LAM–TS complex.

Smoking can contribute to distal airway damage, exacerbating air trapping, and chance of pneumothorax. Additionally, pregnancy is associated with estrogen and progesterone swings, each negatively affecting the course of the disease. LAM recurrence in transplanted lung (presumably due to migration or in vivo metastasizing from native to donor lung) is rare.

The main differentials based on imaging are as follows: (1) PLCH—bizarre-shaped cysts with upper/mid lung predominance, interspersed with centrilobular nodules in a smoking host; (2) LIP—most often in autoimmune disorders and AIDS, can manifest solely with lower lung–predominant thin-walled cysts in perivascular distribution; and (3) *P. jiroveci* pneumonia—scattered cystic lesions in an immunocompromised host.

References: Abbott GF, Rosado-de-Christenson ML, Frazier AA, et al. Lymphangioleiomyomatosis: radiologic-pathologic correlation. *Radiographics* 2005;25:803–828.

Avila NA, Dwyer AJ, Moss J. Imaging features of lymphangioleiomyomatosis: diagnostic pitfalls. *AJR Am J Roentgenol* 2011;196(4):982–986.

Seaman DM, Meyer CA, Gilman MD, et al. Diffuse cystic lung disease at high-resolution CT. *AJR Am J Roentgenol* 2011;196(6):1305–1311.

4a **Answer C.**

4b **Answer D.**

4c **Answer B.** On radiographs, bilateral partially cavitating nodules and subtle changes of bronchiectases are present. Elevation of the right hemidiaphragm with partial atelectasis (best seen on lateral view) is responsible for the right lung base opacity and lateral silhouetting of the hemidiaphragm on frontal projection. No radiographically detectable lymphadenopathy, hydrostatic edema, right-sided pleural effusion, or honeycombing is shown.

Polypoid long segment intraluminal tracheal mass and bilateral cavitary parenchymal lesions are present on CT. Distribution of lesions suggests gravitational effect. Chronic atelectasis and postobstructive consolidation with extensive bronchiectases within the right middle lobe are evident. These findings are most consistent with tracheobronchial papillomatosis with pulmonary involvement. Incidence of recurrent laryngeal papillomatosis is 4.3 and 1.8 per 100,000 in children and adults in United States, respectively. The younger the age, the higher the likelihood of distal spread and severity of the disease. It is caused by human papillomavirus (most common HPV-6 and HPV-11). Children acquire the disease during birth by direct contact with mother's genital lesions. Adults develop the disease due to either reactivation of latent virus or new infection after sexual oral contact.

The most common site of involvement is the larynx with only 5% of patients having tracheal involvement and <1% demonstrating pulmonary disease. Extralaryngeal spread of the infection totals 30% and 16% in pediatric and adult groups, respectively.

Tracheobronchial papillomatosis can present either as a focal mass or as diffuse cobblestone changes of mucosa. Nodular appearance of bronchi can be seen. Pulmonary papilloma lesions begin as asymptomatic, noncalcified, peripheral nodules that tend to enlarge and undergo central cavitation/liquefaction and necrosis, often with an air–fluid level. A dependent distribution is common. Calcification is not characteristic.

No definite cure exists. The rate of malignant transformation into squamous cell carcinoma is 14% regardless of age, associated with irradiation in kids and smoking in adults, and more frequently seen in HPV-16 and HPV-18 infection.

In assessment of large airway lesions, conventional chest radiography still remains the initial imaging test; however, it has a low sensitivity. MDCT is the test of choice for identification, localization, extent, and complications. Stenosis and/or malacia could be assessed with CT dynamic imaging of large airways; MRI would be inferior with unnecessary labor and cost involved. Virtual bronchoscopy is superior to conventional bronchoscopy for infection spread and mapping the extent of the process more safely.

References: Hammoud D, Haddad BE. Squamous cell carcinoma of the lungs arising in recurrent respiratory papillomatosis (case report). *Resp Med* 2010;3(4):270–272.

Marchiori E, Neto CA, Meirelles GS, et al. Laryngotracheobronchial papillomatosis: findings on computed tomography scans of the chest. *J Bras Pneumol* 2008;34(12):1084–1089.

Ngo AV, Walker CM, Chung JH, et al. Tumors and tumorlike conditions of the large airways. *AJR Am J Roentgenol* 2013;201:301–313.

5a   **Answer A.**

5b   **Answer B.**

5c   **Answer C.**   The important observation from the chest radiograph is preserved lung volumes and bilateral mid and lower lung–predominant reticular opacities that warrant correlation with chest CT. Clinical history suggests underlying autoimmune disease and potentially interstitial lung abnormalities, based on radiographic findings. The latter would be best assessed with high-resolution CT chest.

The key CT findings here are perilymphatic cystic lesions, scattered peripheral opacities (some in peribronchovascular distribution), and lung nodules. The constellation of clinical and imaging information is most suggestive of LIP, in the settings of Sjögren disease. Other parenchymal findings include poorly defined centrilobular and subpleural nodules and thickened peribronchovascular bundles and interlobular septa. The most helpful finding in differential diagnosis is presence of thin-walled perivascular cysts (in 80%) that are believed to result from partial airway obstruction by peribronchiolar cellular deposits. Nodules may represent lymphoproliferative foci or amyloid deposits and may calcify. Mediastinal/hilar lymphadenopathy is occasionally seen. Pleural effusions are rare.

LIP is seen in 1% of patients with Sjögren syndrome. Twenty-five percent of patients with LIP have Sjögren syndrome. Females are affected more often than males (2:1), especially in the fourth to sixth decades of life. The disease is rarely isolated, often linked to autoimmune disorders. LIP in children is considered an AIDS-defining illness. Of note, improvement of radiologic findings correlates with immune status decline in this group. Eighty percent of adult patients with LIP have serum dysproteinemias (most common, IgM). Histopathologically, the infiltrates are composed of polyclonal lymphocytes mixed with plasma cells.

The onset is usually insidious with mild hypoxemia, cough, and progressive respiratory distress over a period of several years. Tissue diagnosis requires thoracoscopic or open lung biopsy. The course of the disease is unpredictable. Improvement or resolution of symptoms is seen in 50% to 60% of patients treated with corticosteroids and/or cytostatics. Thirty-three to fifty percent of patients succumb within 5 years of diagnosis, from infection due to either immunosuppression or lung fibrosis related to treatment of underlying disorder. Five percent of cases progress into low-grade B-cell lymphoma. Radiologically, cysts are seen only in 2% of patients with lymphoma, whereas air–space consolidation and nodules larger than 1 cm are more common in patients with lymphoma (66% and 41%) than LIP (18% and 6%). Pleural effusions can be seen in up to 25% of malignant lymphoma cases but would be very unusual in LIP.

References: Johkoh T, Muller N, Pickford HA, et al. Lymphocytic interstitial pneumonia: thin-section CT findings in 22 patients. *Radiology* 1999;212:567–572.

Lynch DA, Travis WD, Muller NL, et al. Idiopathic interstitial pneumonias: CT features. *Radiology* 2005;236:10–21.

Mueller-Mang C, Grosse C, Schmid K, et al. What every radiologist should know about idiopathic interstitial pneumonias. *Radiographics* 2007;27:595–615.

Swigris JJ, Berry GJ, Raffin TA, et al. Lymphoid interstitial pneumonia: a narrative review. *Chest* 2002;122(6):2150–2164.

6 Answer A. The chest radiograph demonstrates significant enlargement of the cardiac silhouette. This could be related to cardiomegaly or pericardial effusion but is confirmed as cardiomegaly on the CT. Additionally, the interlobular septal thickening is smooth, diffuse, and bilateral with a mild degree of lower lung ground-glass opacity as well. The appearance is classic for cardiogenic interstitial pulmonary edema. Pleural effusions are common and more often right-sided, if small.

Lymphangitic carcinomatosis would be more likely to present with nodular thickening. Similarly, there is no architectural distortion to suggest an underlying fibrotic lung disease. Lymphangiectasia is frequently fatal in infancy but can be seen in adults. The interlobular septal thickening in those cases is generally accompanied by pleural thickening and significant mediastinal abnormality such as lymphangiomas (not seen here). Other mimics of smooth interlobular septal thickening would include sarcoidosis, Niemann-Pick, and lymphangiomatosis (not to be confused with lymphangioleiomyomatosis).

Reference: Oikonomou A, Prassopoulos P. Mimics in chest disease: interstitial opacities. *Insights Imaging* 2013;4(1):9–27.

7a **Answer A.**

7b **Answer A.** Images show upper and mid lung extensive bilateral cavitary/cystic lesions with varying degrees of wall thickness and septations within areas of ground-glass opacities. Lesions are intraparenchymal and peribronchial rather than perivascular. There is no centrilobular emphysema, pulmonary edema, or peripheral fibrosis.

Given the history and imaging findings, the most likely diagnosis is chronic *Pneumocystis jiroveci* pneumonia. The main imaging manifestations of chronic *P. jiroveci* pneumonia include interlobular thickening, bronchiectasis, and a variable degree of fibrosis.

PLCH is upper lung predominant but does not usually manifest as such large cysts. Septic emboli demonstrate more randomly distributed peripheral nodular opacities with variable degrees of cavitation rather than the central and upper lung–predominant abnormality shown. Cysts in LAM are more diffusely distributed and thin walled.

P. jiroveci pneumonia is the most common OPPORTUNISTIC infection among people with HIV/AIDS. However, the most common infection among patients with HIV/AIDS is bacterial pneumonia (20- to 40-fold increase).

Approximately one-third of patients have normal radiographic findings on initial evaluation and radiologic abnormalities lag behind the symptoms in the acute phase. Classic appearance is bilateral perihilar or interstitial opacities (reticular, reticulonodular, or ground glass). If no treatment is given, progressive alveolar consolidation may occur over several days. With treatment, the disease has a tendency to improve within a couple of weeks, with some patients developing irreversible coarse reticular opacities due to fibrosis.

The first-line treatment is generally trimethoprim–sulfamethoxazole. Corticosteroids given within 72 hours from the onset of the disease are found to improve survival. Patients with HIV and PJP infection have higher survival rates than do patients without HIV (86% to 92% vs. 51% to 80%, respectively), likely due to decreased inflammatory response in patients with HIV.

The primary CT finding in the acute phase is geographic ground-glass attenuation (90% of cases). This finding has high predictive value in a patient with HIV in the appropriate clinical scenario and, by itself, sufficient enough to start an empirical treatment. Atypical manifestations are seen in 10% of cases and include isolated focal or asymmetric dense consolidation, adenopathy, and various size nodules that may cavitate or calcify. Pneumothorax is seen in 50% of cases. Up to 38% of patients have thin-walled cystic lesions that are believed to represent pneumatoceles, usually multiple with upper lobe predilection. The cysts usually resolve within a year following treatment but may persist permanently.

As stated before, the majority of HIV/AIDS-infected patients demonstrate CD4 T-lymphocyte count <200 to 100 cells/mm^3 with only 10% to 15% patients having T-helper count >200 cell/mm^3.

References: Allen CA, Al-Jahdali HH, Irion KL, et al. Imaging manifestations of HIV/AIDS. *Ann Thorac Med* 2010;5(4):201–216.

David MH, David AL, McAdams HP, et al. *Imaging of diseases of the chest.* Philadelphia, PA: Elsevier Mosby, 2009.

Kanne JP, Yandow DR, Meyer CA. Pneumocystis jiroveci pneumonia: high-resolution CT findings in patients with and without HIV infection. *AJR Am J Roentgenol* 2012;198: W555–W561.

8a   **Answer B.**

8b   **Answer A.**

8c   **Answer C.**   The most significant findings in this case are bilateral small dense pulmonary nodules (most abundant in upper and mid lungs) in a perilymphatic distribution. Some of the nodules coalesce in the upper lobes and form elongated opacities with distortion of pulmonary architecture. Differential considerations include pneumoconiosis or sarcoidosis; given the history of foundry work, pneumoconiosis is more likely. Diffuse interstitial thickening is most often seen in edema due to heart failure, with associated cardiac enlargement. Healed varicella classically presents with scattered miliary calcified pulmonary nodules; distortion of pulmonary architecture is not characteristic. Granulomatosis with polyangiitis would not produce this constellation of findings. Miliary fungal infection is seen in immunocompromised patients, with lower lung–predominant random nodules. Calcified pleural plaques are seen in asbestos exposure. In silicosis, calcification of mediastinal lymph nodes ("eggshell" calcifications) is present in 5% of cases. The latter is not specific and could be observed in other conditions such as sarcoidosis and histoplasmosis.

Classic silicosis is a chronic form of silicosis that occurs due to inhalation of lower dose dust containing crystalline silicon dioxide. Disease usually manifests after 10 to 20 years of exposure. When changes occur within 10 years from exposure, the form is called accelerated. On CT, 1- to 10-mm nodules are present in a perilymphatic distribution. Geographic and confluent ground-glass opacities with interlobular septal thickening in silica exposure are features of acute silicosis and silicoproteinosis due to inhalation of a large quantity of particles. Patients present with progressive dyspnea, with frequently fatal outcome usually within 1 year. Besides silica particles deposition, alveolar filling with acid-Schiff–positive proteinaceous material is seen, similar to that in alveolar proteinosis, explaining imaging findings.

In the complicated form of chronic silicosis, opacities initially form in upper and mid lungs and gradually migrate toward the hila, distorting architecture and producing adjacent cicatricial emphysema as they evolve into perihilar confluent soft tissue conglomerates (progressive massive fibrosis), which may partially calcify. Internal foci of low attenuation due to necrosis of mass-like tissue can be observed. Occasionally, cavitation with or without pleural thickening develops, which should raise a suspicion of mycobacterial infection. Susceptibility to TB in silicosis is increased by 2 to 30 times.

Coal worker's pneumoconiosis (CWP) and silicosis are distinct entities, despite similar imaging findings and inhalational exposure to inorganic dust. In CWP, workers are exposed to washed coal, which is nearly free of silica or mixed with smaller amount of kaolin, mica, or silica. CWP is seen in coal miners, whereas silicosis has wider range of professional exposure (sandblasters, miners, tunnelers, potters, glassmakers, foundry/quarry/dental/construction workers). Clinically, patients with CWP and PMF tend to do better than patients with silicosis and PMF, and the first group has more frequent mismatch between clinical severity and imaging findings.

References: Chong S, Lee KS, Chung MJ, et al. Pneumoconiosis: comparison of imaging and pathologic findings. *Radiographics* 2006;26(1):59–77.

Cox CW, Rose CS, Lynch DA. State of the art: imaging of occupational lung disease. *Radiology* 2014;270(3):681–696.

Hansell DM, Armstrong P, Lynch DA, McAdams HP. *Imaging of the diseases of the chest*, 4th ed. Philadelphia, PA: Elsevier Mosby, 2005.

9a **Answer A.**

9b **Answer C.**

9c **Answer C.**   On radiographs, well-defined bizarre-shaped dense opacities, different in appearance on the lateral view, are of an extraparenchymal origin. In contrast, parenchymal lesions have smudgy or less defined margins and, if seen on both frontal and lateral radiographs, do not drastically change their appearance between the projections. The density of opacities higher than bone implies calcium with linear coarse calcifications present on diaphragmatic and pericardial surfaces. The appearance is nearly pathognomonic of prior asbestos exposure and represents advanced calcified pleural plaques.

The most common manifestation of asbestos exposure is in the pleura with unilateral reactive pleural effusion (latency of 10 years, from chronic irritation by asbestos fibers). Calcium deposition on parietal pleura is detected in 25% on CXR and 60% on CT, most commonly between the fourth and eighth ribs, 20 years after exposure. Visceral pleural calcifications could occur in interlobar fissures. Dense white edges along the plaque margin are called a rolled edge. When a plaque is soft, it is seen as an irregular, smooth elevation of pleura with single indistinct margin (since it blends with normal pleura). Round atelectasis, either solitary or multifocal, is not unique but common among patients with asbestos exposure and pleural thickening.

The earliest parenchymal change in asbestosis is curvilinear subpleural lines in the lower lungs. These could be subtle and obscured by dependent atelectasis. Therefore, prone images are pivotal to early diagnosis. Later, parenchymal bands and fibrosis with mild or more extensive honeycombing and bronchiectases can occur (seen on provided CT images).

Asbestosis spreads centrifugally from terminal bronchioles and alveolar ducts. As in the case here, it has lower and basal lung predilection. Histologically, it is indistinguishable from usual interstitial pneumonia. The fibrosis tends to progress despite exposure removal.

None of the features of fibrosis in asbestosis are specific. Fibrosis related to drug reaction more frequently manifests with organizing pneumonia or NSIP pattern and would not result in bilateral pleural plaques. ARDS-related fibrosis has anterior upper/mid lung predominance, possibly related to anterior lung barotrauma or hyperoxygenation in a mechanically ventilated host. IPF diagnosis requires excluding other causes of pulmonary fibrosis, and the presence of pleural plaques in these cases strongly points to prior asbestos exposure.

The diagnosis of asbestosis requires occupational history or potential environmental exposure, clinical findings (nonresolving lower lung crackles, clubbing, dyspnea), abnormal pulmonary function tests (reduced vital and diffusion capacity), and radiologic findings. One of the indications for HRCT is identification of asbestosis in symptomatic workers with normal parenchyma on chest radiographs. Other indications for CT use are identification of pulmonary fibrosis as distinct from emphysema and diffuse pleural disease, detection of pulmonary fibrosis for compensation purpose (when chest radiograph does not support abnormal pulmonary function tests), and further workup of suspected pleural or parenchymal mass. When the appearance is classic and no worrisome radiographic/clinical findings are present, HRCT is not needed.

Lung cancer and mesothelioma are estimated to occur in 20% to 25% of patients with heavy exposure to asbestos. Asbestos-related lung cancer manifests as either adenocarcinoma or squamous cell carcinoma, with up to 100× increased incidence in asbestos-exposed smokers over nonsmoking unexposed patients. Pleural mesotheliomas, on the other hand, do not demonstrate clear association with smoking but with type of asbestos particles, occurring mostly due to crocidolite deposition. Malignant pleural mesothelioma is a spectrum of asbestos-related disease and characterized by nodular or diffuse pleural thickening (thickness >1 cm). Small pleural effusions could be present. The disease has a 10% lifetime occurrence in asbestos workers (with latency of 30 years or more) and could also occur in their household members or residents living near asbestos mines and plants.

References: Chong S, Lee KS, Chung MJ, et al. Pneumoconiosis: comparison of imaging and pathologic findings. *Radiographics* 2006;26(1):59–77.

Hansell DM, Armstrong P, Lynch DA. Inhalational lung disease pneumoconiosis. In: *Imaging of diseases of the chest*, 4th ed. Elsevier Mosby:458–462.

Kim KL, Kim CW, Lee MK, et al. Imaging of occupational lung disease. *Radiographics* 2001;21(6):1371–1391.

Webb W, Müller N, Naidich D. *High Resolution CT of the lung*, 5th ed. Philadelphia, PA: Lippincott Williams & Wilkins, 2005.

10a **Answer C.**

10b **Answer A.**   On CT, rapid progression in bilateral cystic disease is evident. Some of the lesions are clearly subpleural, responsible for pneumothorax. Thickened bronchovascular bundles, foci of parenchymal consolidation, scattered ill-defined various size nodules, and pleural effusions are seen on follow-up. Given the history, cystic or cavitary metastasis is the most likely diagnosis. The rest of the provided choices are unlikely: (1) Emphysema classically lacks walls; (2) pulmonary Langerhans cell histiocytosis manifests with smoking-related small and bizarre-shaped cysts, centrilobular micronodules, and no pleural effusions or interstitial thickening; and (3) Birt-Hogg-Dube syndrome is an autosomal dominant disease with lower lung–predominant thin-walled large septated cysts, positive dermatologic findings (fibrofolliculomas), and renal tumors.

Multiple variable-sized peripheral round nodules and thickened interstitium are typical manifestations of lung parenchymal metastatic disease. Atypical features are listed as the alternative choices and also include calcification, perinodular ground-glass attenuation, tumor embolism, endobronchial metastasis, dilated vessels within a mass, and a sterilized metastasis (PET-negative CT-persistent nodule, histologically represented by necrotic or fibrotic cells with no viable tumor cells).

Incidence of cavitation is higher in primary bronchogenic carcinoma than in metastatic disease, 9% versus 4%, respectively. Cavitary primary lung carcinomas are represented by squamous cell and adenocarcinomas. Among secondary lung malignancies, 70% of cavitary mets are represented by squamous cell carcinomas (most common, head and neck origin). Urogenital transitional cell carcinomas, colorectal carcinomas, melanoma, and sarcoma metastases are also known for cystic transformation. This may relate to a check-valve mechanism and peripheral tumor necrosis with rupture into the pleural cavity.

References: Lee KH, Lee JS, Lynch DA, et al. The radiologic differential diagnosis of diffuse lung diseases characterized by multiple cysts or cavities (pictorial essay). *J Comput Assist Tomogr* 2002;26(1):5–12.

Seo JB, Im JG, Goo JM, et al. Atypical pulmonary metastases: spectrum of radiologic findings. *Radiographics* 2001;21:403–417.

Tateishi U, Hasegawa T, Kusumoto M, et al. Metastatic angiosarcoma of the lung: spectrum of CT findings. *AJR Am J Roentgenol* 2003;180:1671–1674.

11a **Answer B.**

11b **Answer B.** Unlike the case presented, UIP-related fibrosis has peripheral and basal predilection with key findings of subpleural reticulations and honeycombing. In this case, conglomerate mass-like fibrosis, peribronchovascular and subpleural nodularity, and upper and midvolume loss with hilar retraction are not the features of UIP and IPF but could be seen in advanced stages of sarcoidosis, chronic beryllium disease, and other pneumoconioses. However, beryllium exposure is specifically associated with ceramics manufacture, nuclear weapon production, and the aerospace industry and is seen in up to 16% of workers in some studies.

The pathologic hallmark of chronic beryllium disease is noncaseating granulomas indistinguishable from granulomas in sarcoidosis. It is thought to result from initial macrophage-initiated response to inhaled beryllium that is presented to CD4 T cells initiating chronic inflammation. The pathologic and imaging findings are indistinguishable from those in sarcoidosis. Therefore, the presence of noncaseating granulomas is not characteristic. Mononuclear cellular infiltrate with documented exposure and positive beryllium lymphocyte proliferation testing are generally considered adequate to establish a diagnosis. The latter test is positive in 90% with chronic disease (highest sensitivity is from bronchial lavage). Clinical findings are similar to those in sarcoidosis including extrathoracic manifestations with skin lesions (most frequent). Lymphadenopathy (up to 40%), hypercalcemia, hepatosplenomegaly, and renal calcinosis are also reported.

According to workplace standards, maximum permissible level of beryllium is 2 μg/m^3 over 8-hour period, with a peak level of 25 μg/m^3. Any potential exposure to beryllium dust or fumes is enough to raise practical concern for chronic disease as the presence and severity of disease are not related to the exposure dose, but to the individual's immune response.

References: Cox CW, Rose CS, Lynch DA. State of the art: imaging of occupational lung disease. *Radiology* 2014;270(3):681–696.

Hansell DM, Armstrong P, Lynch DA. Inhalational lung disease pneumoconiosis. In: *Imaging of diseases of the chest*, 4th ed. Elsevier Mosby:465–466.

Sharma N, Patel J, Mohammed TL. Chronic beryllium disease: computed tomographic findings. *J Comput Assist Tomogr* 2010;34(6):945–948.

Webb WR, Muller NL, Naidich DP. Chapter 9: Pneumoconiosis. Occupational and environmental lung disease. In: *High-resolution of the lung*, 4th ed. Philadelphia, PA: Lippincott Williams & Wilkins, 2014:329–330.

12a **Answer A.**

12b **Answer B.**

12c **Answer A.**

12d **Answer D.** The radiographic images show bilateral basal and posterior predominant reticular pattern. No cardiomegaly, lymphadenopathy, or pleural effusions are identified. Decreased lung volumes and relatively symmetric posterior basal predominant reticulations suggest that this is related to the presence of lung fibrosis.

On the CT images, there is peripheral and lower lung–predominant reticular abnormality with development of significant honeycomb cyst formation over time. This is classic for the UIP pattern of fibrosing interstitial pneumonia.

The pattern of fibrosis in NSIP demonstrates more ground-glass abnormality (especially in a bronchovascular pattern) and more traction bronchiectasis. Honeycomb cyst formation can be seen in NSIP but is generally a very late finding indicative of end-stage fibrosis. Organizing pneumonia is characterized by peripheral and lower lung–predominant consolidation and ground glass. LIP is characterized by lower lung–predominant cysts in a perivascular distribution rather than the subpleural honeycomb cysts found here.

A number of conditions could present with features of UIP (connective tissue disease such as rheumatoid arthritis, chronic hypersensitivity pneumonitis, or drug toxicity). It is crucial to exclude any of these identifiable causes to diagnosis idiopathic pulmonary fibrosis (IPF) and guide optimal treatment.

Based on the current official ATS/ERS/JRS/ALAT clinical practice guideline, interstitial lung diseases (ILD) by CT imaging can be summarized into several categories: (1) consistent with UIP—presenting with honeycombing in usual (lower lung subpleural predominant) distribution and no other excluding features such as micronodularity, air trapping, dominant ground-glass opacities, cysts, pleural effusions; (2) probable UIP—as (1) but instead of honeycombing peripheral reticulations and peripheral traction bronchiectasis/bronchioloectasis, with possible mild peripheral ground-glass opacities; (3) indeterminate for UIP—pulmonary fibrosis distribution is not characteristic of any specific etiology or too mild to further characterize; and (4) alternative diagnosis to IPF—pulmonary fibrosis with characteristic findings of an alternative diagnosis such as upper lobe predominance, presence of marker mosaic attenuation, or pleural plaques. The last set of images has classic features that suggest an alternative diagnosis to UIP—peribronchovascular/perilymphatic micronodularity, scattered ground-glass opacities, centroaxial extent of the lung changes, and lack of peripheral honeycombing. These images would be most characteristic for chronic hypersensitivity pneumonitis or sarcoidosis.

Reference: Raghu G, Remy-Jardin M, Myers JL, et al. Diagnosis of idiopathic pulmonary fibrosis. An Official ATS/ERS/JRS/ALAT Clinical Practice Guideline. *Am J Respir Crit Care Med* 2018;198(5):e44–e68.

13a **Answer B.**

13b **Answer C.**

13c **Answer B.**

13d **Answer D.** Radiographic images show diffuse airspace disease with scattered air bronchograms and normal heart in an intubated patient. Small left-sided pleural effusion, small right apical pneumothorax, and subcutaneous air within upper chest/lower neck are present. Several thin vertical lucencies within the upper mediastinum are suspicious for mild pneumomediastinum. The appearance would be highly unlikely to represent cardiogenic edema. Presence of pneumothorax and subcutaneous air and possible mild pneumomediastinum raise a question of barotrauma in a mechanically ventilated patient, which is frequently seen in causes of noncardiogenic edema due to acute respiratory distress syndrome (ARDS). Aspiration tends to be either central (perihilar) or lower lung predominant and not as diffuse as this process is but can transition to ARDS. Similarly, lobar pneumonia refers to infection in a single lobe.

This is a case of acute interstitial pneumonia (AIP). AIP is an idiopathic condition that is histologically and radiographically similar to acute respiratory distress syndrome. The latter could be caused by multiple factors that include but are not limited to viral infection, aspiration, sepsis, shock, trauma, or drug reaction. On CT, bilateral ground-glass opacities are present with gradual appearance of more dense foci of consolidation in dependent distribution. Note the relative absence of septal thickening normally seen in pulmonary edema. Bilateral pleural effusions are evident. The underlying pathology is that of diffuse alveolar damage (DAD). In the acute phase, a combination of airspace exudates, noncardiogenic interstitial edema, inflammation, and alveolar collapse in the dependent portions of the lungs is characteristic. The organizing phase of ARDS is first seen in the beginning of the 2nd week after an insult and depends on the ability of denuded alveoli and exposed epithelial membranes to reorganize and repair, resulting in increased consolidation. Upper and anterior lung–predominant fibrosis results from this fibroproliferative phase. Anterior fibrosis is thought to result from barotrauma and oxygen toxicity in mechanical ventilation to the anterior lungs, whereas the dorsal lungs are relatively protected by the gravity-dependent atelectasis and consolidation. The survival in the acute phase is lower than in the chronic phase, with an average reported difference of 10% to 20% in favor of chronic ARDS.

References: Kligerman SJ, Franks TJ, Galvin JR. From the radiologic pathology archives: organization and fibrosis as a response to lung injury in diffuse alveolar damage, organizing pneumonia, and acute fibrinous and organizing pneumonia. *Radiographics* 2013;33(7): 1951–1975.

Lynch DA, Travis WD, Muller NL, et al. Idiopathic interstitial pneumonias: CT features. *Radiology* 2005;236:10–21.

Webb WR, Muller NL, Naidich DP. Chapter 4: The idiopathic interstitial pneumonias. In: *High-resolution of the lung*, 4th ed. Philadelphia, PA: Lippincott Williams & Wilkins, 2014:206–209.

14a   **Answer A.**

14b   **Answer A.**

14c   **Answer B.**

14d   **Answer D.**

CT images on the first set of CT images show advanced traction bronchiectases, most abundant in the lower lungs, with relative subpleural sparing in the dorsal lower lobes but extension into cardiophrenic angles. Similarly, bilateral peripheral ground-glass opacities demonstrate relative sparing of the most peripheral lung. Patchy consolidation and small pleural effusion are seen on the left. The imaging findings are most indicative of fibrotic nonspecific interstitial pneumonia (NSIP). Multifocal consolidation on the left could represent foci of organizing pneumonia.

NSIP is a chronic interstitial lung disease that accounts for 40% of pathologically proven interstitial lung diseases. The most common etiologies include connective tissue diseases, drug exposure, hypersensitivity pneumonitis, and occupational exposure.

On the second set of images, the dominant abnormality is bilateral asymmetric but basal predominant ground-glass opacities, with the pattern of NSIP and/ or organizing pneumonia. Lack of significant traction bronchiectasis suggests cellular or more acute phase.

The primary findings of NSIP include (1) extensive ground-glass opacities with absent or mild reticulation, (2) traction bronchiectases, (3) absent or minimal honeycombing, (4) basal predominance, and (5) subpleural sparing. Among these criteria, ground-glass opacities with minimal or absent reticulation is considered the cellular type of NSIP. Remainder of the findings corresponds to fibrotic NSIP. Since CT features of NSIP can overlap with organizing pneumonia and desquamative interstitial pneumonia; in these cases, surgical biopsy may be warranted, with sampling of more than one lobe.

Fibrotic NSIP carries worse survival than cellular NSIP, 6 to 14 years in fibrotic NSIP versus complete resolution in nearly all cases. However, fibrotic NSIP is not as poor of a prognosis as IPF (2.5 to 3.5 years average survival from initial diagnosis). Idiopathic NSIP has at least an 80% 5-year survival. Response to corticosteroids and cytotoxic agents is nonuniform in NSIP and depends on the type. Cellular NSIP frequently responds to corticosteroids but is less frequent type of NSIP. Corticosteroids and cytotoxic agents are less effective in fibrotic NSIP.

References: Lynch DA, Travis WD, Muller NL, et al. Idiopathic interstitial pneumonias: CT features. *Radiology* 2005;236:10–21.

Poletti V, Romagnoli M, Piciucchi S, et al. Current status of idiopathic nonspecific interstitial pneumonia. *Semin Respir Crit Care Med* 2012;33:440–449.

Raghu G, Remy-Jardin M, Myers JL, et al. Diagnosis of idiopathic pulmonary fibrosis. An Official ATS/ERS/JRS/ALAT Clinical Practice Guideline. *Am J Respir Crit Care Med* 2018;198(5):e44–e68.

Silva CI, Muller NL, Hansell DM, et al. Nonspecific interstitial pneumonia and idiopathic pulmonary fibrosis: changes in pattern and distribution of disease over time. *Radiology* 2008;247(1):251–259.

Webb WR, Muller NL, Naidich DP. Chapter 4: The idiopathic interstitial pneumonias. In: *High-resolution of the lung*, 4th ed. Philadelphia, PA: Lippincott Williams & Wilkins, 2014:189–198.

15a Answer C.

15b Answer D.

15c Answer C.

15d Answer A. Frontal chest radiograph shows unilateral (right) reticular and reticulonodular pattern, in addition to a focal nodular opacity with peripheral right upper lobe. Differential considerations favor lymphangitic carcinomatosis (LC) or atypical infection (viral pneumonia). Subsequent CT images show unilateral variable (smooth and nodular) septal thickening, thickening of centrilobular core structures, and preservation of normal lobular architecture. Spiculated lung lesion with adjacent pleural reaction is evident, enriching a possibility of malignancy. Emphysema would manifest as hyperinflation and upper lung increased lucency. Pulmonary edema presents with interstitial findings as well, but usually is bilateral, and associated with cardiac enlargement.

When reticular or reticulonodular opacities are unilateral and seen in the presence of an upper lung suspicious lesion, it is often due to bronchogenic carcinoma (as in the case here). Secondary malignancies associated with LC are adenocarcinomas, especially those originating from the breast, stomach, colon, and prostate. However, these have bilateral findings in 80% to 90% of the time. Lymphangitic carcinomatosis generally indicates stage IV disease, and wedge resection would not address the more extensive disease. Importantly, radiographic findings are negative in half of the cases of LC. On CT, reticular pattern corresponds to thickening of interlobular septa that is most frequently nodular or beaded in appearance.

Pathogenesis most commonly reflects initial hematogenous dissemination to the lungs with subsequent invasion or the interstitium and lymphatics. The tumor spreads from the peripheral lung centrally via the interstitium around the lymphatics. In a minority of patients, the spread occurs retrograde from tumor-laden hilar lymph nodes. LC is associated with poor prognosis, with demise frequently seen within 6 months.

References: Johkoh T, Ikezoe J, Tomiyama N, et al. CT findings in lymphangitic carcinomatosis of the lung: correlation with histologic findings and pulmonary function tests. *AJR Am J Roentgenol* 1992;158:1217–1222.

Prakash P, Kalra MK, Sharma A, et al. FDG PET/CT in assessment of pulmonary lymphangitic carcinomatosis. *AJR Am J Roentgenol* 2010;194:231–236.

Scheafer-Prokop C, Prokop M, Fleischman D, et al. High-resolution CT of diffuse interstitial lung disease: key findings in common disorders. *Eur Radiol* 2001;11:373–392.

16a　Answer B.

16b　Answer C.　Bilateral extensive ground-glass opacities (GGO) are present that significantly improved on follow-up imaging with treatment and smoking cessation. Differential considerations would include hypersensitivity pneumonitis (exposure to an extrinsic allergen), desquamative interstitial pneumonia—DIP (history of smoking), and nonspecific interstitial pneumonia. In this patient, hypersensitivity pneumonitis is less likely in the setting of smoking (one of the few diseases actually inhibited by smoking). Usual interstitial pneumonia manifests with subpleural reticulations, intralobular lines, and honeycombing, which are not seen. Pulmonary edema manifests first as vessel distension and interlobular septal thickening, which are not seen in this case.

Imaging features of DIP include bilateral confluent or patchy ground-glass opacities, frequently with small parenchymal cysts in the areas of ground glass. Mild reticulation could be present owing to minimal septal fibrosis.

RB-ILD (respiratory bronchiolitis–interstitial lung disease) is also predominantly a smoking-related illness, but the distribution and findings are somewhat different: diffuse or geographic areas of ground-glass opacities with lower lung predominance in DIP and upper lung–predominant ground-glass nodules in RB-ILD. Some authors believe that RB-ILD and DIP represent continuum in smoking-related injury. Pathologically, RB-ILD is centrilobular peribronchiolar pathologic process whereas DIP represents intra-alveolar accumulation of macrophages with some giant cells. The term "desquamative" is a misnomer and originates from a prior belief that pneumocyte desquamation was occurring.

Up to 40% of DIP presents in nonsmoking patients, generally associated with exposure to inhaled occupational inorganic particles (beryllium, aluminum, diesel fumes) and aflatoxin, drugs (nitrofurantoin, busulfan), viral illnesses, and autoimmune disease. However, the usual occurrence is in smoking males (male: female ratio is 2:1), 40 to 60 years old, who present with exertional dyspnea and/or mild nonproductive cough. On physical exam, basal crackles and cyanosis are frequently seen. The most frequent abnormal pattern on pulmonary functional test is a restrictive pattern. Severe obstruction on spirometry (FEV1 < 70%) is not characteristic and, when present, likely reflects concomitant chronic bronchitis or emphysema.

Survival from DIP is estimated to be between 68% and 98%. Smoking cessation (or removal of an offending agent in nonsmoking-related DIP) is pivotal. About 20% of patients show spontaneous improvement with cessation of exposure. A large number of patients require corticosteroids. Without treatment, 60% patients deteriorate clinically. About 25% of patients will progress despite the treatment.

References: Attili A, Kazerooni E, Gross BH, et al. Smoking-related interstitial lung disease: radiologic-clinical-pathologic correlation. *Radiographics* 2008;28:1383–1398.

Godbert B, Wissler M, Vignaud J. Desquamative interstitial pneumonia: an analytic review with an emphasis on aetiology. *Eur Respir Rev* 2013;22(128):117–123.

Hobbs S, Lynch D. The idiopathic interstitial pneumonias: an update and review. *Radiol Clin North Am* 2014;52(1):105–120.

7 Diffuse Alveolar Disease and Inflammatory Conditions

Christian W. Cox, MD

QUESTIONS

1a What radiographic pattern best describes the CXR appearance?

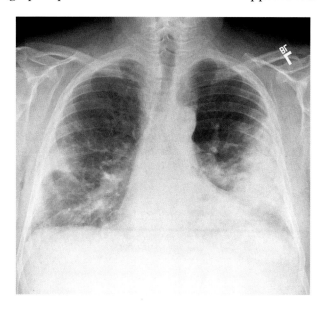

A. Reticular
B. Nodular
C. Pleural thickening
D. Consolidation

1b Chest CT on the same patient obtained 6 months later. Which of the following causes would best explain the imaging findings?

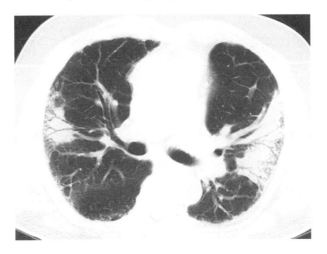

A. Lipoid pneumonia
B. Acute respiratory distress syndrome (ARDS)
C. Bacterial pneumonia
D. Pulmonary embolism

1c What is the preferential treatment for exogenous lipoid pneumonia?

A. Bronchoalveolar lavage
B. Removal of the offending agent
C. Corticosteroids
D. Broad-spectrum antibiotics

2a Which radiographic finding best supports characterizing the pulmonary opacities below as consolidation?

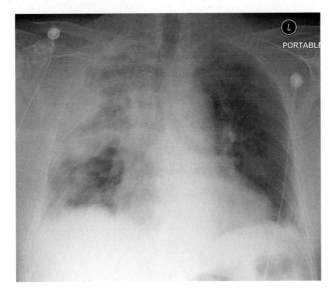

A. Volume loss
B. Outlines minor fissure
C. Presence of "tram-track" opacities
D. Peripheral distribution

2b   A follow-up CT is obtained. Which lobe demonstrates the greatest degree of pulmonary consolidation?

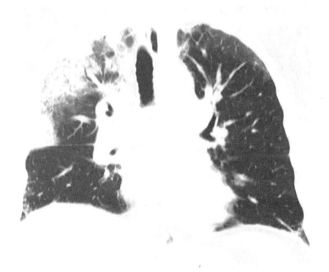

    A. Right middle lobe
    B. Left upper lobe
    C. Lingula
    D. Right upper lobe

2c   Patient condition resolves spontaneously after 1 month, and the patient undergoes follow-up chest radiograph (left). Months later, the patient's symptoms return with repeat chest radiograph (right). What would be the most likely finding on pathology from bronchoscopic alveolar lavage?

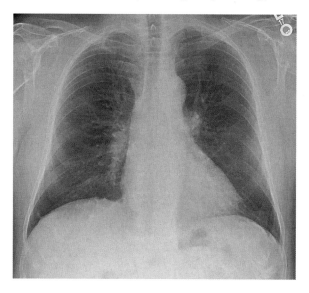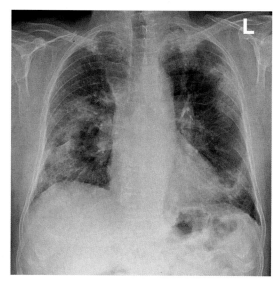

    A. Poorly differentiated adenocarcinoma
    B. Lipid-rich material
    C. Lymphoma
    D. Eosinophils

2d What characteristic finding best differentiates simple eosinophilic pneumonia from chronic eosinophilic pneumonia?

    A. Pulmonary distribution
    B. Time course
    C. Symptoms
    D. Blood eosinophilia

3a A 63-year-old male status post heart transplant. Which diagnostic test result would best characterize the disease as pulmonary alveolar proteinosis?

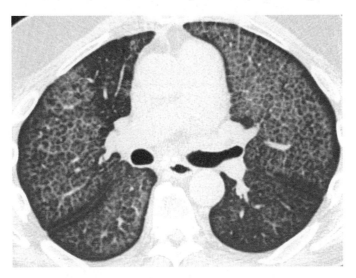

    A. Elevated brain natriuretic peptide blood test
    B. Positive pneumocystis polymerase chain reaction test
    C. Lipoproteinaceous material on bronchoscopic alveolar lavage
    D. Histopathologic acute lung injury on transthoracic lung wedge resection

3b What is the most common cause of pulmonary alveolar proteinosis?

    A. Idiopathic
    B. Drug reaction
    C. Silica exposure
    D. Hematologic malignancy

3c Which group of medications has most commonly been described to cause pulmonary alveolar proteinosis?

    A. Chemotherapy
    B. Bacterial antibiotic
    C. Antihypertensive
    D. Immunosuppressive

4 Chest radiograph following blood product transfusion. The clinical team is worried about the possibility of transfusion-related acute lung injury (TRALI). How long after blood product transfusion does TRALI typically develop?

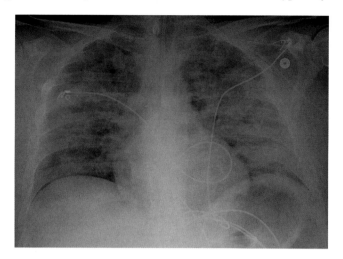

A. Immediately
B. 1 to 6 hours
C. 12 to 24 hours
D. 24 to 48 hours

5a In this 67-year-old male with multifocal peripheral pulmonary consolidations on noncontrast chest CT, the imaging finding is most concerning for which disease process?

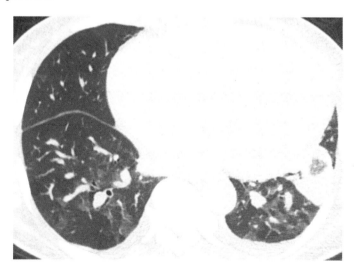

A. Bacterial pneumonia
B. Pulmonary infarct
C. Pulmonary metastases
D. Pulmonary lymphoma

5b A follow-up chest CT angiogram was obtained. Of the selected CT images, which confirms the diagnosis?

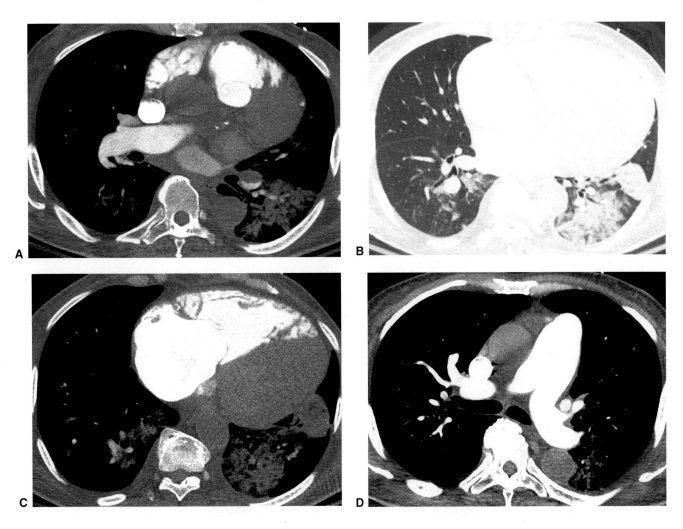

A

B

C

D

6 What is the likely diagnosis in this patient with a long-standing history of recurrent urinary tract infections?

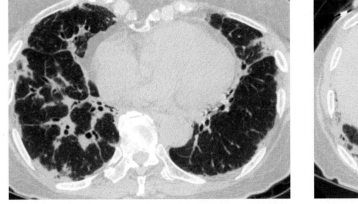

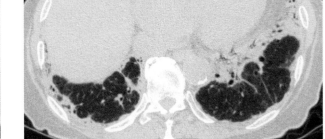

A. Organizing pneumonia
B. Septic emboli
C. Pulmonary hemorrhage
D. Usual interstitial pneumonia

7a What is the most likely etiology of these pulmonary opacities given corresponding symptoms and history of asthma, polyneuropathy, and sinus disease?

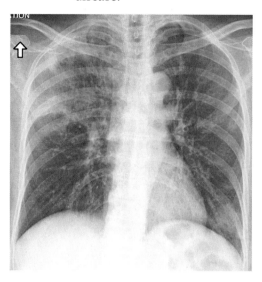 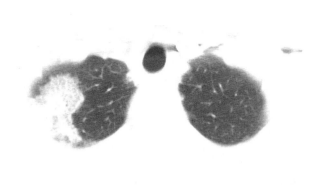

A. Churg-Strauss syndrome (eosinophilic granulomatosis with polyangiitis)
B. Organizing pneumonia
C. Granulomatosis with polyangiitis (Wegener granulomatosis)
D. Microscopic polyangiitis

7b What biomarker is most strongly associated with this disease?

A. c-ANCA
B. p-ANCA
C. Rheumatoid factor
D. Antiphospholipid antibodies

8a What radiologic sign is present on this expiratory CT?

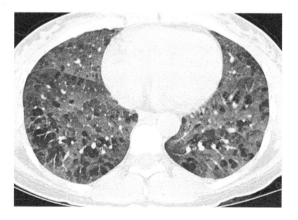

A. Head cheese sign
B. Comet tail
C. Reverse halo
D. Galaxy sign

8b With what disease is this sign most highly associated?

A. Hypersensitivity pneumonitis
B. Organizing pneumonia
C. Eosinophilic pneumonia
D. Desquamative interstitial pneumonia

9   This previously healthy 36-year-old male experienced acute-onset worsening shortness of breath after traveling to the mountains for a hiking trip. No fever or chills are present. What is the likely pathology?

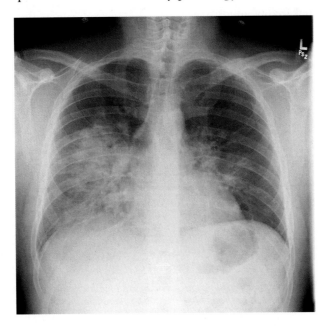

A. Bronchopneumonia
B. Noncardiogenic pulmonary edema
C. Pulmonary hemorrhage
D. Cardiogenic pulmonary edema

10a   Patient presents with a history of chronic renal disease, positive MPO blood test, recent anemia, and the provided chest radiograph. What is the most likely diagnosis?

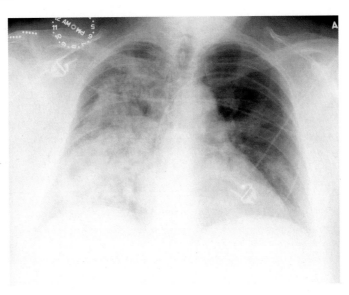

A. Noncardiogenic pulmonary edema
B. Hyperthermal inhalational injury
C. Microscopic polyangiitis
D. Hematologic malignancy

10b Which patient characteristic would best predict subsequent respiratory failure in the setting of diffuse alveolar hemorrhage from antineutrophil cytoplasmic antibody–associated vasculitis?

A. Active renal involvement
B. Degree of hypoxemia at presentation
C. Hemoptysis at presentation
D. History of current or former smoking

11 What is the likely diagnosis given these inspiratory (left) and expiratory (right) CT images?

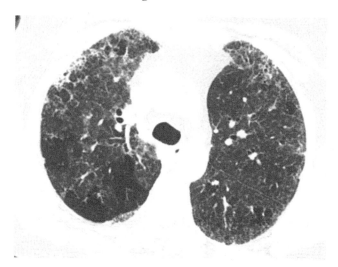 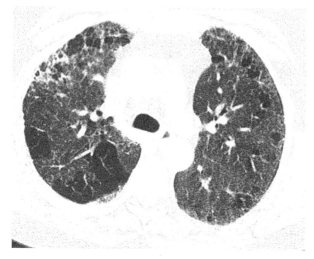

A. Chronic hypersensitivity pneumonitis
B. Idiopathic pulmonary fibrosis
C. Sarcoidosis
D. Progressive massive fibrosis

ANSWERS AND EXPLANATIONS

1a   Answer D.

1b   Answer A.

1c   Answer B.   Initial presentation on chest radiograph is consistent with consolidation supported by the homogeneous opacities with air bronchograms. The peripheral distribution could raise concern for pleural thickening although the poorly defined inner margins, outlining of the horizontal fissure, and air bronchograms contradict a pleural-based process. Interstitial opacities, such as reticular and nodular patterns, can be peripheral but would not produce the homogenous opacities, air bronchograms, or clear outline of the fissure.

Of the options provided, only lipoid pneumonia would produce a static consolidation for 6 months. Although many frequently think of lipoid pneumonia only in the case of low (fat)-density alveolar consolidation, that is not always seen. As the name implies, ARDS is an acute process and one would expect signs of respiratory distress, such as intubation, before suggesting the diagnosis radiographically. Incomplete treatment of bacterial pneumonia could produce a persistent consolidation, but the static nature in this case suggests against it as one would expect progression over time. Infectious pneumonia can convert into an organizing pneumonia, but this is not given as an option. Finally, pulmonary embolism can produce peripheral consolidation due to infarct, but again, the static nature excluded this diagnosis at 6 months. Additionally, hemorrhage as the cause of consolidation in pulmonary infarcts tends to fill the airways, causing a notable absence of air bronchograms.

In terms of treatment, Gondouin et al. reported a multicenter case study of exogenous lipoid pneumonia including 44 patients. In this study, and in others, corticosteroids and bronchoalveolar lavage demonstrated no significant benefit in the treatment of lipoid pneumonia. As the disease is not infectious, antibiotics have no use in the treatment, but patients often fail antibiotics early due to a presumed infectious etiology at initial presentation. Of the 44 cases studied by Gondouin, 13 improved with removal of offending agent, 7 stabilized, and 5 patients experienced ongoing progression and deterioration to include pulmonary fibrosis, recurrent infection, and *Aspergillus*-related complication.

Reference: Gondouin A, et al. Exogenous lipid pneumonia: a retrospective multicentre study of 44 cases in France. *Eur Respir J* 1996;9:1463–1469.

2a   Answer B.

2b   Answer D.

2c   Answer D.

2d   Answer B.   The initial chest radiograph demonstrates a right upper lobe–predominant consolidation that outlines the minor fissure. Classic findings of consolidation on chest radiograph include poorly defined margins, air bronchograms, contained by fissures, and maintained lung volume. While these opacities do prove to be peripherally predominant, this characteristic does not help categorize these opacities as consolidation. Volume loss is not significant on this initial chest radiograph, nor is it a finding of consolidation. Finally, "tram-track" opacities are an axial interstitial finding relating to thickening of the bronchial wall and therefore not a finding of consolidation.

Localizing pulmonary disease can be a challenge on single CT images, and therefore, understanding the relationship with fissures can be helpful. The anatomic position on CT is the same as chest radiograph with the patient position facing the viewer with the patient's right on the left side of the image. That places the consolidations on the provided CT in the patient's right lung. The consolidation along the superior aspect of the minor fissure localizes the findings to the right upper lobe. Interestingly, this patient also has an accessory left horizontal fissure.

When the disease recurs, it demonstrates a classic distribution for eosinophilic pneumonia with peripheral patchy consolidations, often with an upper lobe predominance. This appearance has been described as the "photographic negative on pulmonary edema." Bronchoalveolar lavage revealing eosinophils in the setting of pulmonary consolidation is diagnostic of eosinophilic pneumonia, and secondary causes such as infection or drug toxicity should be excluded. The spontaneous resolution and disease recurrence remove neoplastic etiologies from the differential, such as bronchogenic carcinoma or lymphoma. Lipid-rich pneumonias such as lipoid pneumonia and alveolar proteinosis can cause chronic consolidation, but the recurrent pattern and peripheral upper lobe distribution would favor eosinophilic pneumonia.

Initial time course of disease in this patient, spontaneously resolving after 1 month, is consistent with simple eosinophilic pneumonia, also known as Loeffler syndrome, and helps differentiate from chronic eosinophilic pneumonia, which generally requires steroid treatment and/or identification of an underlying process. Simple eosinophilic pneumonia also typically causes "shifting consolidations," where chronic eosinophilic pneumonia will produce more static homogenous consolidations. Otherwise, both of these types of eosinophilic lung disease may produce similar peripheral consolidations, symptoms, and blood eosinophilia.

References: Jeong YJ, et al. Eosinophilic lung diseases: a clinical, radiologic, and pathologic overview. *Radiographics* 2007;27:617–639.

Webb WR, Higgins CB. *Thoracic imaging.* Philadelphia, PA: Lippincott Williams & Wilkins, 2010.

3a Answer C.

3b Answer A.

3c Answer D.   The provided CT image demonstrates a characteristic "crazy-paving" appearance in the lung, to include septal thickening and ground-glass opacity in a patchwork distribution amongst normal areas of lung. While initially described associated with pulmonary alveolar proteinosis (PAP) and the characteristic appearance of this disease process, the "crazy-paving" pattern has multiple potential causes. Pulmonary edema, atypical infection, and pulmonary hemorrhage are a few of the more common alternative causes of the "crazy-paving" pattern. Of the tests provided, PAS-positive lipoproteinaceous materials on bronchoscopic alveolar lavage confirms the diagnosis of PAP. The other provided options aim at diagnosing one of the alternative causes of crazy paving.

The majority of pulmonary alveolar proteinosis cases are primary/idiopathic and present in mid to late adulthood with progressive dyspnea or cough. There are secondary causes of PAP, to include inhalational exposures, such as silica, hematologic malignancies, and immunosuppression. As a subgroup, immunosuppressive therapies, such as sirolimus in the case provided, are the primary mediations associated with secondary PAP.

References: Frazier AA, Franks TJ, Cooke EO. From the archives of the AFIP: pulmonary alveolar proteinosis. *Radiographics* 2008;28:883–899.

Suzuki T, Trapnell BC. Pulmonary alveolar proteinosis syndrome. *Clin Chest Med* 2016;37(3):431–440.

4 **Answer B.** TRALI is a serious and potentially life-threatening complication of blood product transfusion. The mechanism is not entirely understood, but the clinical presentation is similar to that of ARDS and noncardiogenic edema. Onset is most frequently within 1 to 2 hours with most cases manifesting under 6 hours. Resolution normally occurs within 2 to 4 days with supportive measures. Separating this disease process from fluid overload related to the transfusion (transfusion-associated circulatory overload—TACO) is critical as the use of diuretics should be avoided in TRALI. This was a case of TRALI. Note the lack of features to support cardiogenic edema and TACO including normal cardiac size, lack of effusions, and lack of a more diffuse or lower lung gradient.

Reference: Carcano C, Okafor N, Martinez F, et al. Radiographic manifestations of transfusion-related acute lung injury. *Clin Imaging* 2013;37(6):1020–1023.

5a **Answer B.**

5b **Answer A.** Diagnosis of pulmonary infarct from pulmonary embolism on noncontrast chest CT is a challenge. In a study from 2007, Revel et al. compared 150 peripheral consolidations of variable etiologies on noncontrast chest CT to identify any features that may assist in identifying pulmonary infarction. Only the presence of central lucencies, such as those demonstrated in this case, proved statistically significant in pulmonary infarct as opposed to other causes. Occasionally the central lucencies may form into an "atoll" sign in the setting of pulmonary infarcts. Air bronchograms decrease the likelihood of pulmonary infarcts as the hemorrhage associated with infarcts tends to fill the associated airways.

Several images provided include portions of the pulmonary arteries, but only image "A" of the left lower lobe segmental arteries in soft tissue window confirms the presence of a filling defect from pulmonary embolism as the cause of the peripheral infarct. The other images demonstrate additional left lower lobe consolidation from infarct in lung window, an enlarged right atrium in soft tissue window, and a mildly dilated main pulmonary artery in soft tissue window, respectively.

Reference: Revel MP, et al. Is it possible to recognize pulmonary infarction on multisection CT images? *Radiology* 2007;244(3):875–882.

6 **Answer A.** The CT images demonstrate lower lung predominant peribronchovascular and perilobular consolidation with a mild degree of resulting fibrosis. Of the choices listed, the pattern is most consistent with organizing pneumonia. The history of chronic UTI should specifically draw to mind the possibility of drug toxicity. This was a case of nitrofurantoin-related organizing pneumonia. Cessation of the drug resulted in significant improvement.

Septic emboli would be expected to be more nodular and cavitary (although peripheral opacities are common). Pulmonary hemorrhage would be more diffuse without a specific peripheral predominance. The features of UIP including subpleural reticular abnormality and honeycomb cyst formation are not seen here. Nonspecific interstitial pneumonia (NSIP) would be a consideration for this appearance, but the degree of consolidative abnormality is much more than typically seen without concurrent organizing pneumonia.

A good website to evaluate if a drug has potential pulmonary toxicity and how it might manifest is www.pneumotox.com.

Other manifestations of drug toxicity include eosinophilic pneumonia, diffuse alveolar damage, pulmonary edema, pulmonary hemorrhage, fibrosing interstitial pneumonias, lupus, vasculitis, hypersensitivity pneumonitis, and constrictive bronchiolitis.

References: Rossi SE, Erasmus JJ, McAdams HP, et al. Pulmonary drug toxicity: radiologic and pathologic manifestations. *Radiographics* 2000;20(5):1245–1259.

Webb WR, Higgins CB. *Thoracic imaging*. Philadelphia, PA: Lippincott Williams & Wilkins, 2010.

7a   Answer A.

7b   Answer B.   Churg-Strauss syndrome, now called eosinophilic granulomatosis with polyangiitis, demonstrates a triad of eosinophilia, necrotizing vasculitis, and asthma. The rheumatologic guidelines for diagnosis include having at least four of the following six findings: (1) asthma, (2) mono- or polyneuropathy, (3) migratory pulmonary opacities, (4) paranasal sinus disease, (5) extravascular eosinophils, and (6) peripheral eosinophilia on CBC. The histology is that of both a necrotizing small-vessel vasculitis and eosinophilic inflammatory infiltrate (which accounts for the new naming convention).

The most common radiographic findings are transient bilateral areas of consolidation. There is a predilection for the lung periphery and some evidence of a slightly upper lung predominance (as opposed to organizing pneumonia with a lower lung predominance). Bronchial wall thickening and small centrilobular nodules are also common features, especially given the association with asthma. Upward of 70% of patients will be p-ANCA positive.

Granulomatosis with polyangiitis, previously known as Wegeners Granulomatosis, does not have any specific association with asthma although other features of vasculitis and sinus disease can be present. It has a much stronger association with c-ANCA. Organizing pneumonia also has no specific association with the clinical picture shown but can be due to a variety of connective tissue disease or drug toxicities. Microscopic polyangiitis is a nongranulomatous necrotizing systemic vasculitis and the most common cause of pulmonary renal syndrome (concurrent pulmonary hemorrhage and glomerulonephritis); however, the manifestations are much more commonly renal with 90% of patients having rapidly progressive glomerulonephritis but pulmonary hemorrhage in only up to 30%.

Reference: Castañer E, Alguersuari A, Gallardo X, et al. When to suspect pulmonary vasculitis: radiologic and clinical clues. *Radiographics* 2010;30(1):33–53.

8a   Answer A.

8b   Answer A.   The head cheese sign reflects adjacent low, normal, and high attenuation in adjacent secondary pulmonary lobules. It reflects a combination of airspace disease (high attenuation) and obstructive disease (low attenuation). The low-attenuation small airway disease component reflects mosaic attenuation, and the high-attenuation component reflects ground-glass opacity.

The disease is most highly associated with subacute hypersensitivity pneumonitis and was initially considered pathognomonic. However, other diseases including sarcoidosis, atypical infections (such as *Mycoplasma*), respiratory bronchiolitis, and DIP have demonstrated this feature. Additionally, this sign can manifest in patients with multiple pathologic processes, such as constrictive bronchiolitis and pulmonary hemorrhage.

Reference: Chong BJ, Kanne JP, Chung JH, et al. Headcheese sign. *J Thorac Imaging* 2014;29(1):W13.

9   **Answer B.**   The radiograph demonstrates asymmetric, right greater than left airspace disease in an alveolar pattern. The airspace disease is greatest in the central lungs, and there are no identifiable effusions. Also, the heart is not enlarged. Given patient age and the lack of cardiac findings and effusions, cardiogenic edema is less likely. The other three considerations are possible; however, the history of recent high-altitude travel should make one strongly suspicious of high-altitude pulmonary edema (HAPE), a noncardiogenic pulmonary edema.

HAPE is a potentially fatal condition that occurs after traveling to a low-oxygen and low–atmospheric pressure environment (generally found at high altitudes). Most frequently, it occurs in young male patients 1 to 2 days after rapid ascent to elevations above 3,000 m. The mechanism is not well understood but likely is related to vasoconstriction and acute-onset pulmonary hypertension with resulting capillary leak. Treatment is supportive with return to normal altitude being critical.

Reference: Gluecker T, Capasso P, Schnyder P, et al. Clinical and radiologic features of pulmonary edema. *Radiographics* 1999;19(6):1507–1531.

10a   **Answer C.**

10b   **Answer B.**   From a pulmonary alveolar perspective, acute consolidation has a relatively limited differential, most commonly fluid (pulmonary edema), inflammatory cells and debris (pneumonia), and occasionally red blood cells (hemorrhage). Therefore, the clinical presentation and other diagnostic tests are key in further differentiating the potential causes.

In this case with asymmetric but bilateral acute pulmonary consolidation, several clues point towards diffuse alveolar hemorrhage. The myeloperoxidase (MPO) or proteinase 3 (PR3) tests are recognized as the preferred screening tests for antineutrophilic cytoplasmic antibody (ANCA)-associated vasculitides. MPO specifically is most commonly associated with microscopic polyangiits (MPA). The additional findings of a recent drop in hematocrit/anemia and prior history of chronic sinusitis create a classic picture for diffuse alveolar hemorrhage from ANCA-associated vasculitis.

When specifically examining patients presenting with diffuse alveolar hemorrhage from ANCA-associated vasculitis, Cartin-Ceba found that the degree of hypoxemia at presentation was one of three measures that predicted respiratory failure with statistical significance. Concurrent active renal disease, smoking history, and associate hemoptysis did not demonstrate a statistically significant increase in respiratory failure in these patients.

References: Cartin-Ceba R, et al. Diffuse alveolar hemorrhage secondary to antineutrophil cytoplasmic antibody-associated vasculitis. *Arthritis Rheumatol* 2016;68(6):1467–1476.

Lichtenbuerger JP, et al. Diffuse pulmonary hemorrhage: clues to diagnosis. *Curr Probl Diagn Radiol* 2014;43:128–139.

11   **Answer A.**   The pattern of disease is almost identical on inspiration and expiration. There is diffuse ground glass with some areas of geographic sparing and mosaic attenuation (air trapping) as well as peripheral reticular abnormality and fibrosis. One common cause of upper lung predominant fibrosis with this degree of mosaic air trapping is chronic hypersensitivity pneumonitis (findings of subacute HP with superimposed fibrosis). Although sarcoidosis does cause upper lung fibrosis and can have air trapping, the pattern is generally more bronchovascular, radiating from the hilum with bronchiectasis being a significant feature. Progressive massive fibrosis can also cause upper lung fibrosis but is more similar to sarcoid-related fibrosis with the addition of mass-like perihilar consolidation. Idiopathic pulmonary fibrosis is the idiopathic form of usual interstitial pneumonitis generally producing lower lung–predominant, subpleural, and reticular fibrosis, with or without honeycomb cyst formation.

Reference: Silva CI, Churg A, Müller NL. Hypersensitivity pneumonitis: spectrum of high-resolution CT and pathologic findings. *AJR Am J Roentgenol* 2007;188(2):334–344.

8

Airway Disease

Carlos A. Rojas, MD

QUESTIONS

1a A 62-year-old female with chronic cough. What are the most salient imaging findings?

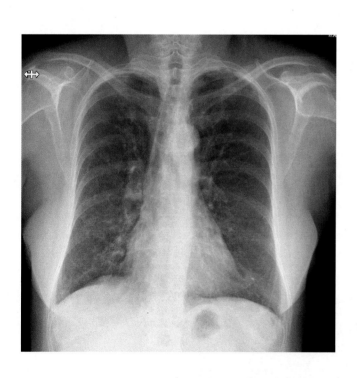
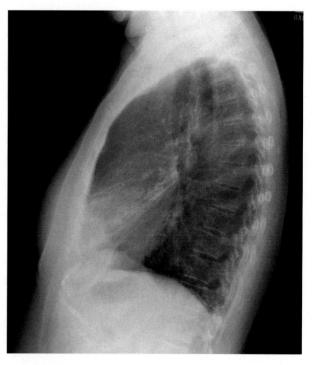

A. Bronchiectasis and nodularity
B. Airspace consolidation and scarring
C. Pleural effusions and hyperinflation
D. Emphysema and linear atelectasis

1b   A CT is shown of the same patient. Which of these imaging findings is absent?

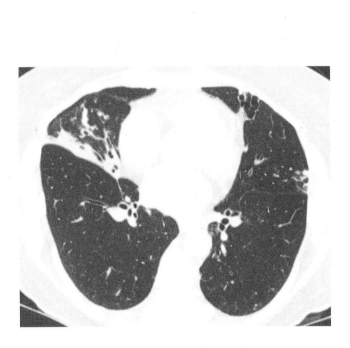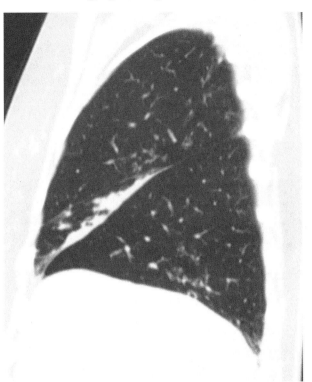

    A. Tree-in-bud nodularity
    B. Bronchiectasis
    C. Mucous plugging
    D. Cavitation

1c   What is the most likely diagnosis in this patient?

    A. Aspiration
    B. *Mycobacterium avium*-intracellulare (MAI)
    C. Allergic bronchopulmonary aspergillosis (ABPA)
    D. Cystic fibrosis

2a   What type of anatomic variant is demonstrated on the image below?

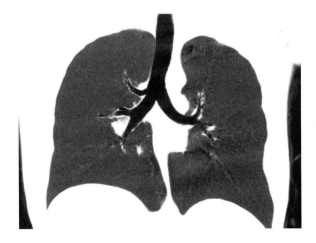

    A. Accessory right upper lobe bronchus
    B. Supernumerary right upper lobe bronchus
    C. Abnormal origin of the right upper lobe bronchus
    D. Abnormal segmental subdivision of the right upper lobe bronchus

2b What is the most specific term for the anatomic variant depicted?

    A. Tracheal bronchus

    B. Pig bronchus

    C. Cardiac bronchus

    D. Tracheal diverticulum

3a Inspiratory and dynamic expiratory CT images are provided. What is the diagnosis?

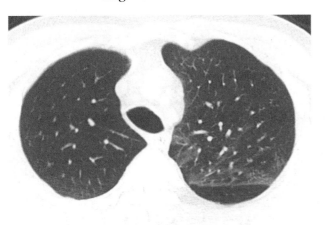 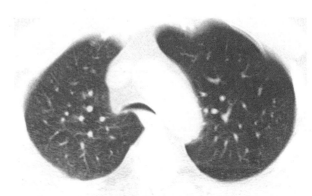

    A. Saber sheath trachea

    B. Tracheal diverticulum

    C. Tracheobronchitis

    D. Tracheomalacia

3b On inspiratory CT images, which is highly specific of tracheobronchomalacia?

    A. Saber-sheath trachea

    B. Lunate trachea

    C. Tracheal wall thickening

    D. Frown sign

4 The patient presents with shortness of breath. Based on the image below, which one of the following is the most likely diagnosis?

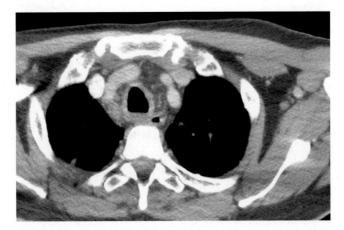

    A. Granulomatosis with polyangiitis

    B. Postintubation stenosis

    C. Tracheal neoplasm

    D. Tracheobronchopathia osteochondroplastica

5a   Based on the imaging findings below, what would be the most likely diagnosis?

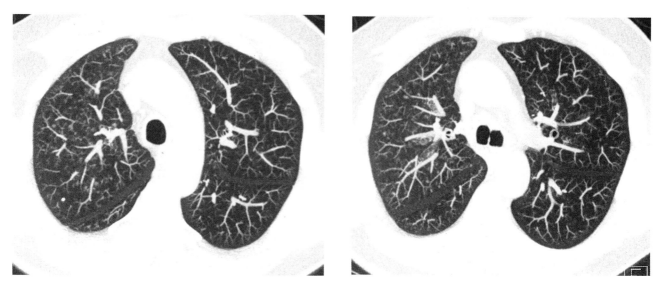

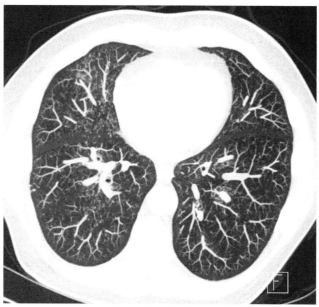

    A. Aspiration-related lung disease
    B. Lung contusions
    C. Endobronchial masses with postobstructive changes
    D. Cystic fibrosis

5b   Which of the following are not considered imaging findings on CT of aspiration-related lung disease?

    A. Airway thickening and airway opacification
    B. Tree-in-bud nodularity
    C. Centrilobular ground-glass opacities
    D. Randomly distributed lung nodules

6 What is the most likely diagnosis of the imaging findings below?

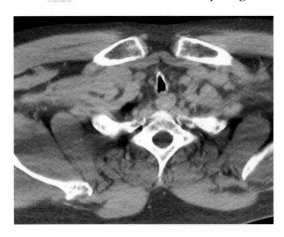 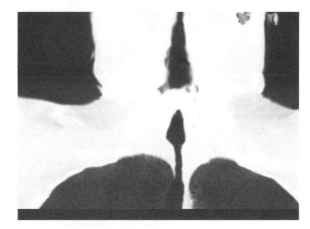

A. Postintubation tracheal stenosis secondary to prior tracheostomy
B. Granulomatosis with polyangiitis
C. Tracheobronchopathia osteochondroplastica
D. Squamous cell carcinoma

7a What imaging findings are present below?

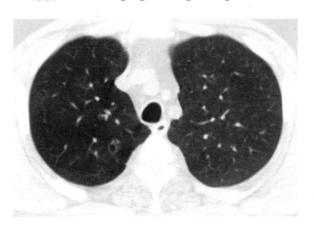 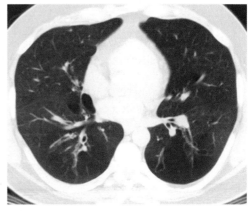

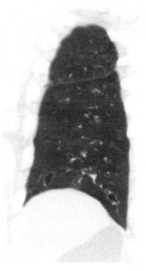 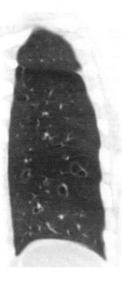

A. Bronchiectasis and mosaic attenuation pattern of the lungs
B. Lung cysts and mosaic attenuation pattern of the lungs
C. Bronchiectasis and tree-in-bud opacities
D. Lung cysts and nodules

7b Which one of the following is the most likely diagnosis?

    A. Cystic fibrosis

    B. Asthma

    C. Bronchiolitis obliterans

    D. Allergic bronchopulmonary aspergillosis

8a What imaging finding is present on this exam?

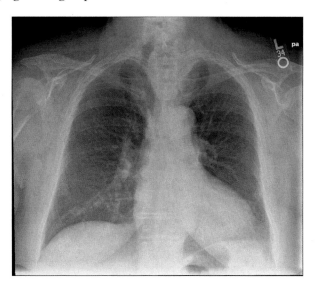

    A. Postintubation tracheal stenosis

    B. Bronchiectasis

    C. Tracheobronchomegaly

    D. Extrinsic compression of the trachea

8b Given the corresponding CT, what is the most likely diagnosis?

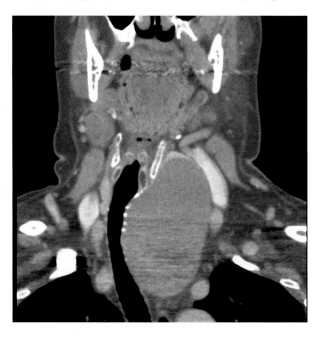

    A. Thyroid cyst/nodule

    B. Squamous cell carcinoma of the trachea

    C. Foregut duplication cyst

    D. Left common carotid artery aneurysm

9a What is the most common primary malignant neoplasm of the trachea?

   A. Squamous cell carcinoma
   B. Mucoepidermoid carcinoma
   C. Adenoid cystic carcinoma
   D. Carcinoid

9b What is the most common hematogenously spread metastatic lesion to involve the trachea?

   A. Thyroid cancer
   B. Esophageal cancer
   C. Lung cancer
   D. Melanoma

10a What is the likely diagnosis in this patient?

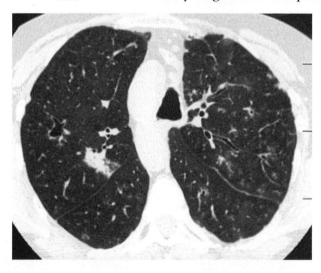 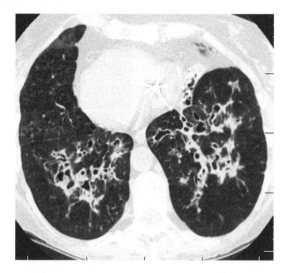

   A. Common variable immunodeficiency (CVID)
   B. Kartagener syndrome
   C. Sarcoid
   D. Diffuse panbronchiolitis

10b What percentage of patients with immotile cilia syndrome have situs inversus totalis?

   A. 10%
   B. 25%
   C. 50%
   D. 100%

11a In the setting of cystic fibrosis, what vessels are the typical source of hemoptysis?

   A. Pulmonary arteries
   B. Hypertrophied bronchial arteries
   C. Internal thoracic (mammary) arteries
   D. Intercostal arteries

11b What treatment is typically recommended for treatment of recurrent hemoptysis in the setting of bronchiectasis with hypertrophied bronchial arteries?

   A. Bronchial artery embolization
   B. Antimicrobial therapy
   C. Steroid therapy
   D. Surgical resection

12a Characterize the radiographic appearance:

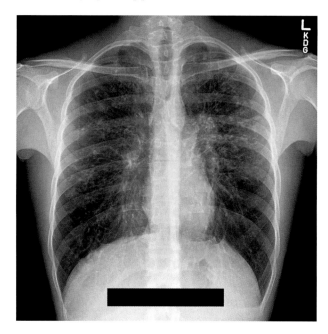

A. Airway pattern, lower lobe predominant
B. Nodular pattern, lower lobe predominant
C. Consolidation, upper lobe predominant
D. Airway pattern, upper lobe predominant

12b What is the most likely diagnosis on CT in this 27-year-old female (different patient)?

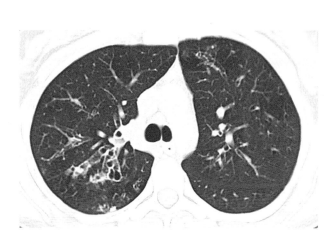 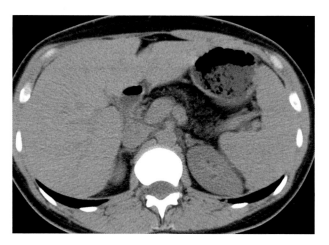

A. Allergic bronchopulmonary aspergillosis
B. Cystic fibrosis
C. Kartagener syndrome
D. Common variable immunodeficiency

13a Given this chest radiograph, what pattern of emphysema is most likely?

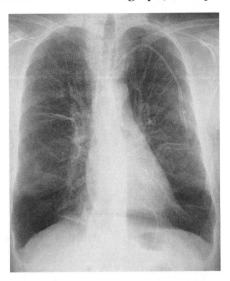 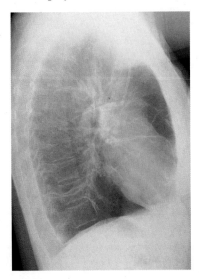

   A. Paraseptal
   B. Centrilobular
   C. Panlobular
   D. Cicatricial

13b Which of the following causes of emphysema is most likely?

   A. Alpha-1 antitrypsin deficiency
   B. Cigarette smoking
   C. HIV infection
   D. Marfan syndrome

13c Besides alpha-1 antitrypsin deficiency, which of the following is most associated with panlobular (panacinar) emphysema?

   A. Marfan syndrome
   B. Smoking
   C. IV methylphenidate abuse
   D. Malnutrition

14a Given the below CT images, what is the most likely diagnosis?

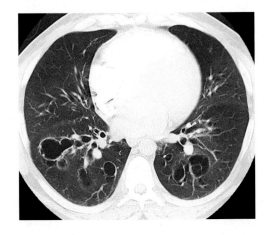 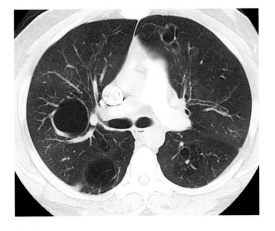

   A. Williams-Campbell
   B. Tracheobronchomegaly (Mounier-Kuhn)
   C. Ciliary dyskinesia
   D. Cystic fibrosis

14b In Williams-Campbell syndrome, what generations of bronchi are affected?

A. 1 to 2
B. 3 to 4
C. 4 to 6
D. 7-terminal

15a What is the most likely diagnosis?

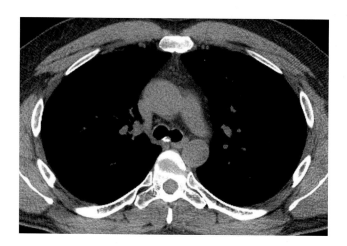
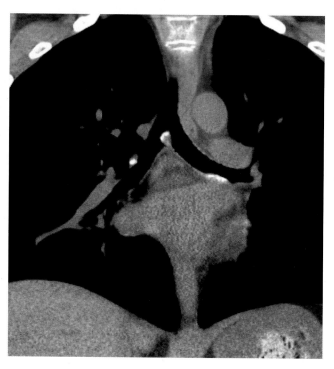

A. Tracheobronchopathia osteochondroplastica
B. Relapsing polychondritis
C. Tracheobronchial amyloidosis
D. Tracheobronchial granulomatosis with polyangiitis

15b What type of amyloid most commonly involves the tracheobronchial tree?

A. Amyloid transthyretin (ATTR)
B. Amyloid light chain (AL)
C. Amyloid A
D. A Lys

16 Given the below CT images, what is the most likely diagnosis?

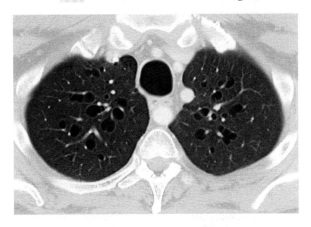 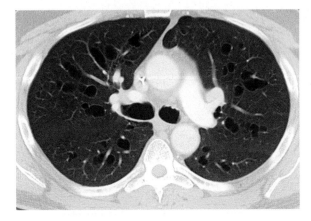

    A. Williams-Campbell
    B. Tracheobronchomegaly (Mounier-Kuhn)
    C. Ciliary dyskinesia
    D. Cystic fibrosis

17 What is the most likely diagnosis?

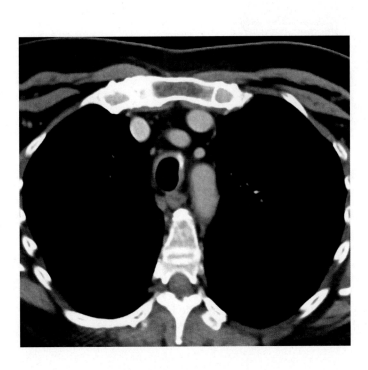 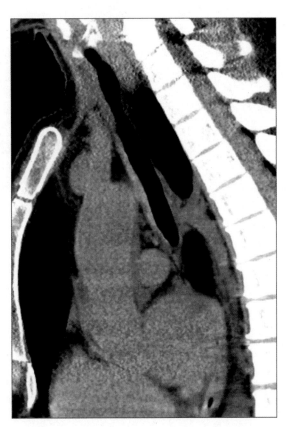

    A. Tracheal amyloidosis
    B. Relapsing polychondritis
    C. Granulomatosis with polyangiitis
    D. Tracheobronchopathia osteochondroplastica

18a Which of the following best describes the imaging findings below?

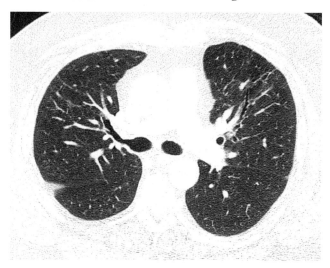
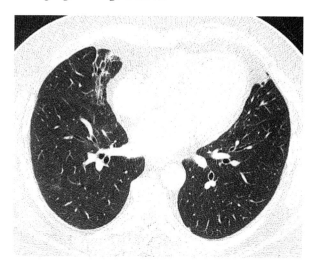

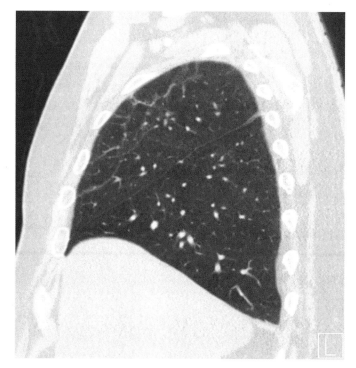

A. Linear scaring and bronchiectasis with anterior distribution
B. Linear scaring with ground-glass opacities and honeycombing in the lower lobes
C. Bronchiectasis with tree-in-bud nodularity in the right middle lobe and lingula
D. Bronchiectasis with upper lung zone distribution and mosaic attenuation pattern

18b What is the most likely diagnosis?

A. Recurrent aspiration
B. Allergic bronchopulmonary aspergillosis
C. Usual interstitial pneumonia (UIP)
D. Bronchiectasis from prior acute respiratory distress syndrome

ANSWERS AND EXPLANATIONS

1a **Answer A.**

1b **Answer D.**

1c **Answer B.**   Tree-in-bud nodularity represents dilated and impacted lobular bronchioles. On CT images, these appear as centrilobular branching structures that resemble a budding tree. Multiple causes have been described such as infectious (mycobacteria, fungal, viral, parasitic), congenital (cystic fibrosis, Kartagener syndrome), idiopathic (obliterative bronchiolitis, panbronchiolitis), aspiration, immunologic (allergic bronchopulmonary aspergillosis), connective tissue disorders, and neoplastic pulmonary embolic phenomenon.

The constellation of imaging findings (tree-in-bud nodularity, bronchiectasis with mucous plugging, and air trapping) predominantly in the right middle lobe and lingula are highly suggestive of MAI infection. This is frequently referred to as Lady Windermere syndrome, which reflects one of the demographic groups frequently affected by NTM infection. The other group is the "classic" form and occurs in older men with emphysema and COPD with an imaging appearance identical to that of postprimary tuberculosis.

Organism diagnosis by culture is important for these cases as it guides antibiotic therapy (which often lasts for years). Culture can be difficult even with appropriate steps, so the suggest of NTM infection by imaging can be important to alert the bronchoscopist prior to the procedure.

Reference: Martinez S, et al. The many faces of pulmonary nontuberculous mycobacterial infection. *AJR Am J Roentgenol* 2007;189(1):177–186.

2a **Answer C.**

2b **Answer B.**   Tracheobronchial anatomic variants can be divided into minor variants in lobar and segmental subdivisions (common) and major variants that include abnormal origin or supernumerary bronchus (rare). The major bronchial abnormalities include accessory cardiac bronchus (ACB) and tracheal bronchus. The ACB is a supernumerary bronchus that arises from the inner wall of the right mainstem bronchus or the intermediate bronchus opposite to the origin of the right upper lobe bronchus.

A tracheal bronchus is an anatomic variant characterized by an abnormal origin of a segmental or lobar bronchus arising within 2 cm of the carina and supplying a portion or the entire upper lobe. This term can also be used to describe an accessory bronchus that arises from the mainstem bronchus and serves the right upper lobe. When it serves the entire right upper lobe, as in this case, it is also known as "pig bronchus" or "bronchus suis." One in 400 normal persons has a tracheal bronchus.

Most of the time this anatomic variant is asymptomatic, however can become symptomatic in the setting of intubation, given the predisposition to develop atelectasis and/or pneumonia.

Reference: Ghaye B, et al. Congenital bronchial abnormalities revisited. *Radiographics* 2001;21(1):105–119.

3a   **Answer D.**

3b   **Answer B.**   Tracheomalacia or tracheobronchomalacia (TBM) is defined as diffuse or segmental tracheal weakness with luminal area narrowing of >70% as criteria on dynamic expiratory CT. Correlation of CT findings with pulmonary functional evidence of airway obstruction is important as the degree of normal can vary. TBM can be divided into primary (congenital) and secondary (acquired) depending on the etiology. Acquired conditions are more common and include severe emphysema in smokers, prolonged intubation, chronic tracheal infections, extrinsic compressions (such as aortic aneurysms), or chronic tracheal inflammation such as relapsing polychondritis. A lunate configuration of the trachea on inspiratory CT images is highly specific for tracheomalacia but low in sensitivity. Tracheomalacia "frown sign" describes the characteristic anterior bowing of the posterior membranous trachea on expiratory CT images resulting in a reversed U-shaped air column. Overlap exists by many authors between tracheomalacia and excessive dynamic airway collapse (EDAC). In EDAC, the posterior membrane is redundant and bulges anteriorly during expiration resulting in tracheal narrowing. Dynamic bronchoscopy remains the gold standard to diagnose tracheomalacia. End inspiratory and forced expiratory imaging of the trachea is needed to diagnose tracheomalacia or EDAC on CT. Quantification of the airway collapse is performed as follows: collapsibility index (CI): area at end inspiration (AEI) − dynamic expiratory area (DEA)/area at end inspiration (AEI) × 100. A CI between 70% to 80% is consistent with mild, 80% to 90% moderate, and >90% severe airway collapse.

References: Chung J, Kanne J, Gilman M. CT of diffuse tracheal diseases. *AJR Am J Roentgenol* 2011;196:w240–w246.

Ridge CA, O'Donnell CR, Lee, et al. Tracheobronchomalacia: current concepts and controversies. *J Thorac Imaging* 2011;26:278–289.

Zhang J, Hasegawa I, Feller-Kopman D, et al. 2003 AUR Memorial Award. Dynamic expiratory volumetric CT imaging of the central airways: comparison of standard-dose and low-dose techniques. *Acad Radiol* 2003;10(7):719–724.

4   **Answer A.**   Granulomatosis with polyangiitis (GPA) is a systemic granulomatous process with necrotizing vasculitis involving the lung, upper respiratory tract, and kidneys. This disease was formerly referred to as Wegener granulomatosis but has now been renamed. Characteristic imaging findings in the chest include pulmonary nodules and ground-glass opacities. Central cavitation occurs in up to 50% of nodules larger than 2 cm. Involvement of the trachea and bronchi is present in 16% to 23% of cases. Circumferential wall thickening is characteristic and helps differentiate from other common tracheal pathologic entities such as tracheobronchopathia osteochondroplastica and relapsing polychondritis, which characteristically spare the posterior membrane. Subglottic location is classic for GPA involvement of the trachea.

Reference: Chung J, Kanne J, Gilman M. CT of diffuse tracheal diseases. *AJR Am J Roentgenol* 2011;196:w240–w246.

5a   **Answer A.**

5b   **Answer D.**   This case depicts asymmetric tree-in-bud nodularity involving the right lung on MIP images in this patient with a history of aspiration and right side sleeping position. Note the metallic device in the esophagus with blooming artifact consistent with an esophageal probe. Aspiration-related lung disease is an underrecognized clinicopathologic entity that is estimated to account for at least 5% to 15% of community-acquired pneumonias. It is also considered the most common cause of death in patients with dysphagia due to neurologic insult. The most common imaging findings of acute aspiration-related lung disease include debris in the airway, lobar airway thickening, tree-in-bud nodularity, ground-glass centrilobular nodularity, and airspace disease. Chronic changes of aspiration-related lung disease include bronchiectasis, parenchymal granulomas, reticulation, and honeycombing.

Reference: Prather AD, et al. Aspiration related lung diseases. *J Thorac Imaging* 2014;29(5):304–309.

6 **Answer A.**   Postintubation tracheal stenosis is the most common cause of focal tracheal stenosis. It can present as a weblike stenosis (<1 cm), membranous concentric stenosis without damage of the cartilage, and the "A"-shaped stenosis, which happens secondary to lateral impacted fracture of the cartilage in patients with prior tracheostomy (as seen in this case). These are referred to as "pseudoglottic stenosis" during bronchoscopy due to their appearance. Critical tracheal narrowing is generally defined as <10 mm by imaging.

Long-segment tracheal wall thickening and/or narrowing may be secondary to saber-sheath trachea, relapsing polychondritis, or tracheobronchopathia osteochondroplastica. Less common causes include amyloidosis, granulomatosis with polyangiitis (Wegner granulomatosis), tumors, inflammatory bowel disease, or thermal injury. Saber-sheath trachea is characterized by a tracheal index <0.6 (transverse dimension of the trachea divided by the anteroposterior dimension). Note that some abnormalities such as relapsing polychondritis and tracheobronchopathia osteochondroplastica tend to spare the posterior membrane (which lacks cartilage), which can help limit the differential diagnosis.

Differential considerations for more short-segment narrowing in the trachea includes granulomatosis with polyangiitis, squamous papillomatosis, rhinoscleroma (Klebsiella rhinoscleromatis), cicatricial pemphigoid, sarcoidosis, and amyloidosis.

References: Chung J, Kanne J, Gilman M. CT of diffuse tracheal diseases. *AJR Am J Roentgenol* 2011;196:w240–w246.

Grenier PA, Beigelman-Aubry C, Brillet PY. Nonneoplastic tracheal and bronchial stenoses. *Radiol Clin North Am* 2009;47(2):243–260.

7a **Answer A.**

7b **Answer C.**   The images demonstrate lower lung predominant findings of cylindrical and varicoid bronchiectasis with significant mosaic attenuation that is likely related to small airway disease. Cysts would not connect with the bronchi as shown, and there is no significant nodularity. Of the diseases listed, asthma can present with significant small airway disease, especially in acute exacerbation, but air trapping predominates in asthma as opposed to mosaic attenuation as seen here. Additionally, the degree of bronchiectasis would be atypical in asthma alone. Both cystic fibrosis and ABPA would be expected to be upper lung predominant and generally exhibit more nodules and mucoid impaction. The mucoid impaction in ABPA can be characteristically high density, which is nearly pathognomonic. Atypical mycobacterial disease has a classic predilection for the right middle lobe and lingular (Lady Windermere syndrome) but can present with the distribution shown. However, there should be evidence of nodules (possibly cavitary or tree-in-bud) to suggest active disease that is not seen. Bronchiolitis obliterans (constrictive bronchiolitis) is the best choice given the images seen. Careful clinical history should be obtained to evaluate for potential causes such as prior infection, inhalational exposures, connective tissue disease (especially rheumatoid arthritis), or drug toxicity. Other causes of lower lung bronchiectasis include chronic/recurrent aspiration, immunodeficiency, and ciliary dyskinesia.

Reference: Hansell DM, Lynch DA, McAdams HP, et al. *Imaging of diseases of the chest*, 5th ed. Maryland Heights, MO: Mosby, 2009.

8a **Answer D.**

8b **Answer A.** The chest x-ray demonstrates severe deviation of the trachea to the right due to a superior mediastinal mass. Subsequent CT confirms the presence of a mass at the thoracic inlet and the extrinsic compression of the trachea. The mass itself is intermediate to low density, but well circumscribed, and despite its large size, does not seem to invade any adjacent structures as would be seen in carcinomas. The location is atypical for a foregut duplication cyst, and there is no contrast enhancement to suggest an aneurysm. However, there does appear to be a claw sign involving the thyroid (noted at the superior margin of the mass) consistent with thyroid etiology.

Reference: Hansell DM, Lynch DA, McAdams HP, et al. *Imaging of diseases of the chest,* 5th ed. Mosby, 2009.

9a **Answer A.**

9b **Answer D.** The most common primary malignant neoplasm of the trachea is squamous cell carcinoma, followed by adenoid cystic cell carcinoma and mucoepidermoid, respectively. The most common metastatic lesion to the trachea is secondary to local extension from thyroid cancer, esophageal cancer, and lung cancer. Hematogenous spread of tumor to the trachea is rare but can be seen in melanoma and breast cancer.

Reference: Hansell DM, Lynch DA, McAdams HP, et al. *Imaging of diseases of the chest,* 5th ed. Mosby, 2009.

10a **Answer B.**

10b **Answer C.** There is significant lower lung predominant bronchial wall thickening and varicoid bronchiectasis with areas of consolidation and tree-in-bud opacity. Considerations for only those findings would include immunodeficiency (such as CVID), ciliary dyskinesia, or diffuse panbronchiolitis. However, this patient also has situs inversus totalis (note the right aortic arch and dextrocardia). This combination is characteristic of Kartagener syndrome, a subtype of primary ciliary dyskinesia, which also features infertility and chronic sinus disease. Fifty percent of patients with immotile cilia syndrome will have situs inversus totalis as the determination of situs during embryologic development requires normal ciliary beating. Nonfunctioning cilia result in situ being determined randomly with half being normal and half inverted.

Other common associations for the other answer choices include splenomegaly with CVID and East Asian heritage with diffuse panbronchiolitis. Sarcoid can present with central bronchiectasis related to fibrosis, but the distribution is typically upper lobe predominant.

Reference: Hansell DM, Lynch DA, McAdams HP, et al. *Imaging of diseases of the chest,* 5th ed. Mosby, 2009.

11a **Answer B.**

11b **Answer A.** In the setting of bronchiectasis (including cystic fibrosis), hypertrophied bronchial arteries are formed with sometimes significant collateralization (>90% of cases). These hypertrophied arteries are prone to recurrent bleeding with sometimes catastrophic consequences. Bronchial artery anatomy is highly variable but typically arises from the descending thoracic aorta at the T5 or T6 level. The pulmonary arteries would be an atypical source of bleeding due to the lower pressure system unless a mycotic aneurysm has formed. The internal thoracic arteries and intercostal arteries form parenchymal collaterals much less frequently.

Surgical resection is a possible therapy, but bronchial artery particle embolization is preferred as a less invasive treatment. Although useful for controlling the underlying parenchymal disease, antimicrobial therapy and steroids do not play a primary role in treating the hemoptysis itself.

References: Bruzzi JF, Rémy-Jardin M, Delhaye D, et al. Multi-detector row CT of hemoptysis. *Radiographics* 2006;26(1):3–22.

Flume PA, Mogayzel PJ Jr, Robinson KA, et al. Cystic fibrosis pulmonary guidelines: pulmonary complications: hemoptysis and pneumothorax. *Am J Respir Crit Care Med* 2010;182(3):298–306.

Yoon W, Kim JK, Kim YH, et al. Bronchial and nonbronchial systemic artery embolization for life-threatening hemoptysis: a comprehensive review. *Radiographics* 2002;22(6):1395–1409.

12a **Answer D.**

12b **Answer B.** Chest radiograph demonstrates upper lobe predominant tram tracking, bronchiectasis, and nodularity consistent with an airway pattern. CT of the chest in another patient with the same disease process reveals airway disease with bronchiectasis, bronchial wall thickening, mucous plugging, and nodularity. Mediastinal kernel through the upper abdomen shows near-complete fatty replacement of the pancreas in this 27-year-old female. The constellation of findings are most consistent with cystic fibrosis. Allergic bronchopulmonary aspergillosis (ABPA) would be a consideration for the pulmonary findings alone but is not associated with pancreatic atrophy. Likewise, Kartagener syndrome and common variable immunodeficiency can cause bronchiectasis and airway disease, but airway disease generally has a lower lobe predominance. Also, these diseases have other characteristic-associated imaging findings.

Cystic fibrosis is increasingly seen in adults due to improvements in disease treatment and recognition of cases of adult-onset cystic fibrosis. It is the "most common life-limiting inherited disease" of Caucasians and results from a genetic mutation on chromosome 7 at the CF transmembrane conductance regulator (CFTR) causing impaired transport of chloride ions across membranes. This results in increased thickening of airway secretions leading to repetitive infections and inflammation followed by progressive bronchiectasis, further perpetuating the cycle. In the abdomen, cystic fibrosis often first manifests in intestinal dysfunction as meconium ileus. Adult manifestations of cystic fibrosis still include intestinal disease but also hepatobiliary, pancreatic, and less commonly renal disease. In the pancreas, proximal duct obstruction from inspissated secretions in cystic fibrosis causes fibrotic and fatty replacement of the pancreas as seen in this case.

References: Helbich TH, Heinz-Peer G, Eichler I, et al. Cystic fibrosis: CT assessment of lung involvement in children and adults. *Radiology* 1999;213:537–544.

Robertson MB, Choe KA, Joseph PM. Review of the abdominal manifestations of cystic fibrosis in the adult patient. *Radiographics* 2006;26:679–690.

13a **Answer C.**

13b **Answer A.**

13c **Answer C.** The pattern of emphysema in alpha-1 antitrypsin deficiency is that of panlobular (panacinar) emphysema, which is typically lower lung predominant (shown). The other forms of emphysema are associated with smoking (centrilobular and paraseptal) or a result of scarring and fibrosis (cicatricial). Interestingly, IV methylphenidate abuse is associated with the development of panlobular emphysema similar to that seen in antitrypsin deficiency. Other rare causes of panlobular emphysema include hypocomplementemic urticarial vasculitis syndrome or Ehlers-Danlos. HIV and Marfan are also rare causes of emphysema but tend to produce apical bullae as the emphysema pattern.

References: Hansell DM, Lynch DA, McAdams HP, et al. *Imaging of diseases of the chest,* 5th ed. Mosby, 2009.

Lee P, Gildea TR, Stoller JK. Emphysema in nonsmokers: alpha 1-antitrypsin deficiency and other causes. *Cleve Clin J Med* 2002;69(12):928–929.

Stern EJ, Frank MS, Schmutz JF, et al. Panlobular pulmonary emphysema caused by i.v. injection of methylphenidate (Ritalin): findings on chest radiographs and CT scans. *AJR Am J Roentgenol* 1994;162(3):555–560.

14a Answer A.

14b Answer C.   The CT demonstrates normal-appearing main bronchi but markedly dilated and bronchiectatic perihilar bronchi bilaterally (cystic bronchiectasis). The process is relatively diffuse involving both the upper lobes and the lower lobes and spars the periphery. There is a component of mosaic attenuation related to airway disease noted as well. These findings are most consistent with Williams-Campbell syndrome. This is a rare congenital cause of bronchiectasis due to abnormal cartilage in the fourth to sixth generations of bronchi. This limited bronchial involvement results in a characteristic appearance of central cystic bronchiectasis. The other choices demonstrate tracheal and main bronchi involvement. Additionally, cystic fibrosis is upper lung predominant, and ciliary dyskinesia demonstrates a lower lung predominance.

Reference: Hansell DM, Lynch DA, McAdams HP, et al. *Imaging of diseases of the chest,* 5th ed. Mosby, 2009.

15a Answer C.

15b Answer B.   Axial and coronal images of the chest demonstrate irregular nodular thickening of the trachea at the carina as well as in the bronchus intermedius and distal left mainstem bronchus. Tracheal amyloidosis is typically characterized by patchy irregular nodular tracheal and bronchial thickening with or without calcifications. No sparing of the posterior tracheal membrane is seen. Secondary narrowing of the airway can result in atelectasis.

Involvement of the airway by granulomatosis with polyangiitis (GPA) is typically characterized by a segment of asymmetric circumferential thickening. The subglottic area of the trachea is most commonly involved. Tracheobronchopathia osteochondroplastica is a benign entity in which there is development of calcified or noncalcified submucosal tracheal nodules sparing the posterior membrane of the trachea. Relapsing polychondritis is an autoimmune inflammatory process of the tracheal and bronchial cartilages, therefore spares the posterior tracheal membrane.

Tracheobronchial amyloidosis is rare. Amyloid light chain (AL) in the most common type of amyloid to deposit in the tracheobronchial tree. It is formed from monoclonal immunoglobulin light chain from plasma cell dyscrasia such as multiple myeloma.

References: Aylwin AC, Gishen P, Copley SJ. Imaging appearance of thoracic amyloidosis. *J Thoracic Imaging* 2005;20(1):41–46.

Chung JH, et al. CT of diffuse tracheal diseases. *AJR Am J Roentgenol* 2011;196(3):W240–W246.

Khoor A, Colby TV. Amyloidosis of the lung. *Arch Pathol Lab Med* 2017;141:247–254.

16 **Answer B.**   Although there is perihilar and central bronchiectasis, there is also dilation of the main bronchi and the trachea. The trachea here is almost as large as the vertebral body. Additionally, there are focal outpouchings and early diverticula formation along the main bronchi. These features are consistent with Mounier-Kuhn disease. The tracheal and main bronchi involvement help distinguish this case from what would otherwise be very similar to Williams-Campbell. Tracheobronchomegaly is most frequently found in 20- to 40-year-old men, and patients frequently have a history of recurrent respiratory infections and chronic cough. The defect is related to a deficiency of smooth muscle and elastic fibers and has an association with other disorders such as Marfan, Ehlers-Danlos, and cutis laxa. A tracheal diameter on frontal radiograph exceeding 25 mm (transverse diameter) should suggest the diagnosis in men, 21 mm in women. Add 2 mm each for the lateral projections (AP diameter). The diameter used on CT is 3 cm, measured 2 cm above the aortic arch. Tracheomalacia is frequently seen in conjunction.

Reference: Webb WR, Higgins CB. *Thoracic imaging*. Philadelphia, PA: Lippincott Williams & Wilkins, 2010.

17 **Answer B.**   Relapsing polychondritis is an autoimmune inflammatory process involving the laryngotracheobronchial cartilage. Disease also involves the nasal and ear cartilages. On imaging, there is thickening and increased attenuation of the cartilaginous tracheal and bronchial walls. This results in sparing of the posterior tracheal membrane.

18a **Answer A.**

18b **Answer D.**   Axial CT chest images demonstrate linear scaring and bronchiectasis with anterior distribution.

Bronchiectasis associated with scaring and fibrosis in an anterior distribution can be seen in the setting of chronic infectious airway disease, such as in atypical mycobacterial infection, and in the setting of healed acute respiratory distress syndrome (ARDS). The mechanism responsible for the parenchymal scaring and bronchiectasis includes both injury to the lung parenchyma by the initial lung insult and barotrauma from prolonged mechanical ventilation that commonly happens in these patients. The dependent portions of the lungs are protected by gravitational consolidation resulting in changes localized in the anterior portions of the lungs.

Reference: Milliron B, et al. Bronchiectasis: mechanisms and imaging clues of associated common and uncommon diseases. *Radiographics* 2015;35(4):1011–1030.

9

Thoracic Manifestations of Systemic Disease

David A. Lynch, MD

QUESTIONS

1a What is the most likely diagnosis given the constellation of findings?

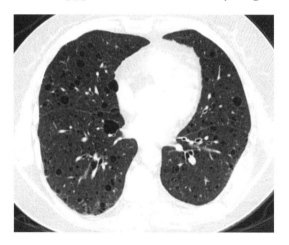 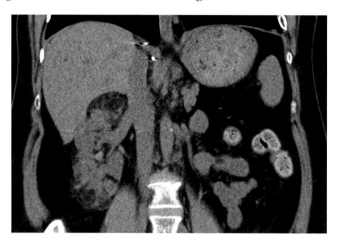

    A. Cystic lymphocytic interstitial pneumonia
    B. Pulmonary Langerhans cell histiocytosis
    C. Tuberous sclerosis
    D. Neurofibromatosis

1b Of the major criteria for tuberous sclerosis, which would be the least common?

    A. Subependymal giant cell tumors
    B. Lymphangioleiomyomatosis
    C. Renal angiomyolipomas
    D. Cardiac rhabdomyomas

2 What is the most common pulmonary manifestation of dermatomyositis–polymyositis interstitial lung disease?

    A. Usual interstitial pneumonia
    B. Nonspecific interstitial pneumonia
    C. Granulomatous lymphocytic interstitial lung disease
    D. Lymphoid interstitial pneumonia

3a What best explains the pulmonary opacities in this patient with chronic renal failure?

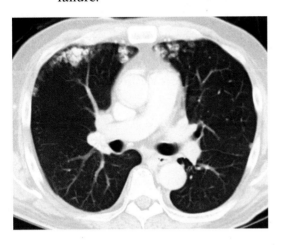 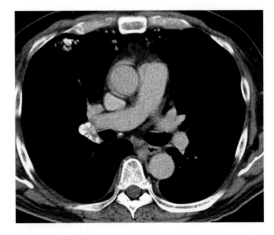

    A. Pulmonary edema
    B. Calcified metastases
    C. Pulmonary fibrosis
    D. Metastatic calcification

3b What percentage of patients who have undergone hemodialysis will have metastatic pulmonary calcification on autopsy?

    A. 10% to 25%
    B. 40% to 55%
    C. 60% to 75%
    D. 95% to 100%

3c Metastatic pulmonary calcification may accelerate in which clinical setting?

    A. Failed renal transplantation
    B. Starting dialysis
    C. Parathyroidectomy
    D. New renal transplantation

4a What is the salient finding on mediastinal windows in this patient with chronic cough?

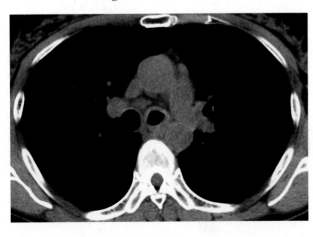 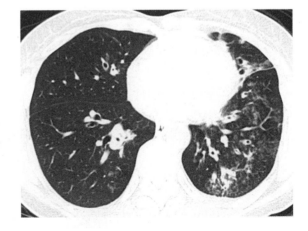

    A. Lymphadenopathy
    B. Enlarged main pulmonary artery
    C. Dilated ascending aorta
    D. Bronchial wall thickening

4b   What systemic conditions could cause the combination of findings in this case?

    A. Rheumatoid arthritis
    B. Ulcerative colitis
    C. Sarcoidosis
    D. Common variable immune deficiency

5   What chest CT finding suggests hepatopulmonary syndrome in the setting of cirrhosis?

    A. Main pulmonary artery enlargement
    B. Pulmonary fibrosis
    C. Interstitial thickening and ground-glass opacities
    D. Dilated peripheral pulmonary vessels

6a   The pulmonary pattern on radiograph is best be described as:

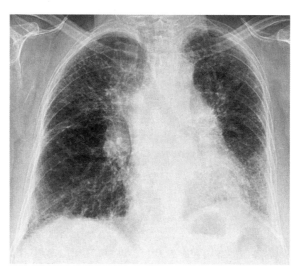

    A. Reticular
    B. Nodules
    C. Consolidation
    D. Bronchiectasis

6b   The pulmonary CT pattern in this patient with rheumatoid arthritis is consistent with:

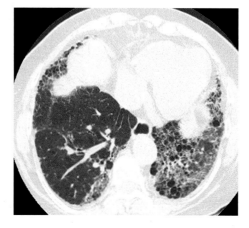

    A. Nonspecific interstitial pneumonia
    B. Usual interstitial pneumonia
    C. Bronchiolitis
    D. Organizing pneumonia

6c What is the most common CT pattern found in patients with rheumatoid arthritis?

    A. Nonspecific interstitial pneumonia
    B. Usual interstitial pneumonia
    C. Bronchiolitis
    D. Organizing pneumonia

7a The pulmonary pattern is

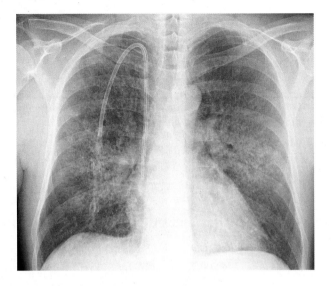

    A. Reticular
    B. Consolidation
    C. Cystic
    D. Nodular

7b Which cause of consolidation would support Goodpasture syndrome?

    A. Pulmonary edema
    B. Aspiration
    C. Alveolar proteinosis
    D. Pulmonary hemorrhage

8a What is the diagnosis?

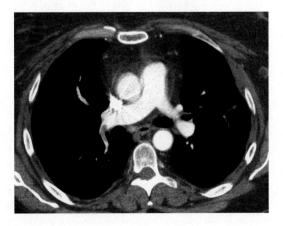

    A. Pulmonary artery hypertension
    B. Pulmonary embolism
    C. Pulmonary edema
    D. Pulmonary hemorrhage

8b Which of the following autoimmune disorders has the highest risk of pulmonary embolism?

A. Sjögren syndrome
B. Systemic lupus erythematosus
C. Systemic sclerosis
D. Wegener granulomatosis

8c Which of the following is the most common thoracic complication of systemic lupus erythematosus?

A. Pulmonary parenchymal disease
B. Pulmonary artery hypertension
C. Pleural effusion
D. Lymphoma

9a What is the most common clinical circumstance associated with death in adult patients with sickle cell anemia?

A. Cerebral vascular accident
B. Myocardial infarction
C. Aortic dissection
D. Acute chest syndrome

9b What medical imaging finding on this CT is required to diagnose acute chest syndrome?

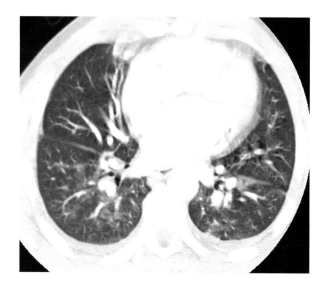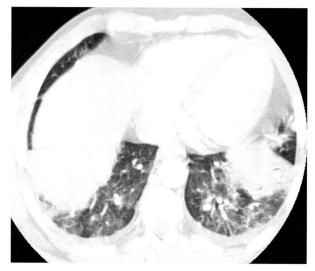

A. New parenchymal opacity
B. Pleural effusion
C. Pulmonary embolism
D. Cardiomegaly

10a Which systemic disease best correlates with the CT findings?

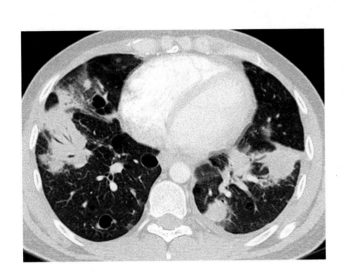
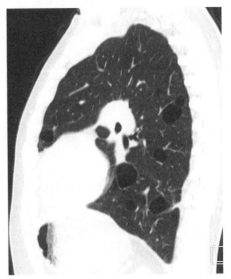

   A. Diabetes mellitus
   B. Granulomatosis with polyangiitis
   C. Hepatopulmonary syndrome
   D. Sjögren syndrome

10b Chronic consolidation in the setting of Sjögren syndrome raises concern for which complication?

   A. Lymphoma
   B. Sarcoidosis
   C. Alveolar proteinosis
   D. Lipoid pneumonia

11a What finding on the chest radiograph suggests granulomatosis with polyangiitis?

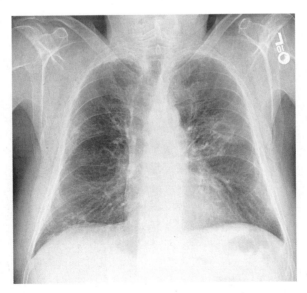

   A. Right apical cap
   B. Pulmonary cavitation
   C. Atherosclerotic aorta
   D. Deviated trachea

11b Cavitation of pulmonary nodules occurs in what percentage of granulomatosis with polyangiitis cases?

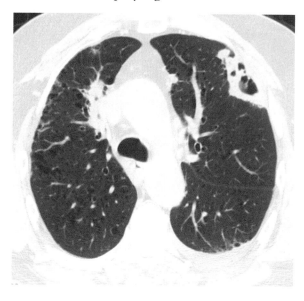 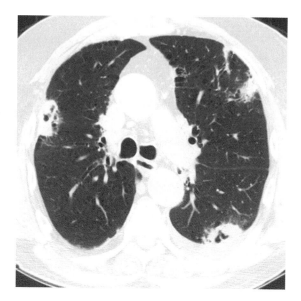

A. 5%
B. 25%
C. 50%
D. 85%

11c What system is the most likely to be involved in granulomatosis with polyangiitis?
A. Upper respiratory tract
B. Lungs
C. Kidneys
D. Liver

12 What is the most likely diagnosis associated with this patient's chronic low lung volumes?

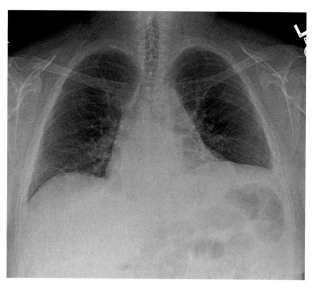 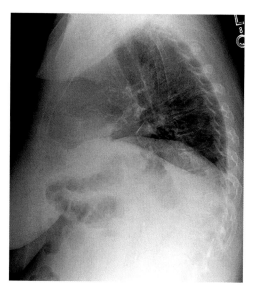

A. Sjögren syndrome
B. Systemic sclerosis
C. Systemic lupus erythematosus
D. Granulomatosis with polyangiitis

13a What CT pattern is present in this patient?

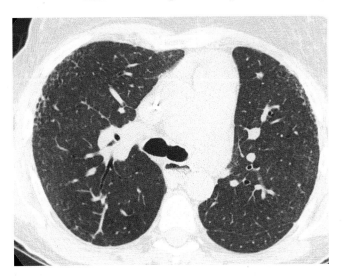
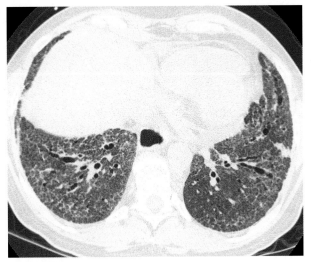
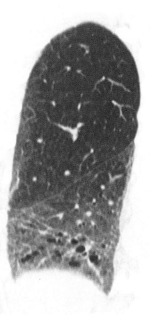
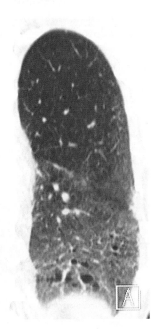

A. Nonspecific interstitial pneumonia
B. Usual interstitial pneumonia
C. Bronchiolitis
D. Organizing pneumonia

13b Which of the following diseases is most likely to be associated with this pattern?

A. Systemic lupus erythematosus
B. Rheumatoid arthritis
C. Sjögren syndrome
D. Systemic sclerosis

14a These inspiratory and expiratory CT images are consistent with which disease?

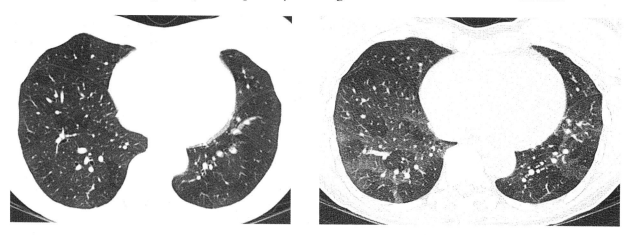

A. Emphysema
B. Nonspecific interstitial pneumonia
C. Obliterative bronchiolitis
D. Organizing pneumonia

14b Obliterative bronchiolitis is most commonly associated with which collagen vascular disease?

A. Rheumatoid arthritis
B. Systemic lupus erythematosus
C. Scleroderma
D. Mixed connective tissue disease

15 Which collagen vascular disease is most likely to cause the CT finding?

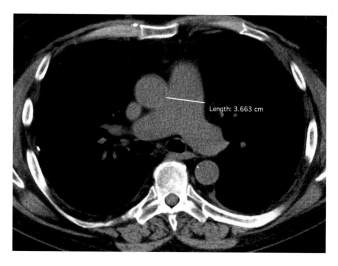

A. Sjögren syndrome
B. Systemic sclerosis
C. Polymyositis–dermatomyositis
D. Systemic lupus erythematosus

16 What systemic disease can cause this combination of CT features?

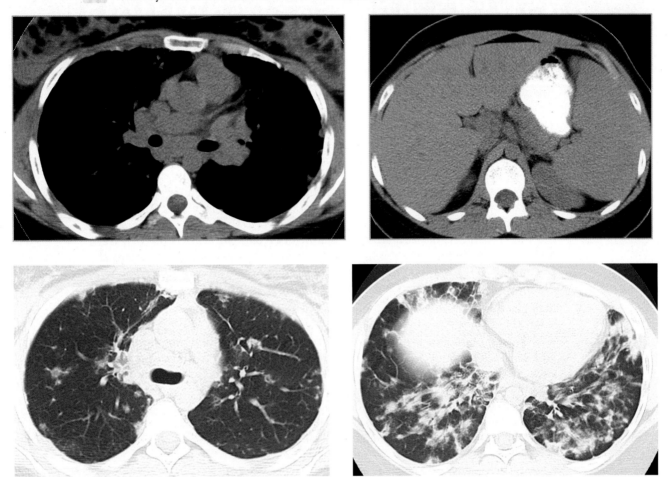

A. Rheumatoid arthritis

B. Sarcoidosis

C. Common variable immunodeficiency

D. Sickle cell disease

ANSWERS AND EXPLANATIONS

1a   Answer C.

1b   Answer A.   Several systemic diseases may develop cystic lung disease, to include but not limited to tuberous sclerosis, neurofibromatosis, Sjögren syndrome, amyloidosis, and Langerhans cell histiocytosis. Of these, tuberous sclerosis will cause a diffuse random distribution of lung cysts, fat-containing renal lesions (AMLs), and cerebral cortical tubers as seen in this patient. Neurofibromatosis, while also a neurocutaneous disorder and able to cause scattered cysts, causes neurofibromas often seen on chest imaging as intercostal nodular soft tissue cords or as cutaneous nodules. Pulmonary Langerhans cell histiocytosis is most commonly a disease localized to the lung in smokers, but the systemic form of Langerhans cell histiocytosis can cause lung disease and lytic bone lesions in a younger population. Lastly, lymphocytic interstitial pneumonia (LIP) is a lymphoproliferative disorder that can result in cystic lung disease, most commonly in the setting of Sjögren syndrome.

Major and minor criteria have been established for the diagnosis of tuberous sclerosis given the highly variable manifestations of the disease both within and between families. Lymphangioleiomyomatosis, renal angiomyolipomas, and cardiac rhabdomyomas are all common major criteria, while only the subependymal giant cell tumors are uncommon although classic manifestations of tuberous sclerosis.

References: Adriaensen ME, et al. Radiological evidence of lymphangioleiomyomatosis in female and male patients with tuberous sclerosis complex. *Clin Radiol* 2011;66:625–628.

Umeoka S, et al. Pictorial review of tuberous sclerosis in various organs. *Radiographics* 2008;28(7):e32.

2   Answer B.   In a study of 973 patients diagnosed with polymyositis–dermatomyositis, 58 demonstrated associated lung disease, and of those, 18 out of 22 patients with lung biopsies were diagnosed with nonspecific interstitial pneumonia (NSIP). Other less common pulmonary manifestations included usual interstitial pneumonia, diffuse alveolar damage, and organizing pneumonia. More recent medical literature will include antisynthetase syndrome with PM-DM as myositis syndromes that cause interstitial lung disease. Also, more recent experience suggests that a combined NSIP–OP pattern is the most common pulmonary manifestation of the myositis syndromes.

Reference: Douglas WW, et al. Polymyositis-dermatomyositis-associated interstitial lung disease. *Am J Respir Crit Care Med* 2001;164:1182–1185.

3a   Answer D.

3b   Answer C.

3c   Answer A.   The CT images provided demonstrate focal nodular opacities that are partially calcified and centered on the secondary pulmonary lobule. Of the options provided, metastatic pulmonary calcification would be the most likely cause in this patient with chronic renal failure. Pulmonary edema would not account for the focal nature, nodularity, or calcification of the opacities. Similarly, pulmonary fibrosis would not cause these findings, but generally result in architectural distortion with reticular opacities. Finally, calcified pulmonary metastases in the setting of osteosarcoma or adenocarcinoma can cause calcified nodules, but the focal cluster and uniform centering on the pulmonary lobule would be very atypical.

While not 95% to 100%, metastatic pulmonary calcification is seen at autopsy in the majority of patients who have required hemodialysis (60% to 75%). The remaining options incorrectly indicate that metastatic pulmonary calcification occurs in the minority of this patient population.

Starting dialysis, parathyroidectomy, and new renal transplantation have all been associated with CT imaging improvement in metastatic pulmonary calcification. Of these choices, only failed renal transplantation correlates with described cases of accelerated metastatic pulmonary calcification.

Reference: Belem LC, et al. Metastatic pulmonary calcification: state-of-the-art review focused on imaging findings. *Respir Med* 2014;108:668–676.

4a **Answer D.** The mediastinal windows show marked concentric thickening of the wall of the left main bronchus, compared with the normal right main bronchus.

4b **Answer B.** The lung windows show marked airway wall thickening and bilateral cylindric bronchiectasis. Mucoid impaction and patchy tree in bud pattern are best seen in the left lower lobe. While there is a lengthy list of causes of lower lung bronchiectasis and tree in bud pattern, the associated thickening of the walls of major bronchi is distinctly unusual. Sarcoidosis or granulomatous polyangiitis could be considered in the differential diagnosis, but neither of these conditions typically results in bronchiectasis or tree in bud pattern. A small percentage of patients with ulcerative colitis develop severe inflammation of the central bronchial tree and/or bronchiectasis. On bronchoscopic visualization, the central airways are often dramatically inflamed, and on CT concentric narrowing of the trachea, right or left main bronchi, or lobar and segmental bronchi may be seen. Bronchiectasis is typically cylindric, and tree in bud pattern reflects a pattern of cellular bronchiolitis or panbronchiolitis. Each of these patterns (large airway thickening/stenosis, bronchiectasis, and small airway features) may occur together or independently of each other.

References: Garg K, et al. Inflammatory airways disease in ulcerative colitis: CT and high-resolution CT features. *J Thorac Imaging* 1993;8(2):159–163.

Wilcox P, et al. Airway involvement in ulcerative colitis. *Chest* 1987;92(1):18–22.

5 **Answer D.** The dilated peripheral vessels seen in hepatopulmonary syndrome directly demonstrate intrapulmonary arteriovenous shunting. Together with an increased A-a gradient and cirrhosis, intrapulmonary shunting defines hepatopulmonary syndrome. Shunting can be confirmed by contrast echocardiography, pulmonary perfusion scintigraphy, or pulmonary angiography.

Main pulmonary artery enlargement suggests pulmonary artery hypertension, which can occur in the setting of chronic liver disease, but is not a defining component of hepatopulmonary syndrome. Likewise, pulmonary fibrosis and mixed pulmonary interstitial and ground-glass opacities are not findings of hepatopulmonary syndrome.

Reference: McAdams HP, et al. The hepatopulmonary syndrome: radiologic findings in 10 patients. *AJR Am J Roentgenol* 1996;166:1379–1385.

6a **Answer A.**

6b **Answer B.**

6c **Answer B.** The chest radiographs provided demonstrate reticular basilar opacities typical of fibrosing interstitial pneumonias and characterized by the fine netlike radiopaque lines over the lower lung fields. The corresponding CT through the lung bases reveals peripheral-predominant, basal-predominant reticular abnormality with honeycombing, a finding that defines the CT pattern of usual interstitial pneumonia and differentiates it from nonspecific interstitial pneumonia, bronchiolitis, and organizing pneumonia.

When studying 63 patients with rheumatoid arthritis–related lung disease, Tanaka et al. found that the most common pulmonary CT findings are ground-glass opacities and reticulation and the most common pattern was usual interstitial pneumonia.

Reference: Tanaka N, et al. Rheumatoid arthritis-related lung diseases: CT findings. *Radiology* 2004;232:81–91.

7a **Answer B.**

7b **Answer D.** Obscuration of the pulmonary vascular marking by hazy poorly defined opacities with associated air bronchograms is consistent with consolidation. Some component of interstitial thickening may be present in this patient with pulmonary hemorrhage, but the other choices of reticular, cystic, or nodular are not the predominant pattern. Additionally, diffuse pulmonary hemorrhage generally spares the lung apices.

With the placement of a dialysis catheter, the radiograph raises concern for a renopulmonary disease. Any one of the options provided can cause consolidation on chest radiograph. Only pulmonary hemorrhage, as demonstrated by hemoptysis or present on bronchoscopy, specifically favors Goodpasture syndrome. Caused by anti–glomerular basement membrane antibodies, Goodpasture syndrome classically results in glomerulonephritis and diffuse pulmonary hemorrhage (DPH). Once diffuse pulmonary hemorrhage has been identified, the differential etiologies are commonly categorized as (1) Goodpasture syndrome/anti–glomerular basement membrane disease, (2) other immunologically mediated diseases such as systemic lupus erythematosus or granulomatosis with polyangiitis, (3) non–immunologically mediated causes such as medications or idiopathic pulmonary hemosiderosis, or (4) immunocompromised conditions with infection such as leukemia, HIV, or transplant.

Reference: Primack SL, Miller RR, Muller NL. Diffuse pulmonary hemorrhage: clinical, pathologic and imaging features. *AJR Am J Roentgenol* 1995;164:295–300.

8a **Answer B.**

8b **Answer B.**

8c **Answer C.** The CT image provided demonstrates a focal pulmonary artery filling defect consistent with pulmonary embolism in a patient also diagnosed with systemic lupus erythematosus (SLE). Approximately one-third of patients with SLE also have antiphospholipid antibody syndrome, placing them at significant risk for recurrent pulmonary embolism and venoocclusive disease, but even SLE patients without antiphospholipid antibody syndrome are at increased risk of pulmonary embolism. In a study of over 500,000 patients hospitalized with autoimmune disorder in Sweden over 44 years, subjects with autoimmune disease had an overall relative risk of 6.38 for subsequent pulmonary embolism within 1 year relative to those without autoimmune disease. The autoimmune conditions with highest risk for pulmonary embolism in this study were polymyositis–dermatomyositis (relative risk 16.44), polyarteritis nodosa (relative risk 13.26), immune thrombocytopenic purpura (relative risk 10.79), and systemic lupus erythematosus (relative risk 10.23). Still, the most common thoracic manifestation of SLE is pleural effusion, followed by pulmonary parenchymal disease, diaphragmatic dysfunction, and pulmonary arterial hypertension.

References: Lalani TA, et al. Imaging findings in systemic lupus erythematosus. *Radiographics* 2004;24:1069–1086.

Zoller B, et al. Risk of pulmonary embolism in patients with autoimmune disorders: a nationwide follow-up study from Sweden. *Lancet* 2012;379:244–249.

9a **Answer D.**

9b **Answer A.** Acute chest syndrome is the most common "circumstance" associated with death in adults with sickle cell anemia in a study of 209 patients older than 20 years who died after study enrollment, followed by stroke, infection, and perioperative complications. Chronic organ failure was a common additional associated condition, but rarely found in the study as the primary cause of death.

By definition, acute chest syndrome patients must exhibit fever or chest pain, pulmonary symptoms such as wheezing, and pulmonary opacities on chest imaging in the setting of sickle cell anemia. Often seen following vasoocclusive crisis, acute chest syndrome may be complicated by infection, fluid overload, splinting from chest wall bone pain, and fat emboli. Recommended treatments for acute chest syndrome include antibiotics, supplemental oxygen, monitoring for bronchospasm, and potential transfusions for anemia.

References: Minter KR, Gladwin MT. Pulmonary complications of sickle cell anemia: a need for increased recognition, treatment and research. *Am J Respir Crit Care Med* 2001;164:2016–2019.

Platt OS, et al. Mortality in sickle cell disease: life expectancy and risk factors for early death. *N Engl J Med* 1994;330(23):1639–1644.

Yawn BP, et al. Management of sickle cell disease: summary of the 2014 evidence-based report by Expert Panel Members. *JAMA* 2014;312(10):1033–1048.

10a **Answer D.**

10b **Answer A.** Lower lung–predominant, perilymphatic cysts are seen in approximately 70% of patients with lymphocytic interstitial pneumonia. Other common CT findings are bilateral ground-glass and centrilobular opacities. Lymphocytic interstitial pneumonia results from bronchus-associated lymphoid tissue (BALT) hyperplasia and is most commonly seen in Sjögren syndrome and other autoimmune diseases. Other diseases associated with LIP can be categorized as immunodeficiencies such as HIV and miscellaneous/idiopathic.

The differential diagnosis for chronic consolidations on chest CT includes chronic infection, sarcoidosis, and lipoid pneumonia, but in the setting of Sjögren syndrome (SS)–associated lung disease, lymphoma becomes a primary concern. Patients with Sjögren syndrome have 44 times the incidence of lymphoma compared to the equivalent general population. The most common subtype of lymphoma in Sjögren syndrome is MALT lymphoma, an extranodal marginal zone B-cell (non-Hodgkin) lymphoma.

References: Egashira R, et al. CT findings of thoracic manifestations of primary Sjögren syndrome: radiologic-pathologic correlation. *Radiographics* 2013;33:1933–1949.

Johkoh T, et al. Lymphocytic interstitial pneumonia: thin-section CT findings in 22 patients. *Radiology* 1999;212:567–572.

Swigris JJ, et al. Lymphoid interstitial pneumonia: a narrative review. *Chest* 2002;122:2150–2164.

Tonami H, et al. Clinical and imaging findings of lymphoma in patients with Sjögren syndrome. *J Comput Assist Tomogr* 2003;27(4):517–524.

11a **Answer B.**

11b **Answer C.**

11c Answer A.   Each finding is present on the provided chest radiograph, but of the provided choices, only pulmonary cavitation suggests granulomatosis with polyangiitis (GPA), formerly known as Wegener granulomatosis. A granulomatous vasculitis, GPA most commonly presents in the lungs as pulmonary nodules or masses. Pulmonary cavitation is seen in 50% of patient with granulomatosis with polyangiitis. Other manifestations on chest CT of GPA include halo nodules, reverse halo nodules, pulmonary hemorrhage with consolidation and ground-glass opacities, and tracheobronchial thickening. The lungs and kidneys are involved in the majority of cases, but the upper respiratory tract is the most common.

References: Comarmond C, Cacoub P. Granulomatosis with polyangiitis (Wegener): clinical aspects and treatment. *Autoimmun Rev* 2014;13(11):1121–1125.

Martinez F, et al. Common and uncommon manifestations of Wegener granulomatosis at chest CT: radiologic-pathologic correlation. *Radiographics* 2012;32:51–69.

12 Answer C.   Shrinking lungs syndrome occurs in the setting of systemic lupus erythematosus with progressive weakening in the diaphragms and/or restricted chest wall expansion. In this patient, no significant reticular opacity is present to suggest volume loss associated with fibrosing interstitial pneumonia as can be seen with systemic sclerosis/scleroderma. Sjögren syndrome classically causes lymphocytic interstitial pneumonia (LIP), and only isolated cases of combined SLE and Sjögren syndrome have been associated with shrinking lungs syndrome. Granulomatosis with polyangiitis generally causes pulmonary hemorrhage or cavitating pulmonary lesions without known association with shrinking lungs syndrome.

Reference: Warrington KJ, Moder KG, Brutinel WM. The shrinking lungs syndrome in systemic lupus erythematosus. *Mayo Clin Proc* 2000;75:467–472.

13a Answer A.   The CT images show lower lung–predominant fine reticular abnormality with marked traction bronchiectasis. Moderate ground-glass abnormality is present, but the prominent associated traction bronchiectasis suggests that this is predominantly related to fine fibrosis rather than inflammatory abnormality. The relative sparing of the subpleural lung, and extension of fibrosis along the bronchovascular bundle are characteristic of NSIP.

13b Answer D.   NSIP is the most common pattern of fibrosis in systemic sclerosis, being found in about 65% to 75% of patients on biopsy, and the CT features of this condition generally reflect an NSIP pattern. Lung fibrosis is relatively uncommon in SLE. Sjögren syndrome is generally associated with an LIP pattern, and rheumatoid arthritis is most commonly associated with UIP.

References: Desai SR, Veeraraghavan S, Hansell DM, et al. CT features of lung disease in patients with systemic sclerosis: comparison with idiopathic pulmonary fibrosis and nonspecific interstitial pneumonia. *Radiology* 2004;232(2):560–567.

Fujita J, Yoshinouchi T, Ohtsuki Y, et al. Non-specific interstitial pneumonia as pulmonary involvement of systemic sclerosis. *Ann Rheum Dis* 2001;60(3):281–283.

Ozkaya S, Bilgin S, Hamsici S, et al. The pulmonary radiologic findings of rheumatoid arthritis. *Resp Med* 2011;4:187–192.

Schreiber J, Koschel D, Kekow J, et al. Rheumatoid pneumoconiosis (Caplan's syndrome). *Eur J Intern Med* 2010;21:168–172.

Tanaka N, Kim JS, Newell JD, et al. Rheumatoid arthritis-related lung diseases: CT findings. *Radiology* 2004;232(81):91.

Travis WD, Hunninghake G, King TE Jr, et al. Idiopathic nonspecific interstitial pneumonia: report of an American Thoracic Society project. *Am J Respir Crit Care Med* 2008;177(12):1338–1347.

14a Answer C.

14b **Answer A.** Obliterative bronchiolitis, also known as bronchiolitis obliterans and constrictive bronchiolitis, most commonly demonstrates mosaic attenuation on inspiratory CT images and air trapping on expiratory CT images, as seen in the case provided. In a series comparing obliterative bronchiolitis and severe asthma, mosaic attenuation in obliterative bronchiolitis proved to be the best differentiator between the two.

Airway disease can occur in multiple autoimmune diseases, but obliterative bronchiolitis is most characteristic of rheumatoid arthritis. Systemic lupus erythematosus is an alternative, but less common, cause in the setting of collagen vascular disease.

References: Jensen SP, et al. High-resolution CT features of severe asthma and bronchiolitis obliterans. *Clin Radiol* 2002;57:1078–1085.

Lynch DA. Lung disease related to collagen vascular disease. *J Thorac Imaging* 2009;24: 299–309.

15 **Answer B.** The normal diameter of the main pulmonary artery is approximately 25 mm. The 90th percentile cutoff value is 29 mm in men and 27 mm in women. A measurement of 37 mm, as found in this case, is highly likely to be associated with pulmonary arterial hypertension. A recent meta-analysis showed that pulmonary arterial hypertension was found in about 13% of subjects with systemic sclerosis, compared with 3% of patients with lupus. The prevalence of pulmonary hypertension in subjects with Sjögren syndrome and polymyositis–dermatomyositis is low. In patients with systemic sclerosis, the NSIP pattern of lung fibrosis is found in 78% of surgical lung biopsies, substantially more common than other pathologies including UIP.

References: Bouros D, Wells AU, Nicholson AG, et al. Histopathologic subsets of fibrosing alveolitis in patients with systemic sclerosis and their relationship to outcome. *Am J Respir Crit Care Med* 2002;165(12):1581–1586.

Truong QA, Massaro JM, Rogers IS, et al. Reference values for normal pulmonary artery dimensions by noncontrast cardiac computed tomography: the Framingham Heart Study. *Circ Cardiovasc Imaging* 2012;5(1):147–154.

Yang X, Mardekian J, Sanders KN, et al. Prevalence of pulmonary arterial hypertension in patients with connective tissue diseases: a systematic review of the literature. *Clin Rheumatol* 2013;32(10):1519–1531.

16 **Answer C.** The CT findings here are subcarinal lymph node enlargement, splenomegaly, perilymphatic nodules in the upper lungs, and peribronchovascular consolidative abnormality in the lower lungs. This is an unusual combination of findings, but is characteristic of granulomatous lymphocytic interstitial lung disease (GLILD), a condition found in common variable immunodeficiency. Sarcoidosis might be considered in the differential diagnosis, but the lower lobe consolidative abnormality and marked splenomegaly would be unusual in sarcoidosis. Rheumatoid nodules are not usually perilymphatic, and rheumatoid arthritis is not usually associated with marked mediastinal lymphadenopathy. Sickle cell disease is usually associated with decreased spleen size and not associated with nodules or lymphadenopathy.

References: Bang TJ, Richards JC, Olson AL, et al. Pulmonary manifestations of common variable immunodeficiency. *J Thorac Imaging* 2018;33(6):377–383.

Torigian DA, LaRosa DF, Levinson AI, et al. Granulomatous-lymphocytic interstitial lung disease associated with common variable immunodeficiency: CT findings. *J Thorac Imaging* 2008;23(3):162–169.

10

Atelectasis and Collapse

Christopher M. Walker, MD

QUESTIONS

1a A 55-year-old man presents with cough and an abnormal chest radiograph. What is the underlying abnormality?

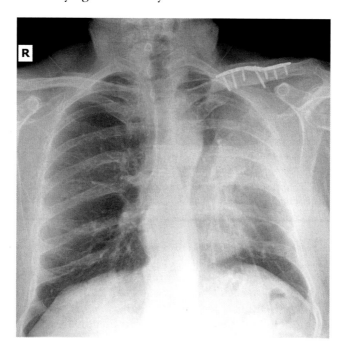

    A. Left upper lobe collapse
    B. Lingular collapse
    C. Pneumonia
    D. Left lower lobe collapse

1b Which sign is shown?

    A. S sign of Golden
    B. Flat waist
    C. Luftsichel
    D. Comet tail

1c Which anatomic structure is represented by the arrow?

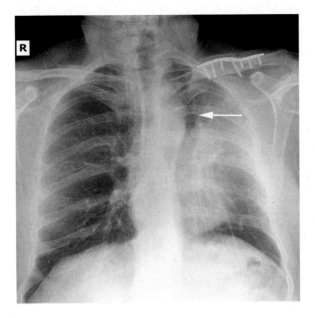

    A. Left upper lobe bronchus
    B. Superior segment of left lower lobe
    C. Anterior segment of left upper lobe
    D. Lingula

1d Which of the following is a direct sign of volume loss?

    A. Fissural displacement
    B. Hemidiaphragm elevation
    C. Shifting granuloma
    D. Juxtaphrenic peak

1e A CT scan was obtained. What is the most likely diagnosis?

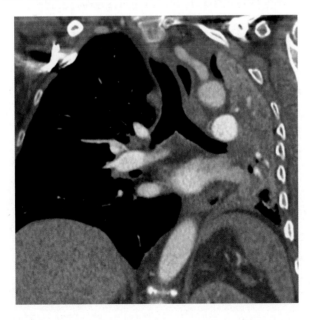

    A. Hamartoma
    B. Foreign body
    C. Mucous plug
    D. Lung cancer

2a A 70-year-old man undergoes chest CT and PET to evaluate a mass (arrow) that was identified on chest radiography. What is the most likely diagnosis?

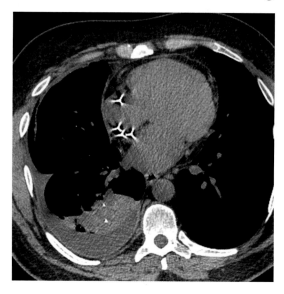 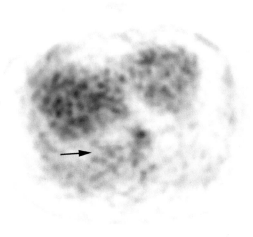

A. Rounded atelectasis
B. Lung cancer
C. Hamartoma
D. Pneumonia

2b Which of the following features is essential to diagnose rounded atelectasis?
A. Pleural plaque
B. FDG activity above mediastinal blood pool
C. Round mass
D. Comet tail sign

3a A 22-year-old woman presented to the emergency department with chest pain, wheezing, and dyspnea. What is the salient abnormality?

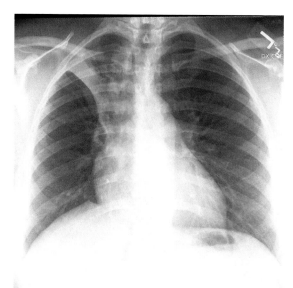

A. Pneumonia
B. Pneumomediastinum
C. Mediastinal mass
D. Right upper lobe atelectasis

3b What is the direct radiographic sign of volume loss?

    A. Displacement of the minor fissure
    B. Pulmonary opacity
    C. Tracheal shift
    D. Right hemidiaphragm elevation

3c What is the most likely cause for this patient's right upper lobe atelectasis?

    A. Hamartoma
    B. Foreign body
    C. Mucous plug
    D. Lung cancer

4 What best describes the role of prone imaging in the evaluation of possible diffuse lung disease by high-resolution CT (HRCT)?

    A. Differentiate honeycomb cyst formation from bronchiolectasis
    B. Separate dependent atelectasis from mild subpleural opacity
    C. Confirm the presence of lower lung traction bronchiectasis
    D. Distinguish round atelectasis from a pulmonary mass

5a An intubated 50-year-old man has a daily portable chest radiograph. What is the most likely cause of the perihilar and basal lung opacities given no fever and a normal white blood cell count?

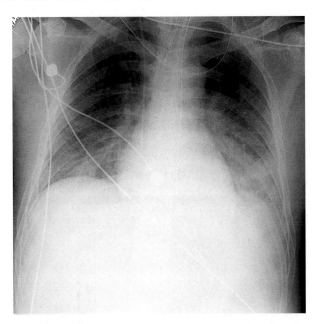

    A. Pulmonary edema
    B. Malignancy
    C. Pleural effusions
    D. Pneumonia

5b Four hours later, a radiograph was obtained for sudden hypoxia. What is the abnormality?

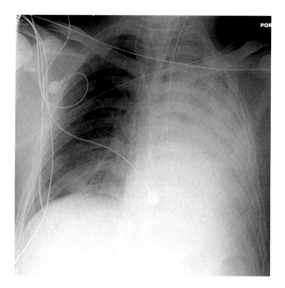

    A. Increasing pulmonary edema
    B. Pneumonia
    C. Pneumothorax
    D. Complete left lung atelectasis

5c What is the most likely cause of atelectasis?

    A. Carcinoid
    B. Foreign body aspiration
    C. Mucous plug
    D. Lung cancer

6a A 45-year-old woman with lupus undergoes CT for chest pain. What is the likely etiology of the opacity adjacent to the pleural effusion?

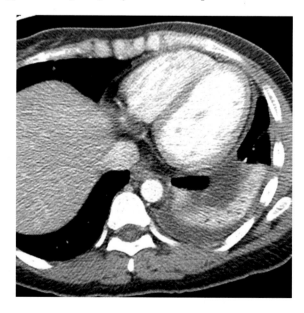

    A. Pneumonia
    B. Lung cancer
    C. Atelectasis
    D. Infarct

6b Which of the following types of atelectasis best characterizes the abnormality?

    A. Relaxation
    B. Adhesive
    C. Cicatricial
    D. Resorption

7a A 68-year-old woman presents with progressive dyspnea and cough. PA and lateral radiographs are obtained. What is the abnormality?

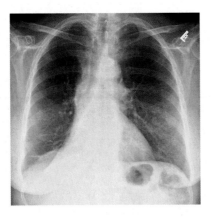 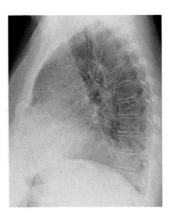

    A. Pneumonia
    B. AP window lymphadenopathy
    C. Loculated pleural effusion
    D. Atelectasis

7b Which lobe or lobes are collapsed?

    A. Right upper lobe
    B. Right lower lobe
    C. Right middle lobe
    D. Right lower and middle lobes

7c Which fissures are visible on the frontal radiograph?

    A. Right minor fissure only
    B. Right major fissure only
    C. Left major fissure only
    D. Right major and right minor fissures

7d A chest CT is obtained. What is the most likely diagnosis?

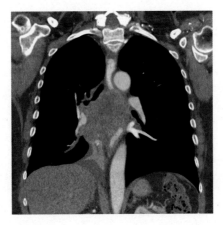

    A. Lung cancer
    B. Foreign body
    C. Mucous plug
    D. Carcinoid

8a   A 55-year-old man presents with dyspnea to his primary care physician and undergoes chest radiography. What is the abnormality?

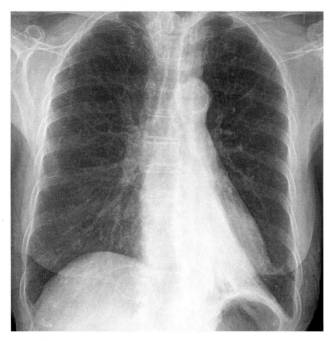
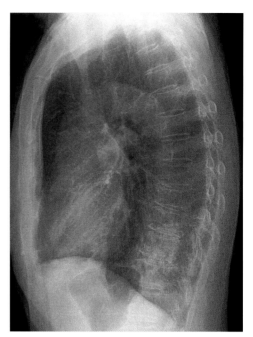

A. Pneumonia
B. Mediastinal mass
C. Loculated pleural effusion
D. Lobar atelectasis

8b   Which sign may be seen with this condition?

A. Comet tail sign
B. Flat waist sign
C. Air crescent sign
D. Luftsichel sign

8c   What sign is present on the lateral radiograph?

A. Spine sign
B. Doughnut sign
C. Fat pad sign
D. Comet tail sign

8d   What is the likely etiology of lobar collapse in an adult who presents to his/her primary care physician?

A. Lung cancer
B. Foreign body
C. Mucous plug
D. Aspiration

9a A 48-year-old man presents with chronic cough to a pulmonologist who orders a chest radiograph. What is the abnormality?

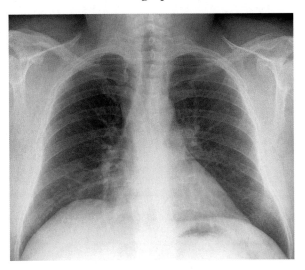 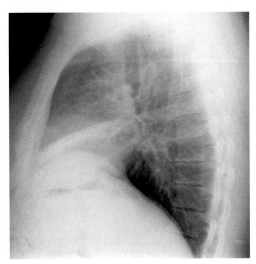

A. Pneumonia
B. Lobar atelectasis
C. Lung mass
D. Mediastinal lymphadenopathy

9b Which anatomic structure abuts the superior portion of the opacity on the lateral chest radiograph?

A. Minor fissure
B. Major fissure
C. Intermediate stem line
D. Right hilar vascular opacity

9c A CT is performed and reveals no centrally obstructing lesion. A review of the patient's abdominal CT from years earlier shows no interval change. What is the most common cause of this condition in adults?

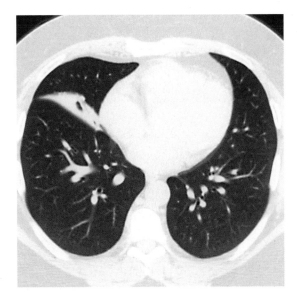

A. Sarcoidosis
B. Pneumoconiosis
C. Benign tumor
D. Nonobstructive inflammatory conditions

9d What is the most common cause of this condition in childhood?

A. Cystic fibrosis
B. Asthma
C. Carcinoid tumor
D. Foreign body aspiration

10a A 55-year-old man presents with dyspnea to his primary care physician and undergoes chest radiography. What is the abnormality?

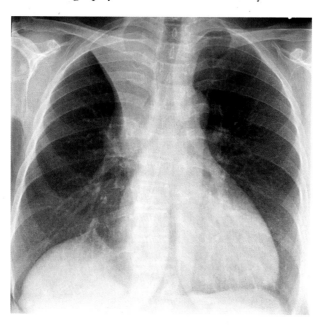

A. Pneumonia
B. Mediastinal mass
C. Loculated pleural effusion
D. Lobar atelectasis

10b What sign is present?

A. S sign of Golden
B. Flat waist sign
C. Comet tail sign
D. Luftsichel sign

10c What is the significance of the S sign of Golden?

A. Central mass
B. Foreign body
C. Mucous plug
D. Pneumonia

10d What is the density of the tumor?

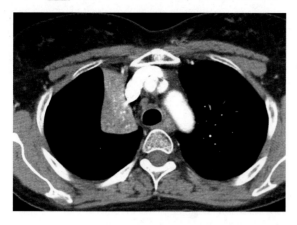
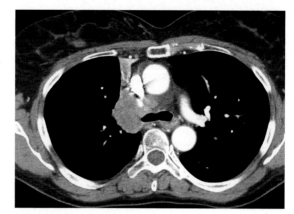

A. Calcified
B. Soft tissue
C. Water
D. Cavitary

11a An intubated premature infant with surfactant deficiency has a daily chest radiograph showing diffuse fine granular airspace opacities (left). Two hours later, a repeat radiograph (right) was performed for sudden desaturation. What is responsible for the imaging appearance?

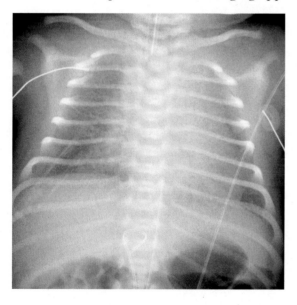
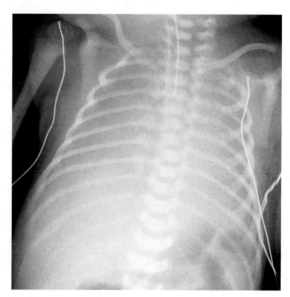

A. Atelectasis
B. Pulmonary edema
C. Pneumonia
D. Aspiration

11b Which of the following types of atelectasis best characterizes the abnormality?

A. Relaxation
B. Adhesive
C. Cicatricial
D. Resorption

12a A 44-year-old man underwent a chest radiograph for hypoxia. What is the cause of the left hemithorax opacity?

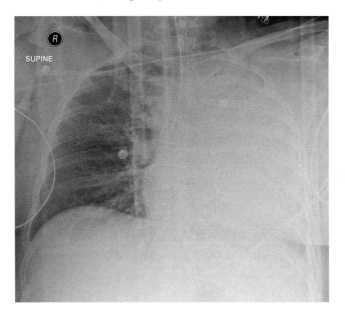

A. Pleural effusion
B. Large mass
C. Hemothorax
D. Complete lung atelectasis

12b What is the most likely cause for this patient's left lung atelectasis?

A. Foreign body
B. Malpositioned endotracheal tube
C. Lung cancer
D. Aspiration

ANSWERS AND EXPLANATIONS

1a **Answer A.**

1b **Answer C.**

1c **Answer B.**

1d **Answer A.**

1e **Answer D.**   The posteroanterior chest radiograph shows a large left hilar mass with left upper lobe collapse. There are several indirect signs of volume loss including leftward tracheal shift, increased opacity, and left hilar elevation as evidenced by outward and upward rotation of the left interlobar pulmonary artery, which is obscured laterally by the hilar mass (silhouette sign).

The Luftsichel or air crescent sign is classically seen in patients with left upper lobe collapse. The sign is produced by a hyperexpanded superior segment of the left lower lobe that interposes between the collapsed left upper lobe and aortic arch. The flat waist sign is seen with left lower lobe collapse, and the S sign of Golden is most commonly seen with right upper lobe collapse. The comet tail sign is seen on CT and represents a swirling of vessels and is used in the diagnosis of rounded atelectasis.

Contrast-enhanced CT scan shows an obstructing mass occluding the distal left main bronchus with a surrounding hypoattenuating mass, most compatible with primary lung cancer. A lung mass may be differentiated from adjacent atelectasis by looking at the enhancement of the parenchyma. Atelectasis results in vascular crowding and generally enhances briskly following contrast administration. However, a lung cancer is generally hypoattenuating or demonstrates heterogeneous enhancement following contrast administration.

Lobar collapse in an adult outpatient is malignancy until proven otherwise, usually from a primary lung cancer. Other causes of lobar collapse include endobronchial tumors such as carcinoid, hamartoma, and metastatic disease. The most common cause of lobar collapse in an intubated or sedated patient is a mucous plug that is optimally treated with aggressive suctioning or bronchoscopy. Foreign body is a frequent cause of lobar collapse in pediatric patients.

References: Molina PL, Hiken JN, Glazer HS. Imaging evaluation of obstructive atelectasis. *J Thorac Imaging* 1996;11:176–186.

Woodring JH, Reed JC. Radiographic manifestations of lobar atelectasis. *J Thorac Imaging* 1996;11:109–144.

2a **Answer A.**

2b **Answer D.**   Noncontrast chest CT scan shows a small to moderate right pleural effusion with pleural thickening and an adjacent masslike opacity in the right lower lobe. There is FDG uptake within the mass equal to mediastinal blood pool, which argues against a diagnosis of primary lung cancer or pneumonia. There is no macroscopic fat to suggest a diagnosis of pulmonary hamartoma. There are four features that are needed to confidently diagnose rounded atelectasis on CT:
1. Volume loss in the affected lobe (usually identified by fissural displacement).

2. Comet tail sign (i.e., curving of ipsilateral bronchovascular structures toward the mass).
3. Adjacent pleural abnormality (e.g., pleural thickening or pleural effusion).
4. Rounded opacity must have significant contact with pleural abnormality.

Rounded atelectasis is frequently metabolically inactive with FDG activity equal to or less than mediastinal blood pool (see arrow). CT follow-up of rounded atelectasis is controversial with some thoracic radiologists advising no follow-up and some suggesting follow-up at intervals (3 to 6 months) to ensure stability. Rounded atelectasis may improve, increase in size, or stay the same size on follow-up examinations.

References: Batra P, Brown K, Hayashi K, et al. Rounded atelectasis. *J Thorac Imaging* 1996;11:187–197.

Gurney JW. Atypical manifestations of pulmonary atelectasis. *J Thorac Imaging* 1996;11: 165–175.

McAdams HP, Erasums JJ, Patz EF, et al. Evaluation of patients with round atelectasis using 2-[18F]-fluoro-2-deoxy-D-glucose PET. *J Comput Assist Tomogr* 1998;22:601–604.

3a **Answer D.**

3b **Answer A.**

3c **Answer C.** The posteroanterior chest radiograph shows right upper lobe atelectasis. The clinical presentation is most suggestive of an asthma attack resulting in an obstructing mucous plug. There are a few direct and several indirect signs of volume loss. The direct signs include fissural displacement and crowding of the bronchovascular structures, the latter is optimally assessed on CT. In this case, there is upward and medial displacement of the minor fissure, a direct sign of volume loss. Indirect signs of volume loss that are present include right hemidiaphragm elevation, rightward tracheal shift, and increased pulmonary opacity.

Reference: Woodring JH, Reed JC. Radiographic manifestations of lobar atelectasis. *J Thorac Imaging* 1996;11:109–144.

4 **Answer B.** Prone imaging is generally part of a standard initial HRCT evaluation for patients suspected to have interstitial lung disease. Prone imaging enhances evaluation of the subpleural dependent lower lungs. Since the peripheral lower lung is frequently the initial site of abnormality for many interstitial pneumonias, the presence of atelectasis can obscure subtle, early ILD. Thus, prone imaging is performed to eliminate any dependent atelectasis and confirm the presence or absence of any mild underlying lung disease.

Reference: Lynch DA, Newell JD, Lee JS. *Imaging of diffuse lung disease.* Hamilton, ON: B.C. Decker, Inc., 2000.

5a **Answer A.**

5b **Answer D.**

5c **Answer C.** The initial chest radiograph shows life support devices in expected locations. There are perihilar and basal lung opacities with vascular indistinctness, which is most consistent with pulmonary edema. The absence of fever and a normal white blood cell count argue against the diagnosis of pneumonia. While there are likely small bilateral pleural effusions, the majority of the opacities are related to pulmonary edema.

A radiograph obtained at the time of hypoxia shows new left lung collapse. There is ipsilateral mediastinal shift with displacement of the gastric tube, endotracheal tube, and right internal jugular central venous catheter. In an intubated or sedated patient, sudden lung collapse is frequently from an obstructing mucous plug. Tumor is more common in outpatients presenting with lobar collapse. There are only a few conditions that change rapidly over a few hours on chest radiography and include atelectasis, pulmonary edema, and aspiration.

References: Woodring JH, Reed JC. Radiographic manifestations of lobar atelectasis. *J Thorac Imaging* 1996;11:109–144.

Woodring JH, Reed JC. Types and mechanisms of pulmonary atelectasis. *J Thorac Imaging* 1996;11:92–108.

6a **Answer C.**

6b **Answer A.** The axial contrast-enhanced chest CT shows densely enhancing left lower lobe surrounded by a left pleural effusion. This is most characteristic of relaxation atelectasis. While pneumonia is not entirely excluded, it is less likely given lack of hypodense enhancement within the collapsed lung.

There are four types of atelectasis related to etiology:

Relaxation or passive atelectasis occurs when a pleural effusion, pneumothorax, or mass allows the lung to collapse to its normal lower volume.

Adhesive atelectasis is seen primarily in premature infants with surfactant deficiency or adults following smoke inhalation and is caused by alveolar collapse secondary to insufficient surfactant production or surfactant dysfunction.

Cicatricial atelectasis occurs in patients with lung fibrosis, which leads to adjacent lung atelectasis.

Resorption atelectasis results from proximal bronchial obstruction and may be seen with tumor, mucous plug, or foreign body aspiration.

Reference: Woodring JH, Reed JC. Types and mechanisms of pulmonary atelectasis. *J Thorac Imaging* 1996;11:92–108.

7a **Answer D.**

7b **Answer D.**

7c **Answer D.**

7d **Answer A.** The posteroanterior chest radiograph shows combined right middle and right lower lobe collapse. The vertically oriented major fissure intersects the inferiorly displaced minor fissure, and the right interlobar pulmonary artery is invisible. There is rightward mediastinal shift and compensatory hyperinflation of the right upper lobe. A mediastinal mass with paratracheal and subcarinal lymphadenopathy is also noted. The lateral radiograph shows a band of opacity extending from anterior to posterior in the expected location of the right middle and right lower lobes.

The coronal contrast-enhanced chest CT confirms collapse caused by a large mediastinal mass, likely lymphadenopathy. In the absence of a primary tumor elsewhere in the lung or body, the leading considerations would include small cell lung cancer or lymphoma. Carcinoid typically is an endobronchial mass, which is often well defined and may contain calcium in about 25% of cases.

Reference: Woodring JH, Reed JC. Radiographic manifestations of lobar atelectasis. *J Thorac Imaging* 1996;11:109–144.

8a **Answer D.**

8b **Answer B.**

8c **Answer A.**

8d **Answer A.** The posteroanterior chest radiograph shows complete left lower lobe collapse manifesting as a triangular-shaped opacity in the retrocardiac region. The flat waist sign represents a flattening of the left heart border and mediastinum with loss of the normal left-sided moguls or contours including the aortic arch, pulmonary trunk, left atrial appendage, and left ventricular border. It occurs from posterior rotation and leftward shift of the heart. The lateral radiograph shows increased opacity posteriorly over the spine resulting in the spine sign. Normally, the spine should become more lucent inferiorly. Other radiographic signs associated with left lower lobe collapse include the "top-of-the-knob" and "Nordenström" signs. The top-of-the-knob sign results in obscuration of the superomedial aspect of the aortic arch due to leftward mediastinal shift and rotation. The Nordenström sign represents lingular subsegmental atelctasis from kinking and reorientation of the lingular bronchi.

The Luftsichel or air crescent sign is classically seen in patients with left upper lobe collapse. The sign is produced by a hyperexpanded superior segment of the left lower lobe, which interposes between the collapsed left upper lobe and aortic arch. The comet tail sign is a CT finding that helps diagnose rounded atelectasis and represents a swirling of vessels into the masslike opacity.

Lobar collapse in an adult outpatient is caused by malignancy until proven otherwise, usually from a primary lung cancer. Other causes of lobar collapse include endobronchial tumors such as carcinoid, hamartoma, and metastatic disease. Foreign body is the most common cause of lobar collapse in pediatric patients. Mucous plug and aspiration are common causes of collapse in intubated or sedated patients.

References: Kattan KR, Wlot JF. Cardiac rotation in left lower lobe collapse. "The flat waist sign." *Radiology* 1976;118(2):275–279.

Woodring JH, Reed JC. Radiographic manifestations of lobar atelectasis. *J Thorac Imaging* 1996;11:109–144.

9a **Answer B.**

9b **Answer A.**

9c **Answer D.**

9d **Answer B.** The frontal chest radiograph shows subtle obscuration of the right heart border. The lateral radiograph confirms right middle lobe collapse. There is inferior displacement of the minor fissure and anterior and superior displacement of the right major fissure, both direct radiographic signs of volume loss. The intermediate stem line is composed of the posterior wall of the bronchus intermedius and right main bronchus and is not responsible for the radiographic abnormality.

The axial chest CT confirms complete right middle lobe collapse. CT is necessary to exclude a centrally obstructing lung mass or endobronchial tumor. Bronchoscopy is often necessary in addition to CT to exclude small endobronchial nodules. The middle lobe syndrome is a condition that describes chronic right middle lobe collapse and may be seen with both obstructive and nonobstructive etiologies. It is more common in middle or elderly adults, usually women. The most common cause of the middle lobe syndrome in adults is nonobstructive inflammatory conditions including tuberculosis infection. When it occurs in children, it is usually associated with asthma or repeated infection.

References: Gudbjartsson T, Gudmundsson G. Middle lobe syndrome: a review of clinicopathological features, diagnosis and treatment. *Respiration* 2012;84:80–86.

Sekerel BE, Nakipoglu F. Middle lobe syndrome in children with asthma: review of 56 cases. *J Asthma* 2004;41:411–417.

Wagner RB, Johnston MR. Middle lobe syndrome. *Ann Thorac Surg* 1983;35:679–686.

10a **Answer D.**

10b **Answer A.**

10c **Answer A.**

10d **Answer B.** The posteroanterior chest radiograph shows right upper lobe atelectasis and the S sign of Golden. The S sign of Golden is classically associated with right upper lobe collapse from a centrally obstructing tumor, usually lung cancer. The central lung cancer causes a convex inferior bulge with the adjacent elevated minor fissure resulting in a reverse S configuration.

The Luftsichel or air crescent sign is classically seen in patients with left upper lobe collapse. The sign is produced by a hyperexpanded superior segment of the left lower lobe, which interposes between the collapsed left upper lobe and aortic arch. The flat waist sign is seen with left lower lobe collapse. The comet tail sign is a CT finding, which helps diagnose rounded atelectasis and represents a swirling of vessels into the masslike opacity.

Lobar collapse in an adult outpatient is malignancy until proven otherwise, usually from a primary lung cancer. Other causes of lobar collapse include endobronchial tumors such as carcinoid, hamartoma, and metastatic disease. The tumor may be differentiated from atelectatic lung by looking at density on postcontrast CT. Atelectatic lung enhances homogeneously and intensely following contrast as the bronchovascular structures are closely opposed, whereas tumor will typically have heterogeneous and hypodense enhancement.

Reference: Woodring JH, Reed JC. Radiographic manifestations of lobar atelectasis. *J Thorac Imaging* 1996;11:109–144.

11a **Answer A.**

11b **Answer B.** The initial chest radiograph shows diffuse fine granular airspace opacities typical of surfactant deficiency. The follow-up radiograph obtained for desaturation shows low lung volumes with complete whiteout of both lungs, most compatible with adhesive atelectasis.

As stated before, but for review, there are four types of atelectasis:

Adhesive atelectasis is seen primarily in premature infants with surfactant deficiency or in adults following smoke inhalation and is caused by alveolar collapse secondary to insufficient surfactant production or surfactant dysfunction.

Relaxation or passive atelectasis occurs when a pleural effusion, pneumothorax, or mass allows the lung to collapse "relax" to its normal lower volume.

Cicatricial atelectasis occurs in patients with lung fibrosis, which leads to adjacent lung atelectasis.

Resorption atelectasis results from proximal bronchial obstruction and may be seen with tumor, mucous plugging, or foreign body aspiration. With proximal bronchial obstruction, the air within alveoli is progressively absorbed by circulating blood in the pulmonary arterial system. In a nonintubated patient, complete air absorption occurs in 24 hours. In an intubated patient receiving a high concentration of oxygen, the air may be absorbed from the alveoli in as little as an hour.

Reference: Woodring JH, Reed JC. Types and mechanisms of pulmonary atelectasis. *J Thorac Imaging* 1996;11:92–108.

12a Answer D.

12b Answer B.   The anteroposterior chest radiograph shows complete left lung atelectasis secondary to right main bronchus intubation. There are several indirect signs of volume loss including increased opacities, approximation of the left-sided ribs, and leftward mediastinal shift evidenced by the gastric tube position.

Reference: Woodring JH, Reed JC. Radiographic manifestations of lobar atelectasis. *J Thorac Imaging* 1996;11:109–144.

11

Pulmonary Physiology

Said Chaaban, MD • Angel O. Coz Yataco, MD, FCCP

QUESTIONS

1a A 67-year-old male with a 50-pack-year smoking history presents for evaluation of shortness of breath. Spirogram was done in the office and shows these results. What is the pattern described in the spirogram?

	Actual	Predicted	% Predicted
FVC (L)	2.42	2.47	98
FEV₁ (L)	1.09	1.82	60
FEV₁/FVC (%)	45		

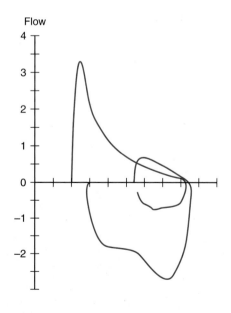

A. Airway obstruction
B. Variable intrathoracic obstruction
C. Restriction
D. Hyperinflation

1b What disease process most likely explains those findings?

    A. Vocal cord dysfunction

    B. Idiopathic pulmonary fibrosis

    C. Chronic obstructive pulmonary disease

    D. Tracheal stenosis

2a A 63-year-old female presents with progressive shortness of breath over the last 4 years. She has smoked 2 packs per day for the past 40 years. Her review of systems is significant for fatigue. She worked in an office for 20 years and only had a dog at home. What is the pattern described in the pulmonary function testing below?

	Actual	Predicted	% Predicted
FVC (L)	1.93	3.86	50
FEV1 (L)	1.45	3.08	47
FEV1/FVC (%)	75		
TLC (L)	1.99	5.00	40
RV (L)	0.61	1.8	32
DLCO (mL/min/mm Hg)	6.21	22.29	28

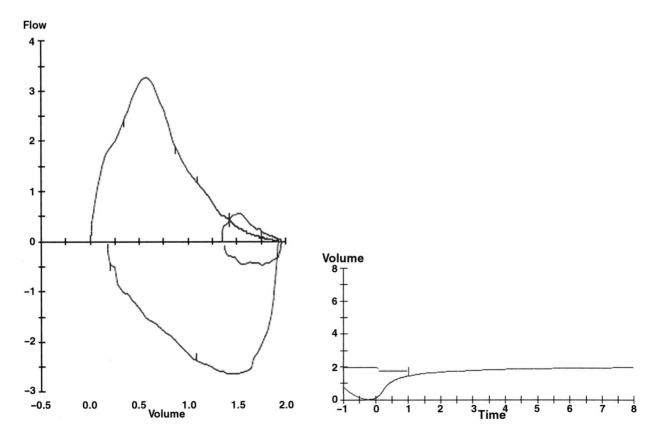

    A. Obstructive lung disease

    B. Restrictive lung disease

    C. Hyperinflation

    D. Combined obstructive and restrictive lung disease

2b The patient had a CT of the chest. What disease process is consistent with the findings on pulmonary function test and imaging?

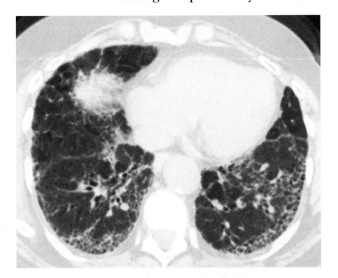 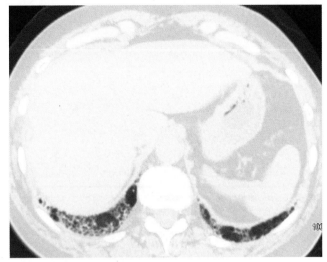

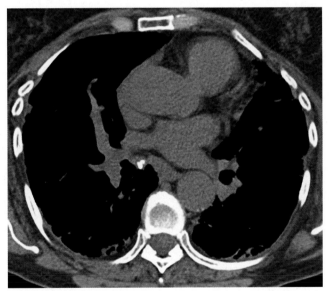

A. Usual interstitial pneumonia (UIP)

B. COPD

C. Asbestosis

D. Hypersensitivity pneumonitis

3 A 32-year-old male undergoes pulmonary function testing as part of a preemployment examination. He has no respiratory complaints. He has never smoked, but he had significant secondhand smoke exposure. The pulmonary function test shows these results.

	Actual	Predicted	% Predicted
FVC (L)	5.25	5.12	103
FEV₁ (L)	3.80	4.04	94
FEV₁/FVC (%)	72		
TLC (L)	6.69	6.83	98
RV (L)	1.52	1.69	90
FRC (L)	3.30	3.36	98
DLCO (mL/min/mm Hg)	18.8	19	99

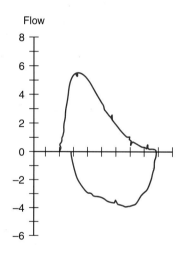

Flow

Which of the following is most consistent with this pulmonary function test?

A. Pulmonary vascular disease
B. Normal study
C. Chronic obstructive pulmonary disease
D. Pulmonary fibrosis

4a A 28-year-old male presents with a 5-year history of progressive dyspnea on exertion that has worsened significantly in the last 3 months. He is a lifelong nonsmoker. On examination, there is bilateral rhonchi and scattered wheezing. His oxygen saturation is 91% on ambient air. A spirogram with bronchodilator administration is performed.

	Pretreatment			Posttreatment		
	Actual	Predicted	% Predicted	Actual	% Predicted	% Change
FVC (L)	4.34	5.57	78	4.40	79	1
FEV$_1$ (L)	1.60	4.61	35	1.76	38	10
FEV$_1$/FVC (%)	37			40		

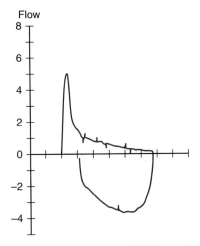

What is the most accurate interpretation of this study?

A. Moderate obstruction with reversibility
B. Moderate obstruction without reversibility
C. Severe obstruction with reversibility
D. Severe obstruction without reversibility

4b What is the most likely diagnosis based on pulmonary function testing and the image shown?

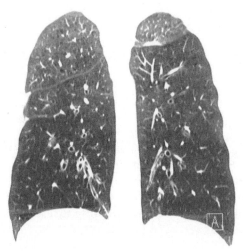

A. Asthma
B. Usual interstitial pneumonia (UIP)
C. Pulmonary hypertension
D. Alpha-1 antitrypsin deficiency

5a A 64-year-old male presents with shortness of breath and cough that has been getting worse over 7 years. He is a lifelong nonsmoker. He owns a farm and raises chickens, ducks, rabbits, goats, cows, and horses. The patient voices no other environmental exposures. There is no history of neurologic impairment, and the patient denies any problems swallowing liquids or solid food. What is the pattern described in the pulmonary function testing below?

	Actual	Predicted	% Predicted
FVC (L)	3.05	4.65	66
FEV1 (L)	2.94	3.48	84
FEV1/FVC (%)	96		
TLC (L)	5.29	7.14	74
RV (L)	2.60	2.51	104
RV/TLC (%)	49		
DLCO (mL/min/mm Hg)	7	24	28

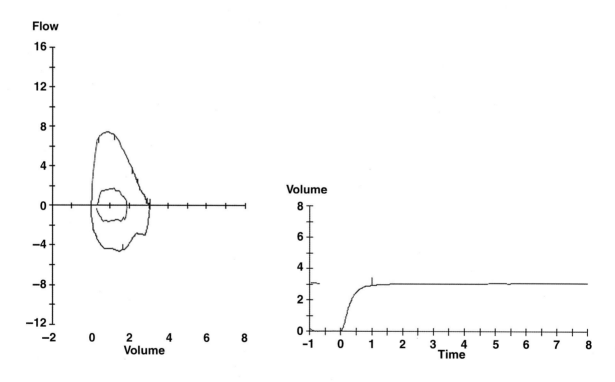

A. Obstructive lung disease with air trapping
B. Restrictive lung disease with air trapping
C. Hyperinflation
D. Combined obstructive and restrictive lung disease

5b The following are representative images of the patient's CT of the chest. What disease process most likely explains the overall findings?

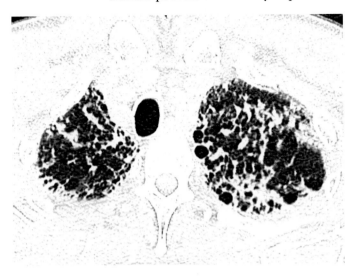
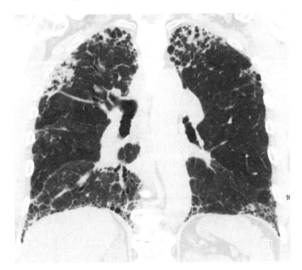

   A. Usual interstitial pneumonia (UIP)
   B. Chronic aspiration
   C. Asbestosis
   D. Hypersensitivity pneumonitis

6 A 35-year-old female is seen in clinic for a 4-month history of shortness of breath and wheezing after climbing one flight of stairs. She has no chest pain or cough but has had intermittent hoarseness. What is the most likely diagnosis?

	Actual	Predicted	% Predicted
FVC (L)	2.78	2.90	96
FEV$_1$ (L)	1.81	2.19	83
FEV$_1$/FVC (%)	65		

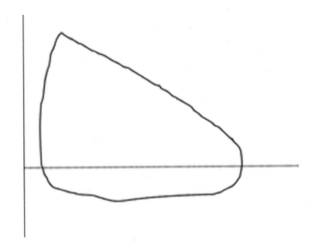

   A. Vocal cord dysfunction
   B. Tracheomalacia
   C. Tracheal stenosis
   D. Emphysema

7 A 45-year-old female presents for evaluation of dyspnea and wheezing. She is a lifelong nonsmoker. She had a motor vehicle accident 3 years ago for which she required prolonged mechanical ventilation and a tracheostomy that was removed several weeks after her recovery. The spirogram and flow–volume loops are shown.

	Actual	Predicted	% Predicted
FVC (L)	1.86	3.10	60
FEV₁ (L)	1.26	2.82	45
FEV₁/FVC (%)	68		

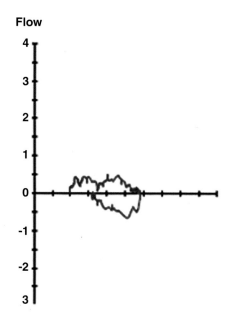

What is the most accurate description of this test?

A. Variable intrathoracic obstruction
B. Fixed airway obstruction
C. Variable extrathoracic obstruction
D. Restriction

8a A 33-year-old female presents on her 30th week of pregnancy complaining of shortness of breath and cough. She is a lifelong nonsmoker. She did not have respiratory symptoms like cough, sputum production, or frequent respiratory infections prior to this pregnancy. On physical examination, she has bilateral wheezing and her oxygen saturation is 92% on room air. A spirogram with bronchodilator administration is performed. What is the most accurate interpretation of this study?

	Pretreatment			Posttreatment		
	Actual	Predicted	% Predicted	Actual	% Predicted	% Change
FVC (L)	2.98	3.63	82	3.41	94	14%
FEV1 (L)	1.87	3.03	62	2.29	76	22%
FEV1/FVC (%)	63			67		

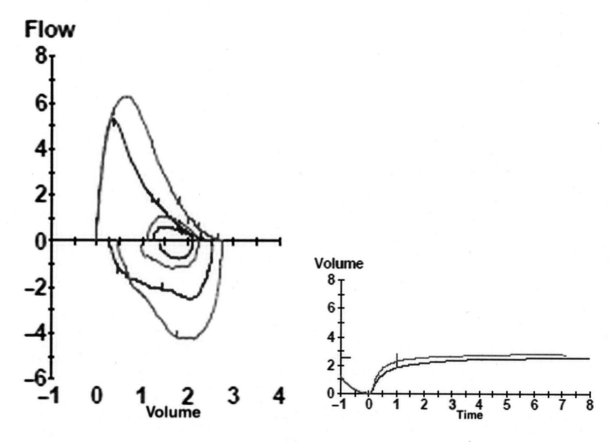

A. Moderate obstructive lung disease with reversibility
B. Moderate obstructive lung disease without reversibility
C. Severe obstructive lung disease without reversibility
D. Severe obstructive lung disease with reversibility

8b What is the most likely diagnosis?

A. Cystic fibrosis
B. Sarcoidosis
C. Asthma
D. Pulmonary hypertension

9a A 54-year-old male presents with a 2-year history of progressive shortness of breath and productive cough. He has a 76-pack-year history of smoking and continues to smoke. On examination, breath sounds are decreased bilaterally. There is no history of sinus disease, epistaxis, or kidney disease. His pulmonary function tests are shown below:

	Actual	Predicted	% Predicted
FVC (L)	3.49	5.70	61
FEV1 (L)	2.28	4.46	51
FEV1/FVC (%)	65		
TLC (L)	8.21	7.89	104
RV (L)	3.10	2.21	140
RV/TLC (%)	38		
DLCO (mL/min/mm Hg)	20.59	36.52	56

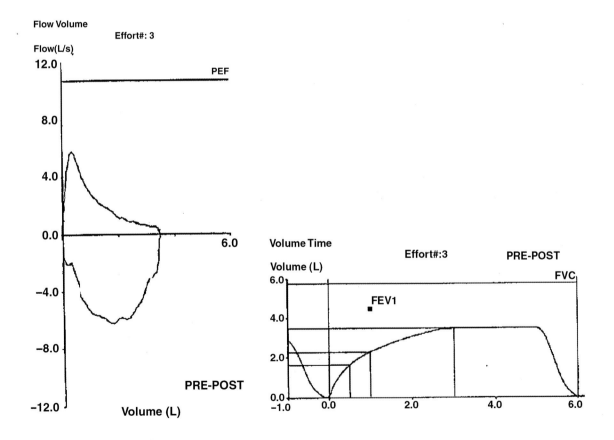

Which of the following best describes this patient's pulmonary function test?

A. Obstructive lung disease with air trapping
B. Restrictive lung disease with air trapping
C. Hyperinflation
D. Combined obstructive and restrictive lung disease

9b The following are representative images of this patient's CT chest. What disease process most likely explains the overall findings?

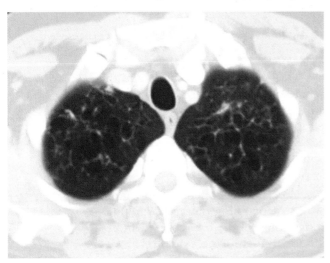 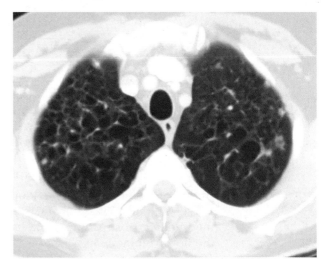

A. Lung metastases
B. Pulmonary Langerhans cell histiocytosis
C. Sarcoidosis
D. Granulomatosis with polyangiitis

10a A 70-year-old male presents for evaluation of dyspnea on exertion. He has a 60-pack-year smoking history. His spirogram and lung volumes are shown.

	Actual	Predicted	% Predicted
FVC (L)	2.06	4.58	45
FEV₁ (L)	0.90	3.60	25
FEV₁/FVC (%)	44		
TLC (L)	8.30	6.41	129
RV (L)	3.00	2.31	130
DLCO (mL/min/mm Hg)	12	24	50

In addition to very severe obstruction, this test shows:

A. Hyperinflation and air trapping
B. Hyperinflation but no air trapping
C. Restriction and air trapping
D. Restriction but no air trapping

10b What disease process is the most likely?

A. Chronic obstructive pulmonary disease
B. Usual interstitial pneumonia (UIP)
C. Sarcoidosis
D. Primary pulmonary hypertension

ANSWERS AND EXPLANATIONS

1a **Answer A.**

1b **Answer C.** The low FEV_1/FVC ratio (<70%) represents obstruction, and the FEV_1 at 60% of predicted indicates moderate obstruction (50% $\leq FEV_1$ < 80% predicted). When evaluating a spirogram, the interpreter must include the numeric values and the flow–volume loops. The latter provide valuable information about different abnormalities in the airway physiology. The arm under the x-axis corresponds to the inspiratory part, whereas the arm above the x-axis corresponds to the expiratory phase of the test.

In this case, the flow–volume loop shows the classic scooped-out appearance in the expiratory phase characteristic of obstructive lung diseases. Variable intrathoracic obstruction would cause a flattening of the expiratory arm of the flow–volume loop. Since the FVC is normal, there is no evidence of a restrictive pattern. However, restriction can only be diagnosed in the presence of a total lung capacity (TLC) lower than 80% of predicted. Hyperinflation can be diagnosed when the TLC exceeds 120% of predicted.

The patient presented in this case has a significant smoking history, and the spirogram shows moderate airflow obstruction with scooped-out pattern. Therefore, the disease that would most likely cause this pattern is chronic obstructive pulmonary disease. Vocal cord dysfunction would cause a variable extrathoracic obstruction pattern on flow–volume loops, affecting the inspiratory phase. Tracheal stenosis would cause a fixed airway obstruction, characterized by an abnormality in both inspiratory and expiratory arms of the flow–volume loops. Idiopathic pulmonary fibrosis would cause a restrictive pattern.

References: Barreiro TJ, Perillo I. An approach to interpreting spirometry. *Am Fam Physician* 2004;69(5):1107–1114. Available at http://www.attud.org/docs/interpretingspirometry.pdf

Kapnadak S, Kreit J. Stay in the loop! *Ann Am Thorac Soc* 2013;10(2):166–171.

Pocket Guide. The global initiative for chronic obstructive disease. Available at https://goldcopd.org/wp-content/uploads/2018/11/GOLD-2019-POCKET-GUIDE-DRAFT-v1.7-14Nov2018-WMS.pdf

2a **Answer B.**

2b **Answer A.** This patient's FEV_1/FVC ratio is >70% and her FVC is 50% of predicted. The normal FEV1/FVC ratio and FVC < 80% suggest restriction. A total lung capacity (TLC) < 80% is needed to confirm the restrictive pattern on lung function testing. The total lung capacity of 40% (<80%) is consistent with restriction. The diffusion capacity is also decreased (<80% predicted).

The restrictive pattern with low diffusion capacity and honeycombing pattern of peripheral distribution is suggestive of idiopathic pulmonary fibrosis. Idiopathic pulmonary fibrosis produces a restrictive defect, and it does not produce obstruction unless associated with a concomitant obstructive disease. Smoking is a major risk factor. It is more common in males but can also be present in females. About 5% to 10% of cases are familial in nature. CT findings can be sufficient to make a definitive diagnosis in cases with subpleural, basal-predominant reticular abnormalities, with honeycombing, and with or without traction opacities. If the classic CT findings are not present, surgical lung biopsy may be necessary for a definitive diagnosis.

The patient was a smoker but did not show any evidence of obstruction on lung function testing. Asbestos is the largest cause of cancer secondary to occupational exposure. It is the result of inhalation of asbestos fibers that can cause a spectrum of diseases after they reach the lung tissue. While lung function testing is usually restrictive in nature, a mixed obstructive and restrictive impairment can also be seen. CT imaging may show honeycombing and thickening of septa and interlobular fissures (suggesting fibrosis), diffuse pleural thickening and rounded atelectasis (fibrosis of the visceral pleura), and pleural plaques. The patient had no occupational exposure to asbestos, and the lack of pleural plaques makes this diagnosis less likely.

Hypersensitivity pneumonitis (HP) is usually the result of an immune-mediated reaction secondary to a recurrent exposure to an environmental antigen in a genetically predisposed individual. HP usually produces a restrictive ventilatory defect with air trapping on lung function testing. The CT findings vary depending on the chronicity of the process. In the acute form, upper and middle lobe–predominant ground-glass opacities (centrilobular nodules) and air trapping are typical. In the chronic form, the usual findings include upper and middle lobe–predominant fibrosis, peribronchovascular fibrosis, honeycombing, mosaic attenuation, air trapping, and centrilobular nodules with relative sparing of the bases. The imaging and the lung function testing are not consistent with current diagnosis.

References: American Thoracic Society. Diagnosis and initial management of nonmalignant diseases related to asbestos. *Am J Respir Crit Care Med* 2004;170(6):691–715. Available at https://www.atsjournals.org/doi/pdf/10.1164/rccm.200310-1436ST

Barreiro TJ, Perillo I. An approach to interpreting spirometry. *Am Fam Physician* 2004;69(5):1107–1114. Available at http://www.attud.org/docs/interpretingspirometry.pdf.

Kapnadak S, Kreit J. Stay in the loop! *Ann Am Thorac Soc* 2013;10(2):166–171.

Pocket Guide. The global initiative for chronic obstructive disease. Available at https://goldcopd.org/wp-content/uploads/2018/11/GOLD-2019-POCKET-GUIDE-DRAFT-v1.7-14Nov2018-WMS.pdf

Raghu G, Remy-Jardin M, Myers JL, et al. Diagnosis of idiopathic pulmonary fibrosis. an official ATS/ERS/JRS/ALAT clinical practice guideline. *Am J Respir Crit Care Med* 2018;198(5):e44–e68. Available at https://www.thoracic.org/statements/resources/interstitial-lung-disease/diagnosis-IPF-full-length.pdf

Vasakova M, Morell F, Walsh S, et al. Hypersensitivity pneumonitis: perspectives in diagnosis and management. *Am J Respir Crit Care Med* 2017;196(6):680–689. Available at https://areasoci.sirm.org/uploads/Documenti/SDS/d8e25a77005731641b0e0768b0aa2d69dcc07d4e.pdf

3   **Answer B.**   The FEV_1/FVC ratio is normal (>70%); therefore, there is no obstruction. The FVC and FEV_1 are normal and the flow–volume loop does not show significant abnormalities. Total lung capacity (TLC) and residual volume (RV) are normal. A decreased TLC (<80%) indicates a restrictive process, whereas an increased TLC (>120%) indicates hyperinflation. An increased RV (>120%), typically seen in obstructive lung diseases, indicates air trapping. Given the normal FEV1/FVC, FEV_1, FVC, and lung volumes, this is a normal spirogram.

Pulmonary vascular disease typically produces a low diffusion capacity of carbon monoxide (DLCO). Chronic obstructive pulmonary disease causes obstruction pattern with a scooped-out flow–volume loop. Pulmonary fibrosis causes restriction, characterized by a low TLC.

References: Barreiro TJ, Perillo I. An approach to interpreting spirometry. *Am Fam Physician* 2004;69(5):1107–1114. Available at http://www.attud.org/docs/interpretingspirometry.pdf

Kapnadak S, Kreit J. Stay in the loop! *Ann Am Thorac Soc* 2013;10(2):166–171.

Pocket Guide. The global initiative for chronic obstructive disease. Available at https://goldcopd.org/wp-content/uploads/2018/11/GOLD-2019-POCKET-GUIDE-DRAFT-v1.7-14Nov2018-WMS.pdf

4a   Answer D.

4b   Answer D.   This patient has airway obstruction as the FEV_1/FVC ratio is <70%. The FEV_1 at 38% of predicted indicates severe obstruction (30% $\leq FEV_1$ < 50% predicted). Moderate obstruction is defined as an FEV_1 between 50% and 79% of predicted. Following the administration of bronchodilators, there was an increase of 160 mL in FEV_1 and an absolute change of 10% of the baseline FEV_1. However, this change is not enough to be considered significant (>200 mL and >12% of baseline FEV_1).

The disease presented demonstrates obstruction that is not reversible with bronchodilators and is usually seen in chronic obstructive pulmonary disease, either tobacco related or secondary to alpha-1 antitrypsin deficiency. The early onset, lack of history of smoking, and severe obstruction support this diagnosis. The CT confirms this suspicion, demonstrating lower lung panlobular emphysema with bronchial wall thickening and mild bronchiectasis.

Asthma typically gives a significant response to bronchodilators. Pulmonary fibrosis is a restrictive disease and is not consistent with the case presented. Primary pulmonary hypertension typically presents with a normal spirogram and an isolated decrease in DLCO and is not present in this case.

References: Barreiro TJ, Perillo I. An approach to interpreting spirometry. *Am Fam Physician* 2004;69(5):1107–1114. Available at http://www.attud.org/docs/interpretingspirometry.pdf

Kapnadak S, Kreit J. Stay in the loop! *Ann Am Thorac Soc* 2013;10(2):166–171.

Pocket Guide. The global initiative for chronic obstructive disease. Available at https://goldcopd.org/wp-content/uploads/2018/11/GOLD-2019-POCKET-GUIDE-DRAFT-v1.7-14Nov2018-WMS.pdf

5a   Answer B.

5b   Answer D.   This patient's FEV_1/FVC ratio is >70% and the FVC is 66% of predicted. The normal FEV1/FVC ratio and FVC < 80% suggest restriction. A total lung capacity (TLC) < 80% is needed to confirm the restrictive pattern on lung function testing. The TLC is 60% (<80%), consistent with severe restriction. Although the residual volume (RV) is also within normal range (<120%), the RV/TLC is elevated (>35%), consistent with air trapping. The diffusion capacity is decreased.

The restrictive pattern with air trapping and low diffusion capacity on lung function test in the context of significant exposures and the findings on imaging are consistent with hypersensitivity pneumonitis (HP). This entity is usually the result of an immune-mediated reaction secondary to a recurrent exposure to an environmental antigen in a genetically predisposed individual. HP usually produces a restrictive ventilatory defect with air trapping on lung function testing. The CT findings vary depending on the chronicity of the process. In the acute form, upper and middle lobe–predominant ground-glass opacities (centrilobular nodules) and air trapping are typical. In the chronic form, the usual findings include upper and middle lobe–predominant fibrosis, peribronchovascular fibrosis, honeycombing, mosaic attenuation, air trapping, and centrilobular nodules with relative sparing of the bases.

Idiopathic pulmonary fibrosis produces a restrictive defect, and it does not typically produce obstruction or air trapping. The upper lobe predominance of the findings on CT makes this diagnosis unlikely.

Asbestos lung disease is the result of inhalation of asbestos fibers. While lung function testing is usually restrictive in nature, a mixed obstructive and restrictive impairment can also be seen, and CT imaging may show honeycombing and thickening of septa and interlobular fissures, suggestive of fibrosis, diffuse pleural thickening, and rounded atelectasis that is fibrosis in the visceral pleura and pleural plaques. While this patient's lung function testing is suggestive of restriction, there was no occupational exposure to asbestos, and the imaging is not consistent with this diagnosis.

References: American Thoracic Society. Diagnosis and initial management of nonmalignant diseases related to asbestos. *Am J Respir Crit Care Med* 2004;170(6):691–715. Available at https://www.atsjournals.org/doi/pdf/10.1164/rccm.200310-1436ST

Barreiro TJ, Perillo I. An approach to interpreting spirometry. *Am Fam Physician* 2004;69(5):1107–1114. Available at http://www.attud.org/docs/interpretingspirometry.pdf

Pocket Guide. The global initiative for chronic obstructive disease. Available at https://goldcopd.org/wp-content/uploads/2018/11/GOLD-2019-POCKET-GUIDE-DRAFT-v1.7-14Nov2018-WMS.pdf

Raghu G, Remy-Jardin M, Myers JL, et al. Diagnosis of idiopathic pulmonary fibrosis. An official ATS/ERS/JRS/ALAT clinical practice guideline. *Am J Respir Crit Care Med* 2018;198(5):e44–e68. Available at https://www.thoracic.org/statements/resources/interstitial-lung-disease/diagnosis-IPF-full-length.pdf

Vasakova M, Morell F, Walsh S, et al. Hypersensitivity pneumonitis: perspectives in diagnosis and management. *Am J Respir Crit Care Med* 2017;196(6):680–689. Available at https://areasoci.sirm.org/uploads/Documenti/SDS/d8e25a77005731641b0e0768b0aa2d69dcc07d4e.pdf

6 **Answer A.** This patient has airway obstruction as the FEV_1/FVC ratio is <70%. The FEV_1 at 83% of predicted indicates mild obstruction ($FEV1 \geq 80\%$ predicted). The flow–volume loop shows flattening in the inspiratory phase with a preserved expiratory phase, a characteristic of variable extrathoracic obstruction.

Variable lesions are characterized by changes in airway lesion caliber during breathing. Depending on their location (intrathoracic or extrathoracic), they tend to behave differently during inspiration and expiration. Airway abnormalities located above the thoracic inlet (extrathoracic) are affected during inspiration because there is an increased flow of air from the atmosphere toward the lungs, resulting in a decreased intraluminal pressure respective to the atmosphere. The decrease in intraluminal pressure during inspiration causes a limitation of inspiratory flow seen as a flattening in the inspiratory limb of the flow–volume loop. During expiration, the positive pressure generated to force the air out expands the narrowed extrathoracic airway. Therefore, the maximal expiratory flow–volume curve is usually normal. Causes of variable extrathoracic lesions include vocal cord paralysis, vocal cord adhesions, vocal cord constriction, laryngeal edema, glottic strictures, and tumors.

Tracheomalacia is an intrathoracic problem, and tracheal stenosis is a fixed defect that would not produce the described change in the flow–volume loop. Emphysema would produce obstruction and a scooped-out configuration in the flow–volume loop.

References: Barreiro TJ, Perillo I. An approach to interpreting spirometry. *Am Fam Physician* 2004;69(5):1107–1114. Available at http://www.attud.org/docs/interpretingspirometry.pdf

Kapnadak S, Kreit J. Stay in the loop! *Ann Am Thorac Soc* 2013;10(2):166–171.

Pocket Guide. The global initiative for chronic obstructive disease. Available at https://goldcopd.org/wp-content/uploads/2018/11/GOLD-2019-POCKET-GUIDE-DRAFT-v1.7-14Nov2018-WMS.pdf

7 **Answer B.** This patient has airway obstruction as the FEV_1/FVC ratio is <70%. The FEV_1 at 45% of predicted indicates severe obstruction ($30\% \leq FEV_1 < 50\%$ predicted). The flow–volume loop shows flattening in both the inspiratory and expiratory phases. This is characteristic of fixed airway obstruction given the lack of changes in the obstructed airway caliber during inspiration or expiration producing a constant degree of airflow limitation during the entire respiratory cycle. A fixed lesion may be extrathoracic or intrathoracic, but the changes in the flow–volume loop are similar. Given the patient's history, the diagnosis is consistent with tracheal stenosis. Other possible causes could include goiter and tracheal tumors.

Variable intrathoracic obstruction is characterized by a flattening of the expiratory phase, whereas variable extrathoracic obstruction presents with a flattening in the inspiratory phase of the flow–volume loop. Although there is a low FVC, a low TLC is required to diagnose restriction. The flow–volume loop does not support a restrictive process.

References: Barreiro TJ, Perillo I. An approach to interpreting spirometry. *Am Fam Physician* 2004;69(5):1107–1114. Available at http://www.attud.org/docs/interpretingspirometry.pdf

Kapnadak S, Kreit J. Stay in the loop! *Ann Am Thorac Soc* 2013;10(2):166–171.

Pocket Guide. The global initiative for chronic obstructive disease. Available at https://goldcopd.org/wp-content/uploads/2018/11/GOLD-2019-POCKET-GUIDE-DRAFT-v1.7-14Nov2018-WMS.pdf

8a   Answer A.

8b   Answer C.   This patient has postbronchodilator airway obstruction as the $FEV1/FVC$ ratio is <70%. The postbronchodilator FEV_1/FVC is <70% suggesting obstruction. The FEV_1 is 76%, consistent with moderate obstruction ($50\% \leq FEV_1 < 80\%$ predicted). Significant reversibility is present following the administration of bronchodilators as there was an increase of 420 mL (>200 mL) in FEV_1 and an absolute change of 22% (>12%) of the baseline FEV_1. This study does not show a restrictive pattern.

The presence of obstruction with airway reversibility is suggestive of asthma. Asthma is the most common lung disease in pregnancy. Asthma can get worse in one-third of pregnant patients, remain unchanged in one-third, or get better in the remaining third of pregnant patients.

Primary pulmonary hypertension is a cause of low diffusion capacity but is not typically a cause of obstruction, hyperinflation, and air trapping.

The lungs are involved in more than 90% of patients who have sarcoidosis. Patients with sarcoidosis often have an abnormal pulmonary function test. Restriction is usually seen, but obstruction can be present secondary to endobronchial involvement, airway stenosis, reactivity, or distortion from parenchymal involvement.

Cystic fibrosis (CF) is a multisystemic disease and is characterized by bronchiectasis with recurring lung infections. Patients with CF usually have a fixed obstructive defect with airway reversibility.

References: Barreiro TJ, Perillo I. An approach to interpreting spirometry. *Am Fam Physician* 2004;69(5):1107–1114. Available at http://www.attud.org/docs/interpretingspirometry.pdf

Baughman RP, Culver DA, Judson MA. A concise review of pulmonary sarcoidosis. *Am J Respir Crit Care Med* 2011;183(5):573–581. Available at https://www-atsjournals org.ezproxy.uky.edu/doi/pdf/10.1164%2Frccm.201006-0865CI

Boyle MP. Adult cystic fibrosis. *JAMA* 2007;298(15):1787–1793.

Galiè N, Humbert M, Vachiery JL, et al. 2015 ESC/ERS guidelines for the diagnosis and treatment of pulmonary hypertension: the Joint Task Force for the Diagnosis and Treatment of Pulmonary Hypertension of the European Society of Cardiology (ESC) and the European Respiratory Society (ERS): Endorsed by: Association for European Paediatric and Congenital Cardiology (AEPC), International Society for Heart and Lung Transplantation (ISHLT). *Eur Heart J* 2016;37(1):67–119. Available at https://orbi.uliege.be/bitstream/2268/221319/1/ehv317.pdf

Mccallister JW. Asthma in pregnancy: management strategies. *Curr Opin Pulm Med* 2013;19(1):13–17.

Pocket Guide. The global initiative for chronic obstructive disease. Available at https://goldcopd.org/wp-content/uploads/2018/11/GOLD-2019-POCKET-GUIDE-DRAFT-v1.7-14Nov2018-WMS.pdf

9a **Answer A.**

9b **Answer B.** The low FEV1/FVC ratio (<70%) represents obstruction. The FEV1 at 51% of predicted indicates moderate obstruction (50% ≤FEV1 < 80% predicted) per GOLD staging. While evaluating a spirogram, the interpreter must interpret the values along with the flow–volume loops. Flow–volume loops offer valuable information that helps identify abnormalities in the airway physiology. The part of the loop under the x-axis corresponds to the inspiratory part, whereas the other part of the loop above the x-axis corresponds to the expiratory phase of the test. In this case, the flow–volume loop shows the classic scooped-out appearance in the expiratory phase that is characteristic of obstructive lung disease.

The total lung capacity, if reduced (<80%), indicates restriction, while hyperinflation is defined as a TLC > 120%. The patient's total lung capacity was 104% of predicted, which is within normal limits.

The CT scan of the chest shows an upper lobe–predominant and reticulonodular pattern with underlying emphysema as well as a few bizarre cysts and small nodules. The combined obstruction and air trapping associated with the findings on CT scan are compatible with pulmonary Langerhans cell histiocytosis (PLCH). This disease is caused by a proliferation of Langerhans cell infiltrates that form multiple bilateral nodules that progressively cavitate and result in bizarre pulmonary cysts, which are most prominent in the upper and middle lung zones. Lung function testing may reveal a restrictive, obstructive, or mixed pattern.

Lung metastasis may present with multiple masses that are typically well circumscribed. While GPA may involve the airways, its presentation in the lung parenchyma can be as focal consolidations, atelectasis, nodules, and cavities most often confused with either infection. Moreover, the patient denies the classic clinical symptoms associated with GPA.

Sarcoidosis presents mainly as a restrictive pattern but also can present as an obstructive or a combined pattern on spirometry. The lungs are involved in more than 90% of patients who have sarcoidosis. Patient with sarcoidosis often have an abnormal pulmonary function test. Restriction is usually seen but obstruction can be present secondary to endobronchial involvement, airway stenosis, reactivity, or distortion from parenchymal involvement. Typically, the findings on CT are upper lobe–predominant disease, but current imaging findings are not supportive of this diagnosis.

References: Barreiro TJ, Perillo I. An approach to interpreting spirometry. *Am Fam Physician* 2004;69(5):1107–1114. Available at http://www.attud.org/docs/interpretingspirometry.pdf

Baughman RP, Culver DA, Judson MA. A concise review of pulmonary sarcoidosis. *Am J Respir Crit Care Med* 2011;183(5):573–581.

Caminati A, Harari S. Smoking-related interstitial pneumonias and pulmonary Langerhans cell histiocytosis. *Proc Am Thorac Soc* 2006;3(4):299–306. Available at https://www. atsjournals.org/doi/pdf/10.1513/pats.200512-135TK

Frankel SK, Schwarz MI. The pulmonary vasculitides. *Am J Respir Crit Care Med* 2012;186(3):216–224. Available at https://www.atsjournals.org/doi/full/10.1164/rccm.201203-0539CI#readcube-epdf

Pocket Guide. The global initiative for chronic obstructive disease. Available at https:// goldcopd.org/wp-content/uploads/2018/11/GOLD-2019-POCKET-GUIDE-DRAFT-v1.7-14Nov2018-WMS.pdf

10a **Answer A.**

10b **Answer A.** This patient has obstruction as the FEV1/FVC ratio is <70%. The FEV1 at 42% of predicted indicates very severe obstruction (FEV1 < 30% predicted). The total lung capacity is markedly increased (>120%), evidencing hyperinflation. The residual volume (RV) is also significantly increased (>120%) showing air trapping. The diffusion capacity is decreased. The combined very severe obstruction, hyperinflation, and air trapping is compatible with chronic obstructive pulmonary disease. Idiopathic pulmonary fibrosis produces a restrictive defect, but it does not produce obstruction unless associated with a concomitant obstructive disease. Sarcoidosis can produce obstruction and can also be associated with restriction, but it is not commonly associated with hyperinflation. Primary pulmonary hypertension is a cause of low diffusion capacity but is not typically a cause of obstruction, hyperinflation, and air trapping.

References: Barreiro TJ, Perillo I. An approach to interpreting spirometry. *Am Fam Physician* 2004;69(5):1107–1114. Available at http://www.attud.org/docs/interpretingspirometry.pdf

Kapnadak S, Kreit J. Stay in the loop! *Ann Am Thorac Soc* 2013;10(2):166–171.

Pocket Guide. The global initiative for chronic obstructive disease. Available at https://goldcopd.org/wp-content/uploads/2018/11/GOLD-2019-POCKET-GUIDE-DRAFT-v1.7-14Nov2018-WMS.pdf

12 Diseases of the Pleura, Chest Wall, and Diaphragm

Andrea Oh, MD

QUESTIONS

1a A 63-year-old female presents with shortness of breath. What is the predominant imaging finding?

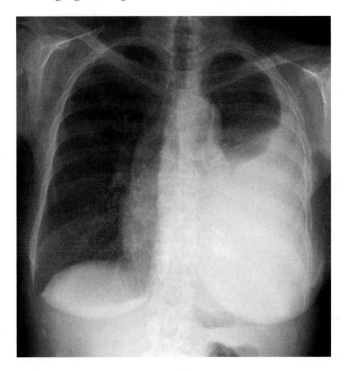

  A. Pneumonia
  B. Pleural effusion
  C. Atelectasis
  D. Cardiomegaly

1b What underlying etiology should be excluded with a massive pleural effusion?
  A. Heart failure
  B. Protein deficiency
  C. Malignancy
  D. Hemorrhage

1c What subtype of pleural effusion would you expect most often with malignancy?

    A. Transudative

    B. Chylous

    C. Hemorrhagic

    D. Exudative

1d What is the most common cause of transudative pleural effusion?

    A. Heart failure

    B. Renal failure

    C. Malignancy

    D. Pneumonia

2a What subtype of pleural effusion would you expect with this diagnosis?

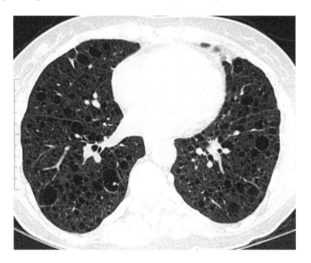

    A. Chylous

    B. Exudative

    C. Transudative

    D. Hemorrhagic

2b What type of renal lesion can be found in up to 50% of individuals with this diagnosis?

    A. Hemorrhagic cyst

    B. Angiomyolipoma

    C. Renal cell carcinoma, clear cell histology

    D. Renal cell carcinoma, papillary histology

3 Chest wall desmoid tumor is most commonly associated with which condition?

    A. Carney triad

    B. Gardner syndrome

    C. Lofgren syndrome

    D. Osler-Weber-Rendu syndrome

4   The patient is asymptomatic and afebrile. What is the most likely diagnosis?

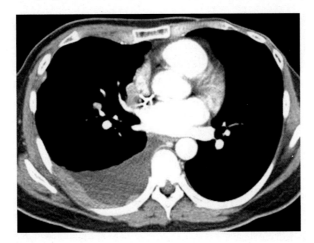

A. Empyema
B. Metastases
C. Fibrous tumor
D. Lymphoma

5a   A 54-year-old male presents with fever and chest pain. What abnormality would most likely account for the radiographic findings?

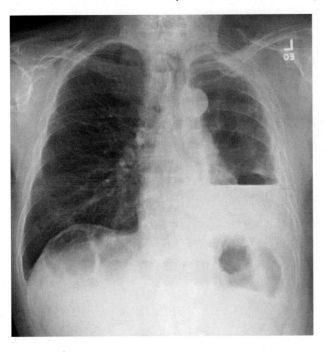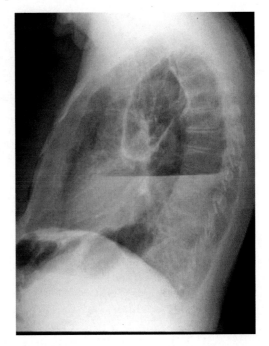

A. Bronchopleural fistula
B. Cardiogenic pulmonary edema
C. Chest wall abscess
D. Interrupted pulmonary artery

5b   Which imaging feature is most suggestive of bronchopleural fistula?

A. Volume loss
B. Exudative effusion
C. Persistent air–fluid level
D. Pleural thickening

5c A chest CT was obtained. What is the most likely diagnosis?

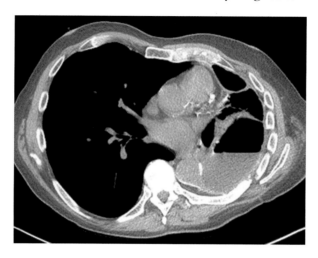

A. Simple effusion
B. Empyema
C. Hemothorax
D. Consolidation

5d What sign is demonstrated?

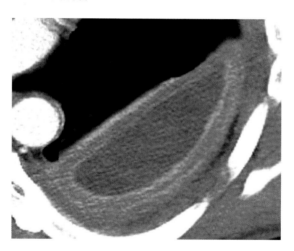

A. Luftsichel
B. Split pleura
C. Bulging fissure
D. Doughnut

5e What is the preferred management of empyema?

A. Antibiotics and close follow-up
B. Aspiration of pleural fluid
C. Antibiotics and drainage
D. Pneumonectomy

6a A 72-year-old male presents for routine evaluation. What are the radiographic findings?

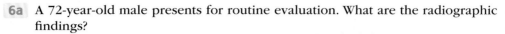

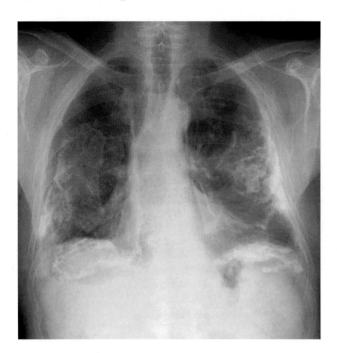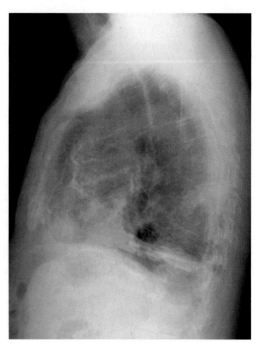

    A. Metastatic disease
    B. Calcified pleural plaques
    C. Multifocal pneumonia
    D. Calcified granulomas

6b A chest CT was obtained. What is the most likely diagnosis?

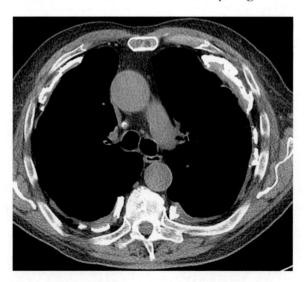

    A. Tuberculous empyema
    B. Asbestos-related pleural disease
    C. Posttraumatic pleural thickening
    D. Metastatic mesothelioma

6c Approximately when do pleural plaques occur after asbestos exposure?

    A. 1 year
    B. 5 years
    C. 20 years
    D. 40 years

7a Another patient with asbestos exposure presents to your clinic with chest pain and hemoptysis. What imaging finding is present?

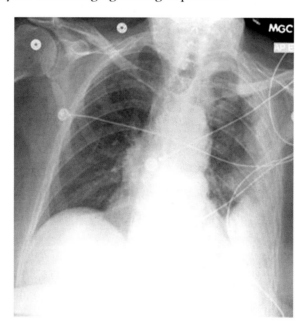

    A. Pneumothorax
    B. Dependent pleural effusion
    C. Peripheral consolidation
    D. Pleural thickening

7b A chest CT was obtained. What is the diagnosis until proven otherwise?

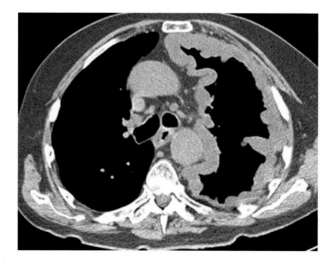

    A. Empyema
    B. Mesothelioma
    C. Hemothorax
    D. Amyloidosis

8a A 45-year-old male presents for routine physical. Where is the primary abnormality located?

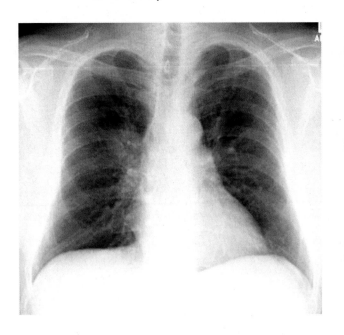 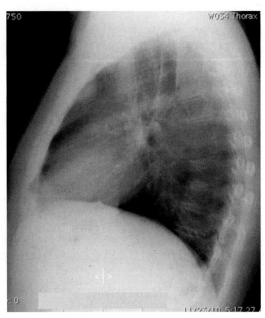

    A. Pulmonary parenchyma
    B. Chest wall or pleura
    C. Mediastinal soft tissues
    D. Osseous structures

8b What sign indicates that this abnormality does not originate within the lung?
    A. Hilum overlay
    B. Comet tail
    C. Incomplete border
    D. Air crescent

8c A chest CT was obtained. What is the diagnosis?

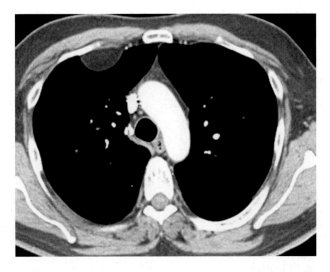

    A. Lipoma
    B. Desmoid tumor
    C. Solitary fibrous tumor
    D. Metastasis

9a An 18-year-old male presents with night sweats, cough, and a painful growing mass along his right anterior chest wall. Where did the chest wall mass originate?

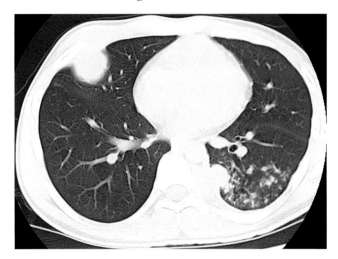 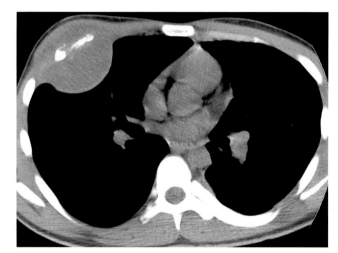

    A. Pleural cavity
    B. Bone
    C. Airway
    D. Muscle

9b What is the most likely causative organism?

    A. *Mycobacterium abscessus*
    B. *Staphylococcus aureus*
    C. *Mycobacterium tuberculosis*
    D. *Streptococcus pneumoniae*

9c What is the diagnosis?

    A. Empyema
    B. Empyema necessitans
    C. Loculated pleural effusion
    D. Lung abscess

10a A 28-year-old female presents with chest pain and shortness of breath. What is the most common thoracic manifestation of this disorder?

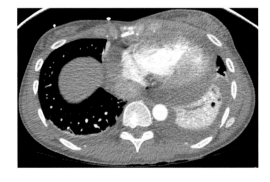 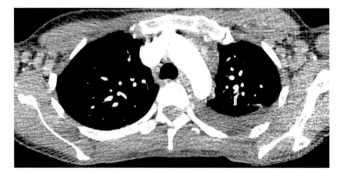

    A. Pulmonary fibrosis
    B. Alveolar hemorrhage
    C. Constrictive bronchiolitis
    D. Pleuritis

10b What type of pleural effusion would you expect?

    A. Exudative

    B. Chylous

    C. Transudative

    D. Hemorrhagic

10c What is the most likely cause of the patient's axillary lymphadenopathy?

    A. Lymphoma

    B. Reactive secondary to underlying autoimmune disease

    C. Breast cancer

    D. Sarcoidosis

11a What is the radiographic finding?

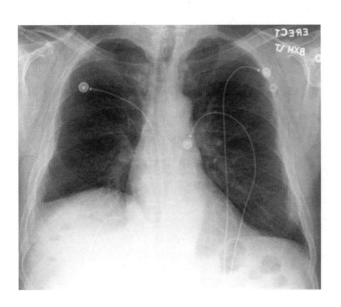
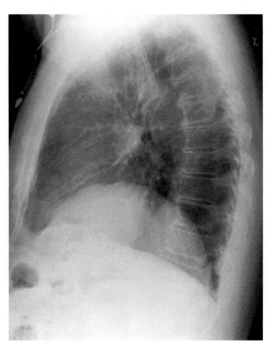

    A. Elevated hemidiaphragm

    B. Deep sulcus sign

    C. Pleural mass

    D. "V" sign of Naclerio

11b What cause of the imaging findings would be your primary consideration if this patient had a history of cardiac surgery with subsequent increased shortness of breath?

    A. Direct injury of the diaphragm

    B. Phrenic nerve injury

    C. Ischemic heart disease

    D. Esophageal rupture

11c What would be the next test of choice to confirm suspected diaphragmatic paralysis?

    A. Ventilation–perfusion scintigraphy

    B. Inspiratory–expiratory chest CT

    C. Nerve conduction studies

    D. Fluoroscopic sniff test

12 What is the finding?

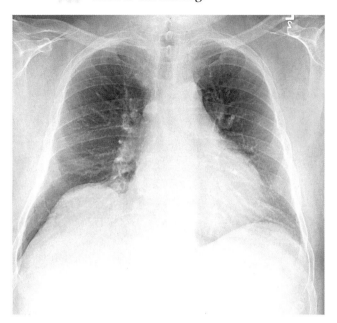 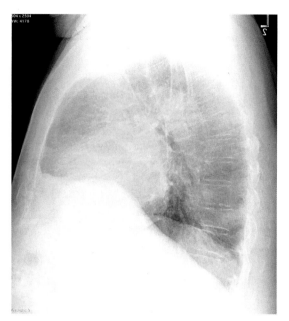

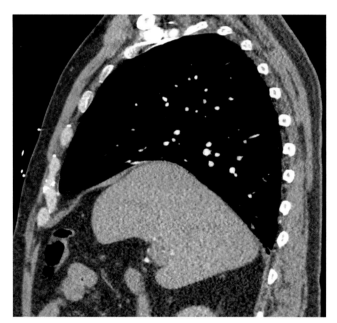

A. Diaphragmatic paralysis
B. Diaphragmatic hernia
C. Diaphragmatic eventration
D. Subpulmonic effusion

13a Having the opacity longer in length in one projection versus the orthogonal view suggests:

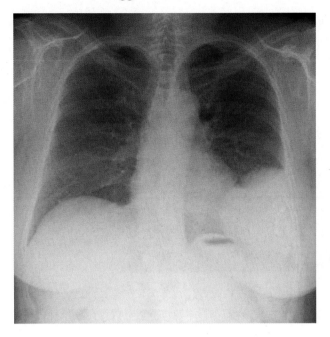
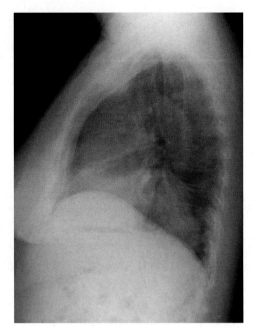

A. Lower lobe pulmonary process
B. Posttraumatic etiology
C. Extrapulmonary location
D. Subdiaphragmatic location

13b A chest CT was obtained. What imaging findings would be exclusive to solitary fibrous tumor of the pleura?

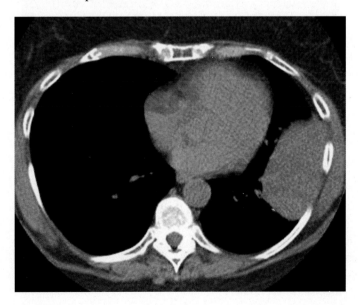

A. Fat
B. None
C. Calcification
D. Fluid

14a A 55-year-old male presents for pulmonary nodule follow-up. What is the diagnosis?

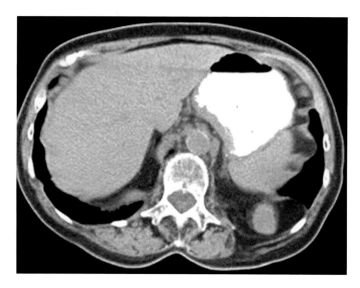

    A. Hiatus hernia
    B. Spigelian hernia
    C. Morgagni hernia
    D. Bochdalek hernia

14b A different 52-year-old male presents for routine checkup. What is the finding?

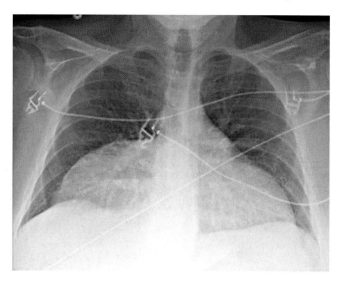

    A. Elevated hemidiaphragm
    B. Pericardial effusion
    C. Lymphadenopathy
    D. Cardiophrenic angle mass

14c A chest CT was obtained. What is the best diagnosis?

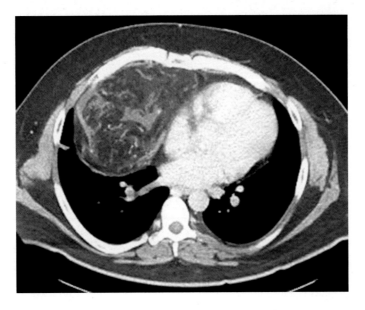

    A. Morgagni hernia
    B. Bochdalek hernia
    C. Hiatal hernia
    D. Hematoma

15a What is the primary abnormality?

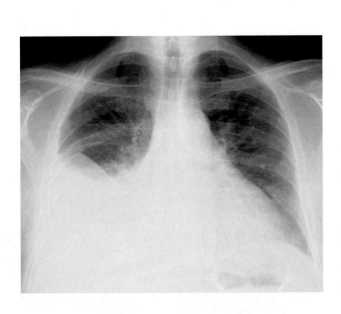
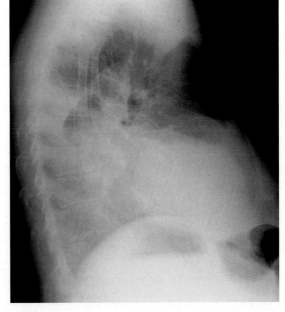

    A. Right lung consolidation
    B. Right pleural effusion
    C. Right pneumothorax
    D. Right hydropneumothorax

15b Given this CT image of the same patient, what is the cause of the right pleural effusion?

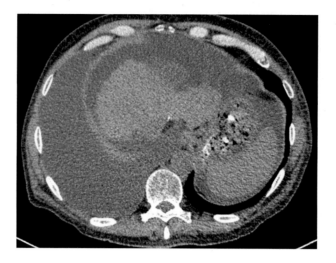

    A. Hepatic cirrhosis
    B. Heart failure
    C. Malignancy
    D. Parapneumonic

15c What percentage of hepatic hydrothoraces are bilateral?
    A. 1% to 2%
    B. 10% to 15%
    C. 50%
    D. >80%

16a A 65-year-old male who previously underwent coronary artery bypass grafting presents with midanterior chest wall pain. One month ago, he had a redo sternotomy for valve surgery. What is the diagnosis?

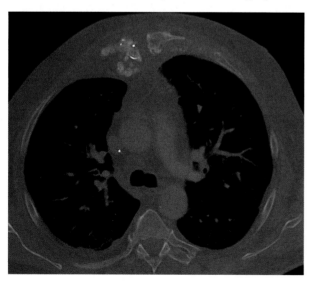
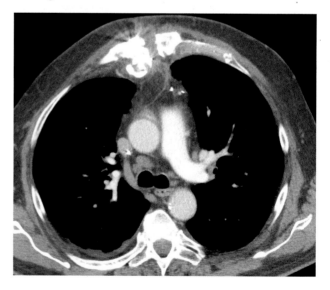

    A. Primary sternal osteomyelitis
    B. Secondary sternal osteomyelitis
    C. Normal postoperative changes
    D. Retrosternal abscess

16b What signal abnormality would a chest MR show in the bone marrow of the affected sternum?

    A. T1 hypointense, T2 hyperintense signal
    B. T1 hypointense, T2 hypointense signal
    C. T1 hyperintense, T2 hyperintense signal
    D. T1 hyperintense, T2 hypointense signal

17a What is the most likely cause of the right rib deformities?

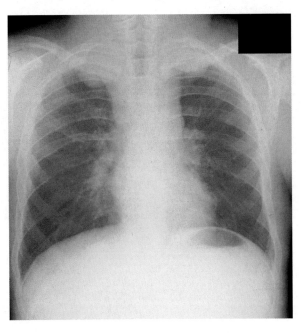

    A. Neurofibromatosis
    B. Aortic coarctation
    C. Posttraumatic fractures
    D. Metastases

17b What abnormality is associated with neurofibromatosis type 1?

    A. Cardiac rhabdomyomas
    B. Lateral meningoceles
    C. Hemiplegia
    D. Choroid plexus papillomas

18 What stage of thymoma is demonstrated?

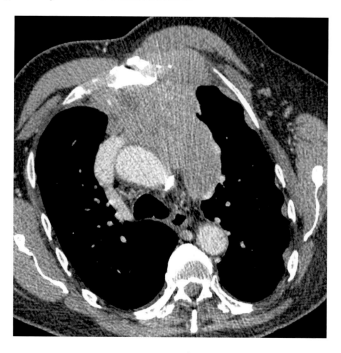

A. Stage I
B. Stage II
C. Stage III
D. Stage IV

19a What does the soft tissue focus represent?

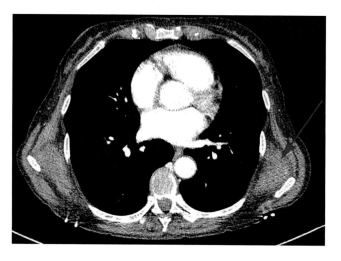

A. Normal muscle
B. Vascular malformation
C. Benign tumor
D. Malignant tumor

19b This was an incidental finding. What is the best recommendation?

    A. No follow-up

    B. Follow-up CT in 6 months

    C. Needle biopsy

    D. Surgical resection

20 CT pulmonary angiography in a 32-year-old female with shortness of breath and 5 days after oocyte retrieval following HCG administration for infertility. What is the most likely cause of the CT findings?

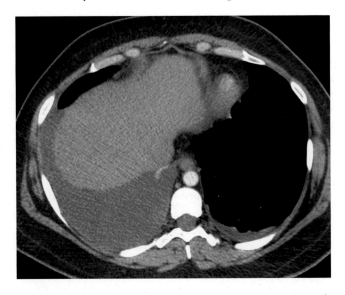

    A. Meadow syndrome

    B. Hepatic failure

    C. Ovarian hyperstimulation syndrome

    D. Meigs syndrome

ANSWERS AND EXPLANATIONS

1a **Answer B.**

1b **Answer C.**

1c **Answer D.**

1d **Answer A.**   The pleural space is composed of inner visceral and outer parietal layers. The pleural space normally holds 10 to 15 mL of fluid and is a potential space. An effusion as small as 50 mL on the lateral and 200 mL on the frontal radiograph can be detected. The most common effusion subtypes are transudative and exudative. Transudative effusions are more common, caused by increased hydrostatic or decreased oncotic pressures. Examples include heart, liver, and renal failure. Exudative effusions result from increased pleural permeability and can be seen with infection or neoplasm.

Of importance, malignancy should be excluded in the presence of a massive pleural effusion. Although only a small number of malignant effusions are massive, most massive effusions are of malignant etiology.

References: Evans AL, Gleeson FV. Radiology in pleural disease: state of the art. *Respirology* 2004;9:300–312.

Kuhlman JE, Singha NK. Complex disease of the pleural space: radiographic and CT evaluation. *Radiographics* 1997;17:63–79.

Maskell NA, Butland RJ. BTS guidelines for the investigation of a unilateral pleural effusion in adults. *Thorax* 2003;58:8–17.

2a **Answer A.**   Chylous effusions are a rare subtype of pleural effusion caused by thoracic duct (or its tributaries) disruption or lymphatic obstruction resulting in leakage of chyle into the pleural space. Causes include lymphangioleiomyomatosis (LAM), lymphangiomatosis, and lymphoma, among others. This case demonstrates the typical appearance of LAM with diffuse cystic lung disease.

References: Evans AL, Gleeson FV. Radiology in pleural disease: state of the art. *Respirology* 2004;9:300–312.

Kuhlman JE, Singha NK. Complex disease of the pleural space: radiographic and CT evaluation. *Radiographics* 1997;17:63–79.

Maskell NA, Butland RJ. BTS guidelines for the investigation of a unilateral pleural effusion in adults. *Thorax* 2003;58:8–17.

2b **Answer B.**   LAM is a rare interstitial lung disease predominantly affecting women and can occur either sporadically or in association with tuberous sclerosis complex (TSC). Abdominal findings may be present in more than 70% of patients with LAM, with the most common finding being a renal angiomyolipoma. Angiomyolipomas are often small (<1 cm), multiple, bilateral, and asymptomatic. They occur in up to 50% of patients with LAM.

References: Abbott GF, Rosado-de-Christenson ML, Frazier AA, et al. Lymphangioleiomyomatosis: radiologic-pathologic correlation. *Radiographics* 2005;25:803–828.

Pallisa E, Pilar S, Roman A, et al. Lymphangioleiomyomatosis: pulmonary and abdominal findings with pathologic correlation. *Radiographics* 2002;22:S185–S198.

3 **Answer B.**   Chest wall desmoid tumor, also called aggressive fibromatosis, is the most common low-grade sarcoma of the chest wall. While this lesion does not metastasize, it is infiltrative and can even invade the intrathoracic cavity. Desmoid tumors have several associations, the most common being Gardner syndrome and trauma. On imaging, desmoid tumors can have variable density on CT, signal lower than muscle on T1, and intermediate signal on T2.

The alternative options have associate thoracic lesions. Carney triad is pulmonary chondromas, extra-adrenal paragangliomas, and gastrointestinal stromal tumors. Lofgren syndrome is sarcoidosis with thoracic adenopathy, erythema nodosum, and arthralgia. Finally, Osler-Weber-Rendu syndrome manifests with multiple arteriovenous malformations and mucocutaneous telangiectasias.

Reference: Tateishi U, Gladish GW, Kusumoto M, et al. Chest wall tumors: radiologic findings and pathologic correlation. *Radiographics* 2003;23:1491–1508.

4   **Answer B.**   This case demonstrates enhancing pleural nodules and pleural thickening in association with the moderate-sized effusion. This is a case of metastatic pleural disease from a breast malignancy. Metastatic disease to the pleura may manifest as effusion, thickening, or nodularity. While pleural soft tissue nodularity may suggest the diagnosis, pleural effusion without nodules does NOT exclude the diagnosis of metastatic pleural involvement. Lung and breast are the two most common origins of metastatic malignancies to the pleura.

Top differentials for pleural nodularity include metastases (most common), lymphoma, fibrous tumor, mesothelioma, and invasive thymoma.

References: Dynes MC, White EM, Fry WA, et al. Imaging manifestations of pleural tumors. *Radiographics* 1992;12:1191–1201.

Hussein-Jelen T, Bankier AA, Eisenberg RL. Solid pleural lesions. *AJR Am J Roentgenol* 2012;198:W512–W520.

5a   **Answer A.**

5b   **Answer C.**

5c   **Answer B.**

5d   **Answer B.**

5e   **Answer C.**   Empyema refers to an infected, purulent collection within the pleural space, which can be life threatening. Empyema often develops secondary to pneumonia with parapneumonic effusion, which later becomes infected. As discussed, infection causes increased pleural permeability, which may result in pleural fluid accumulation.

The split pleura sign is associated with empyema. This sign results from separation of the visceral and parietal pleura, which become thickened and inflamed. Contrast-enhanced imaging often shows pleural enhancement.

Preferred treatment consists of appropriate medical therapy and drainage. This typically consists of antibiotics and thoracostomy tube placement. Complicated empyemas (i.e., internal septation or loculation) may need multiple chest tubes or surgical debridement.

Bronchopleural fistula refers to abnormal communication between the bronchial tree and pleural space. This can be seen with many causes, including infection or empyema as in this case. This abnormality accounts for the air–fluid level seen on imaging and is suspected when attempted drainage fails to clear the pneumothorax component. Another potential complication of empyema is extrathoracic extension, referred to as empyema necessitans.

References: Kraus GJ. The split pleura sign. *Radiographics* 2007;243:297–298.

Kuhlman JE, Singha NK. Complex disease of the pleural space: radiographic and CT evaluation. *Radiographics* 1997;17:63–79.

Stark DD, Federle MP. Differentiating lung abscess and empyema: radiography and computed tomography. *AJR Am J Roentgenol* 1983;141:163–137.

6a   Answer B.

6b   Answer B.

6c   Answer C.   Asbestos-related disease of the lung and pleura may be neoplastic and nonneoplastic. Findings generally take years to manifest, although recent data from asbestos exposures in Libby, Montana, have demonstrated pleural disease in shorter time periods and younger patients. Pleural effusion is one of the earliest findings and may present within 10 years of exposure (effusion may be hemorrhagic). Pleural plaques (with or without calcification) are the most common manifestation, generally occurring 20 to 30 years postexposure. Common distribution sites include the chest wall underlying the ribs and diaphragm.

Important ancillary findings associated with asbestos-related lung disease include rounded atelectasis, asbestosis (parenchymal manifestations of exposure), mesothelioma, and bronchogenic carcinoma. Individuals who smoke have significantly increased risk (50 times or more) of developing primary lung neoplasm.

References: Larson TC, Meyer CA, Kapil V, et al. Workers with Libby amphibole exposure: retrospective identification and progression of radiographic changes. *Radiology* 2010;255(3):924–933.

Roach HD, Davies GJ. Asbestos: when the dust settles—an imaging review of asbestos-related disease. *Radiographics* 2002;22:167–184.

7a   Answer D.

7b   Answer B.   Mesothelioma is the most common primary pleural malignancy and has a delayed presentation, often 35 to 40 years after asbestos exposure. Characteristic imaging shows extensive, circumferential pleural thickening, usually several centimeters thick. Note the extension along the mediastinal pleura as well as the fissural extension, much more common in malignant pleural thickening than benign pleural thickening. Pleural effusion may also be seen, and delayed development (more than 20 years after exposure) of a pleural effusion in the setting of asbestos exposure should raise concern for the diagnosis. Mesothelioma is not thought to arise from preexisting plaques.

Reference: Wang ZJ, Reddy GP. Malignant pleural mesothelioma: evaluation with CT, MR imaging, and PET. *Radiographics* 2004;24:105–119.

8a   Answer B.

8b   Answer C.

8c   Answer A.   Pleural or chest wall lipomas are benign fatty lesions. Radiographs show an abnormality along the anterior chest wall demonstrating the incomplete border sign, indicating this lesion cannot originate with the lung. The lesion creates obtuse margins on the lateral radiograph, also suggesting extraparenchymal origin. Additionally, this case demonstrates a positive hilum overlay sign indicating that the opacity on frontal view does not reside in the hilum, but does not necessarily indicate pleural or chest wall location. CT characterizes this lesion as fat, confirming the diagnosis of lipoma.

Reference: Mullan CP, Rachna M. Radiology of chest wall masses. *AJR Am J Roentgenol* 2011;197:460–470.

9a **Answer A.**

9b **Answer C.**

9c **Answer B.** Empyema necessitans is a complication of pulmonary infection, most frequently secondary to *Mycobacterium tuberculosis* infection, although it can also occur with actinomycosis and pyogenic bacterial infection. It starts with infected pleural fluid (empyema), which then leaks through the parietal pleura with spread of contents into the subcutaneous tissues of the chest wall or, less commonly, into the pericardium, vertebral column, or esophagus. With chest wall involvement, subcutaneous fluid collections and osseous destruction can occur, as demonstrated by this case with abscess formation and rib involvement. Management involves a combination of antituberculous therapy, abscess drainage, and surgical intervention.

References: Jeong YJ, Lee KS. Pulmonary tuberculosis: up-to-date imaging and management. *AJR Am J Roentgenol* 2008;191:834–844.

Nachiappan AC, Rahbar K, Shi X, et al. Pulmonary tuberculosis: role of radiology in diagnosis and management. *Radiographics* 2017;37:52–72.

10a **Answer D.**

10b **Answer A.**

10c **Answer B.** CT images show pericardial and pleural effusions in this patient with systemic lupus erythematosus (SLE), an autoimmune disorder that primarily affects women. One of the diagnostic criteria established by the World Health Organization (WHO) includes serositis (pericardial and pleural effusions). The most common thoracic manifestation of SLE is pleuritis with clinically apparent pleural effusion being reported in up to 50% of patients. Effusions are usually bilateral and are invariably exudative. Exudative pericardial effusions and pericarditis can occur in up to 50% of patients.

CT demonstrates bilateral enlarged axillary lymph nodes. Lymphadenopathy is oftentimes a benign finding in SLE, commonly seen in young patients at the onset of disease or in association with an exacerbation. Biopsies show reactive follicular hyperplasia and necrosis. There is usually a good response to corticosteroids.

References: Keane MP, Lynch JP III. Pleuropulmonary manifestations of systemic lupus erythematosus. *Thorax* 2000;55:159–166.

Kojima M, Motoori T, Asano S, et al. Histological diversity of reactive and atypical proliferative lymph node lesions in systemic lupus erythematosus patients. *Pathol Res Pract* 2007;203:423–431.

Lalani TA, Kanne JP, Hatfield GA, et al. Imaging findings in systemic lupus erythematosus. *Radiographics* 2004;24:1069–1086.

11a **Answer A.**

11b **Answer B.**

11c **Answer D.** Radiographic images show elevation of the right hemidiaphragm (which is normally slightly higher than the left). The diaphragm separates the chest from the abdomen and is the primary muscle of respiration. An elevated hemidiaphragm may have many causes. Phrenic nerve (which innervates the diaphragm) injury is a common etiology, often resulting from surgery, trauma, or tumor invasion. Diaphragmatic eventration refers to asymmetric thinning of diaphragm muscle, typically involving only a segment, producing a focal bulge.

Diaphragmatic paralysis can be confirmed using the fluoroscopic sniff test. A positive exam demonstrates a normal functioning contralateral hemidiaphragm with paradoxical motion of the affected hemidiaphragm as the patient sniffs, which results from negative intrathoracic pressure during rapid inspiration. CT of the chest may be warranted to exclude an underlying process such as malignancy, but does not directly evaluate the hemidiaphragm for paralysis.

Differentials for an apparent elevated hemidiaphragm include normal expiration, congenital hypoplastic lung, decreased lung volume from atelectasis or lung resection, subpulmonic effusion, and mass effect from abdominal neoplasm or organomegaly.

References: Nason LK, Walker CM. Imaging of the diaphragm: anatomy and function. *Radiographics* 2012;32:E51–E70.

Verhey PT, Gosselin MV. Differentiating diaphragmatic paralysis and eventration. *Acad Radiol* 2007;4:420–425.

12   Answer C.   Radiographic images show focal elevation of the right hemidiaphragm. CT of the chest demonstrates thinning of the diaphragm in the region of elevation with normal continuity, confirming the diagnosis of diaphragmatic eventration. True diaphragmatic eventration is a congenital developmental defect in the muscular portion of the diaphragm with preserved attachments to the sternum, ribs, and lumbar spine. Diaphragmatic eventration is rare (incidence <0.05%), is more common in males, and more often affects the left hemidiaphragm. Diaphragmatic eventration can be bilateral, unilateral, total, and localized. Pathologically, the eventrated portion has diffuse fibroelastic changes and a paucity of muscle fibers, whereas patients who have diaphragmatic paralysis have a normal amount of muscle fibers, albeit atrophic. Most adults with eventration are asymptomatic, though some can have exertional dyspnea. Further evaluation is not necessary in asymptomatic patients. Fluoroscopy with sniff testing typically shows normal or slightly reduced diaphragmatic motion on the affected side.

References: Groth SS, Andrade RS. Diaphragmatic eventration. *Thorac Surg Clin* 2009;19:511–519.

Kansal AP, Chopra V, Chahal AS, et al. Right-sided diaphragmatic eventration: a rare entity. *Lung India* 2009;26(2):48–50.

13a   Answer C.

13b   Answer B.   Radiographs show a peripheral, defined mass with an incomplete border and dimension that are much greater in the anteroposterior diameter versus the lateral width on frontal view. The incomplete border sign suggests extrapulmonary origin (obtuse margins also suggest extraparenchymal origin, and acute margins suggest parenchymal origin). The asymmetric dimensions on frontal and lateral are more characteristic of a pleural lesion, and using the same logic with air–fluid levels assists in differentiating pulmonary abscess from empyema. CT demonstrates a well-defined, homogeneous pleural mass. The pathologic diagnosis of fibrous tumor of the pleura was obtained (also known as solitary or localized fibrous tumor).

Fibrous tumor of the pleura is a rare diagnosis most common in adults (fourth through sixth decades). Imaging features depend on size and tumor aggression. Benign and malignant forms exist, benign being more common. Small nonaggressive tumors tend to be homogeneous with obtuse margins and lack chest wall extension. Larger lesions can become heterogeneous and show more acute margins, mimicking pulmonary mass. Malignant forms may have chest wall or bony involvement. Enhancement is typical, and calcifications are rare. Pedunculated forms with fibrovascular stalk can be seen. No imaging finding of the primary lesion is specific for solitary fibrous tumor of the pleura, and no finding differentiates benign versus malignant short of metastatic lesions. Some may demonstrate systemic symptoms in relation to fibrous tumors including hypertrophic osteoarthropathy and in some cases hypoglycemia. Treatment of localized fibrous tumors of the pleura is surgical resection, with a recurrence rate of up to 15%.

PET/CT may demonstrate low-grade FDG uptake in benign forms and more avid uptake in malignant forms. Malignant lesions may be multiple and show a recurrence rate up to 63%. Differentials include metastasis, mesothelioma, and lymphoma.

References: Ginat DT, Bokhari A, Bhatt S, et al. Imaging features of solitary fibrous tumors. *AJR Am J Roentgenol* 2011;196:487–495.

Luciano C, Francesco A, Giovanni V. CT signs, patterns and differential diagnosis of solitary fibrous tumors of the pleura. *J Thorac Dis* 2010;2:21–25.

Rosado-de-Christenson ML, Abbott GF, McAdams HP, et al. From the archives of the AFIP: localized fibrous tumor of the pleura. *Radiographics* 2003;23:759–783.

14a **Answer D.**

14b **Answer D.**

14c **Answer A.**   These cases demonstrate both congenital diaphragmatic hernias, Bochdalek and Morgagni. The first case shows a small Bochdalek hernia containing fat and a small portion of bowel. The second case demonstrates a large cardiophrenic opacity on chest radiograph with subsequent CT, revealing a large Morgagni hernia containing fat and engorged vasculature, likely from omentum.

Bochdalek hernias are far more common, occurring through the foramen of Bochdalek. These are typically unilateral and occur posteriorly on the left. They can also be seen on the right, or may be bilateral. Morgagni hernias occur along the anteromedial right hemidiaphragm. Differentials for right cardiophrenic angle mass on chest radiography include Morgagni hernia, pericardial cyst, lymphadenopathy, and pericardial/mediastinal fat.

References: Mullins ME, Stein J, Saini CC, et al. Prevalence of incidental Bochdalek's hernia in a large adult population. *AJR Am J Roentgenol* 2001;177:363–366.

Sandstrom CK, Stern EJ. Diaphragmatic hernias: a spectrum of radiographic appearances. *Curr Probl Diagn Radiol* 2011;3:95–115.

15a **Answer B.**

15b **Answer A.**

15c **Answer A.**   The chest x-ray demonstrates a large layering right effusion. There is no air–fluid level or pleural line to suggest a pleural air component. The associated CT demonstrates significant liver cirrhosis and ascites, confirming the likely etiology as hepatic hydrothorax.

Hepatic hydrothorax is defined as a significant effusion in the setting of cirrhosis without other identifiable causes. Overall, it is uncommon (5% to 10% of cirrhotic patients), although centers that treat a large number of liver disease patients may see this frequently. The most accepted etiology is leakage of ascitic fluid through small defects in the diaphragm. The majority of hepatic hydrothorax cases are right sided (85%). Only 10% to 15% of causes are left sided with <2% being bilateral. Note that the absence of ascites does not exclude this disease as the normal intra-abdominal and intrathoracic pressure gradient can preferentially fill the pleural space in some cases.

Reference: Kim YK, Kim Y, Shim SS. Thoracic complications of liver cirrhosis: radiologic findings. *Radiographics* 2009;29(3):825–837.

16a **Answer B.**

16b **Answer A.**   CT demonstrates nonunion of the sternum with areas of cortical erosion and destruction of the sternotomy site with bony sequestra and surrounding soft tissue stranding.

Secondary osteomyelitis of the sternum is a rare complication of sternotomy. Up to 2% of patients who undergo sternotomy for heart surgery develop secondary osteomyelitis. This is a potentially severe complication due to the risk of mediastinitis. Risk factors include obesity, diabetes, and internal mammary artery grafts. Organisms involved usually include gram-positive cocci, gram-negative bacilli, and less commonly nontuberculous mycobacteria. This patient had *Mycobacterium abscessus* cultured from his wound.

Primary osteomyelitis of the sternum is uncommon and may occur in patients with a history of intravenous drug abuse, acquired immunodeficiency syndrome, or other immune deficiency states.

MR imaging in sternal osteomyelitis include a lack of signal hypointensity in cortical bone and hypointense signal on T1-weighted images and hyperintense signal on T2-weighted images in the affected bone marrow.

References: Hota P, Dass C, Erkmen C, et al. Poststernotomy complications: a multimodal review of normal and abnormal postoperative imaging findings. *AJR Am J Roentgenol* 2018;211:1194–1205.

Restrepo CS, Martinez S, Lemos DF, et al. Imaging appearances of the sternum and sternoclavicular joints. *Radiographics* 2009;29:839–859.

Sarma S, Sharma S, Baweja UK, et al. *Mycobacterium abscessus* bacteremia in an immunocompetent patient following a coronary artery bypass graft. *J Cardiovasc Dis Res* 2011;2:80–82.

17a **Answer A.**

17b **Answer B.**   While many indolent conditions can cause resorptive changes of the ribs, few cause multilevel erosions. Neither traumatic fractures nor metastases would result in the rib changes seen. Aortic coarctation can cause "rib notching" similar to the findings here, but the chest radiograph also reveals biapical mass lesions as well as subpleural lesions along the inner aspects of the lateral ribs. These findings are consistent with "ribbon ribs" of neurofibromatosis.

Neurofibromatosis type 1 (NF1 or von Recklinghausen disease) is the most common phakomatosis, commonly manifesting with cutaneous neurofibromas, café au lait spots, freckling, optic nerve gliomas, sphenoid wing dysplasia, and other characteristic bony changes. Accompanying NF1, the inactivation of tumor suppression results in multiple different potential tumors, although the potential tumors provided as alternative answers are associated with other phakomatoses (cardiac rhabdomyomas–tuberous sclerosis and choroid plexus papillomas–von Hippel-Lindau disease). Hemiplegia is associated with Sturge-Weber syndrome. Finally, dural ectasia and lateral meningoceles are associated with neurofibromatosis type 1, commonly seen with associated scoliosis.

Reference: Rossi SE, Erasmus JJ, McAdams HP, et al. Thoracic manifestations of neurofibromatosis-I. *AJR Am J Roentgenol* 1999;173:1631–1638.

18 **Answer D.**   A large anterior mediastinal mass at the root of the aorta and projecting to one side is demonstrated on CT with multiple associated left pleural lesions representing "drop metastases." The combination is most consistent with thymoma with direct invasion into the left pleural space. By the Masaoka-Koga staging of thymoma, pleural and pericardial disseminations indicate stage IVa disease with hematogenous metastases, representing stage IVb disease. The distinction between stage IVa and IVb diseases is the difference between neoadjuvant chemotherapy and surgical resection (with or without radiation therapy) and palliative chemotherapy, respectively.

Reference: Benveniste MFK, Rosado-de-Christensen ML, Sabloff BS, et al. Role of imaging in the diagnosis, staging, and treatment of thymoma. *Radiographics* 2011;31:1847–1861.

19a **Answer C.**

19b **Answer A.**   Elastofibroma dorsi is a benign tumor of the chest wall that occurs in the infrascapular region deep to the adjacent musculature. In this case, the lesions are relatively symmetric, although they can be asymmetric or unilateral. Elastofibroma dorsi is most common in elderly women, and some have postulated that mechanical friction is the cause of the right-side predominance of unilateral lesions. The characteristic location and CT appearance are sufficient for diagnosis, particularly in bilateral cases such as this, and require no further follow-up in the asymptomatic patient. Some cases of elastofibroma dorsi do cause symptoms of shoulder pain or "snapping" scapula, for which resection may be considered.

References: Naylor MF, Nascimento AG, Sherrick AD, et al. Elastofibroma dorsi: radiologic findings in 12 patients. *AJR Am J Roentgenol* 1996;167:683–687.

Ochsner JE, Sewall SA, Brooks GN, et al. Best cases from the AFIP: elastofibroma dorsi. *Radiographics* 2006;26:1873–1876.

20 **Answer C.**   Right greater than left pleural effusions are shown on CT pulmonary angiogram. With the clinical history and patient symptoms, the constellation is consistent with ovarian hyperstimulation syndrome (OHSS). The syndrome occurs around 6 days following oocyte retrieval and manifests with enlargement of the ovaries with third spacing of fluid. Severity is classified as mild (ovarian enlargement with abdominal symptoms), moderate (evidence of ascites on imaging), and severe (ascites or hydrothorax with respiratory symptoms, hemoconcentration, or coagulopathy). Most cases are uncomplicated with supportive measures provided until resolution around 12 days after HCG administration. More common complications include pulmonary embolism, ARDS, and pulmonary infection.

Reference: McNeary M, Stark P. Radiographic findings in ovarian hyperstimulation syndrome. *J Thorac Imaging* 2002;17:230–232.

13 Mediastinal Disease

Lara Walkoff, MD

QUESTIONS

1a What best explains the radiographic appearance below?

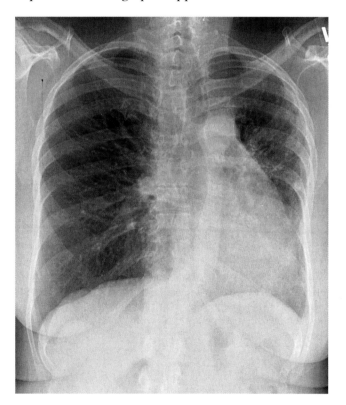

A. Consolidation
B. Cardiomegaly
C. Pulmonary volume loss
D. Pneumothorax

1b Pre- and post-IV contrast CT images provided are oblique MPR contrast images through the right and left pulmonary arteries. What diagnosis best explains the findings?

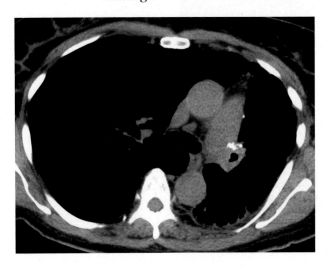
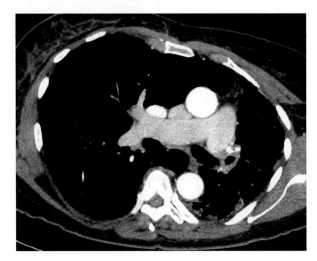

    A. Chronic pulmonary embolism
    B. Fibrosing mediastinitis
    C. Untreated lymphoma
    D. Takayasu arteritis

1c What is the most common cause of fibrosing mediastinitis in the United States?
    A. Histoplasmosis
    B. Idiopathic
    C. Tuberculosis
    D. Radiation

2a Given the CT findings, what is the patient's most likely presenting symptom?

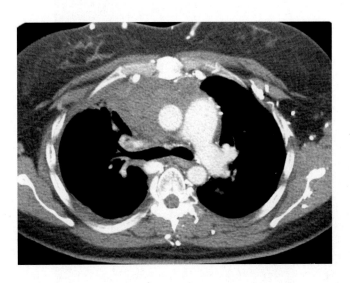
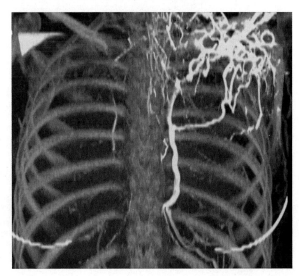

    A. Stridor
    B. Facial swelling
    C. Mental status changes
    D. Nausea

2b Additional CT image from the same study. What is the salient finding?

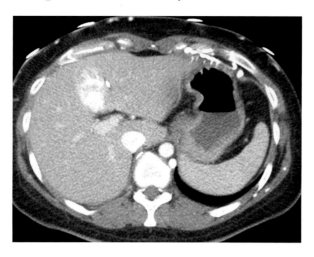

    A. Porcelain gallbladder
    B. Splenic enlargement
    C. Focal hepatic enhancement
    D. Gastric wall thickening

2c What is the most common cause of superior vena cava syndrome?

    A. Cancer
    B. Iatrogenic
    C. Fibrosing mediastinitis
    D. Behcet disease

3a What mediastinal compartment is abnormal?

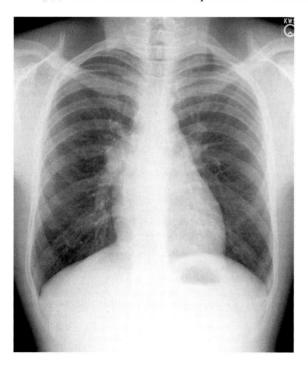
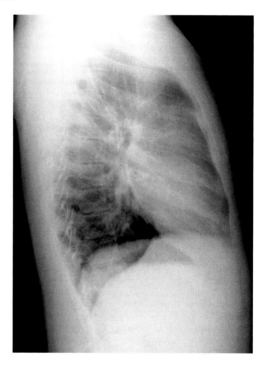

    A. Superior
    B. Anterior
    C. Middle
    D. Posterior

3b Which CT imaging characteristic in this case is typical for thymoma?

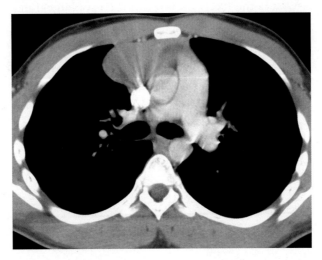

    A. Partial fat attenuation
    B. Pleural metastasis
    C. Projects to one side of the mediastinum
    D. Calcification

3c Excision of the lesion reveals thymoma. Which of the following would be the most common associated condition?

    A. Ischemic heart disease
    B. Hypogammaglobulinemia
    C. Pure red cell aplasia
    D. Myasthenia gravis

4 These two contrast-enhanced CTs were separated in time by 2 weeks (earlier on the left). What is the most likely diagnosis?

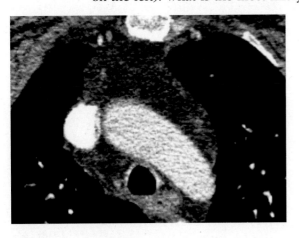 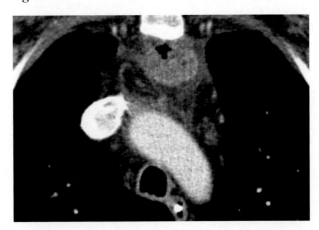

    A. Thymoma
    B. Thymic carcinoma
    C. Mediastinal abscess
    D. Normal thymus

5 What is the most common source of pneumomediastinum in the setting of ARDS?

    A. Alveolar rupture
    B. Extension from pneumothorax
    C. Tracheal rupture from endotracheal tube cuff overinflation
    D. Esophageal rupture

6   An esophageal mass is identified in this patient with a known retroperitoneal liposarcoma. What is the likely etiology of the esophageal mass?

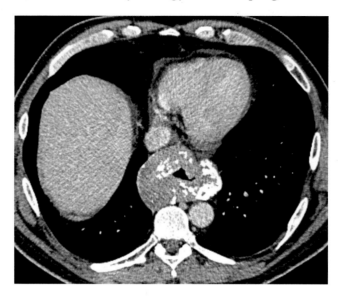

A. Liposarcoma metastasis
B. Primary esophageal carcinoma
C. Esophageal leiomyoma
D. Esophageal lymphoma

7a   In what mediastinal space is the abnormality based on these chest x-rays?

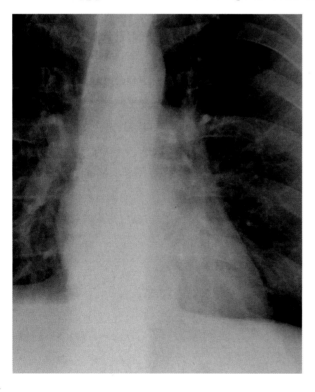
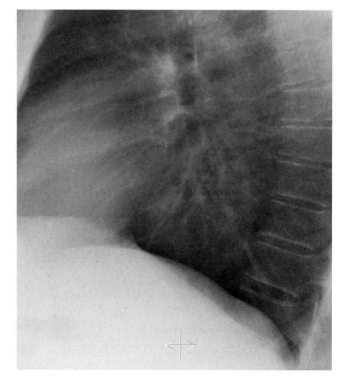

A. Anterior
B. Middle
C. Posterior
D. Superior

7b Based on the corresponding CT, what is the cause of the middle mediastinal opacity on chest x-ray?

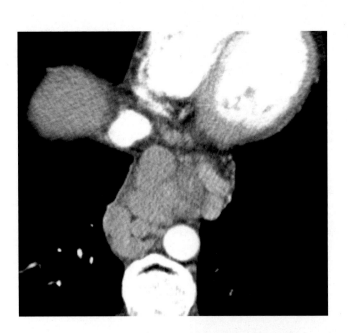
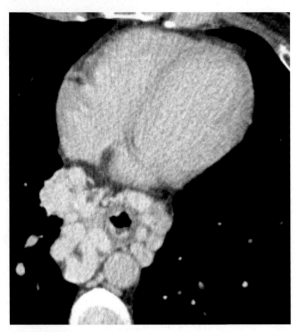
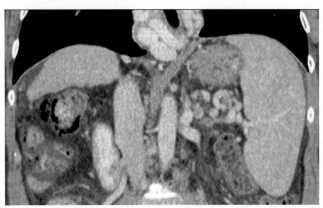

A. Esophageal cancer
B. Esophageal varices
C. Lymphadenopathy
D. Mediastinitis

8a Which of these complications is most common in the setting of a proximal esophageal rupture?

A. Right pleural effusion
B. Left pleural effusion
C. Pneumopericardium
D. Left hydropneumothorax

8b What is the most common feature identified on initial radiograph after esophageal perforation?

A. Mediastinal widening
B. Pneumomediastinum
C. Left pleural effusion
D. Right pleural effusion

9a Based on this CT, what is the most likely diagnosis?

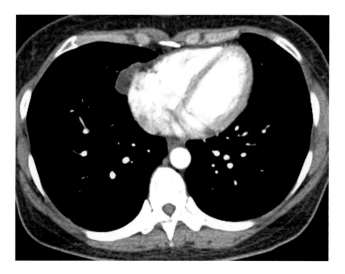

A. Pericardial nodule
B. Pericardial cyst
C. Loculated pleural effusion
D. Pleural implant

9b If clinical scenario warrants, what is the next best imaging modality for confirmation?

A. MRI
B. PET/CT
C. Radiographs
D. Echocardiography

9c An MRI was performed, based on this. What is the likely diagnosis?

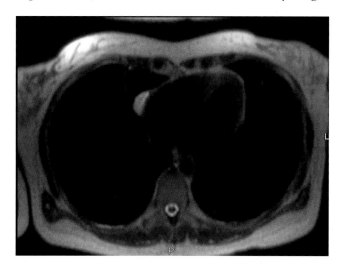

A. Pericardial nodule
B. Pericardial cyst
C. Loculated pleural effusion
D. Pleural implant

10a On the evaluation of these radiographs, what is the best diagnosis?

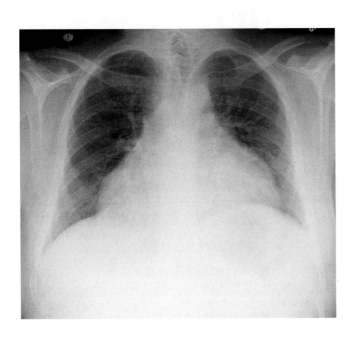
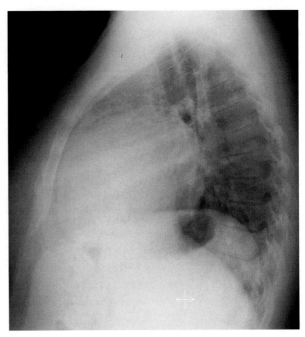

    A. Cardiomegaly
    B. Anterior mediastinal mass
    C. Pneumomediastinum
    D. Pericardial effusion

10b What is the upper limit of normal for volume of pericardial fluid?

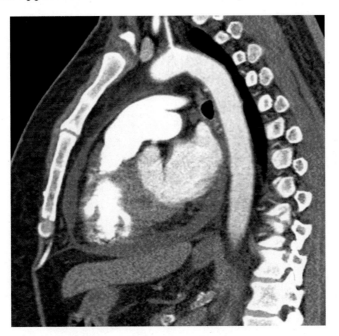

    A. 5 mL
    B. 50 mL
    C. 100 mL
    D. 200 mL

11a What is the most likely diagnosis?

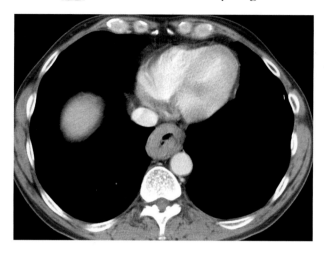
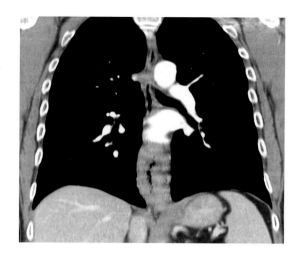

    A. Esophageal duplication cyst
    B. Esophageal varices
    C. Esophageal carcinoma
    D. Barrett esophagus

11b Endoscopy with biopsy confirms esophageal carcinoma. If the CT demonstrates direct invasion of the adjacent lung, what tumor category would it be?

    A. T1
    B. T2
    C. T3
    D. T4

12a Given the salient abnormality on this axial CT, what is the next best step?

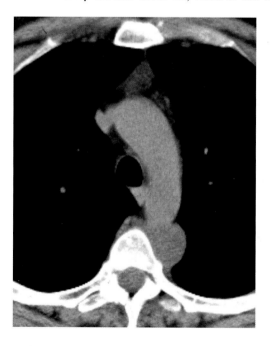

    A. PET/CT
    B. MRI
    C. Follow-up CT in 1 year
    D. CT-guided biopsy

12b An MRI was performed with T1-weighted imaging (left), T2-weighted imaging (middle), and T1 postcontrast imaging (right). What is the likely diagnosis?

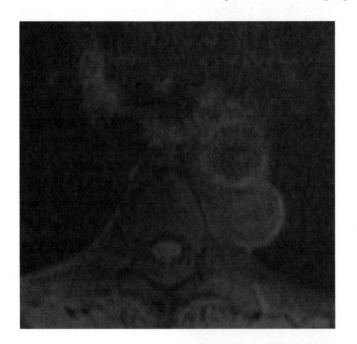

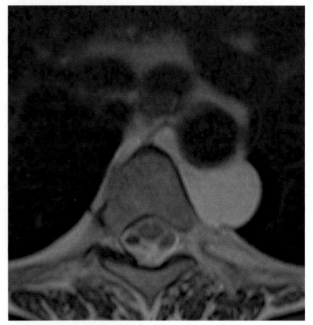

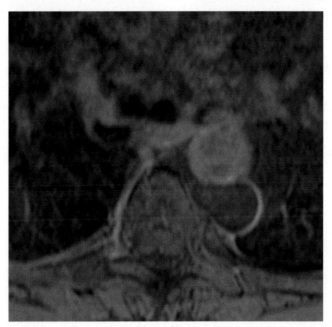

A. Schwannoma
B. Pleural metastasis
C. Foregut duplication cyst
D. Descending aortic pseudoaneurysm

13a In which mediastinal compartment is the lesion?

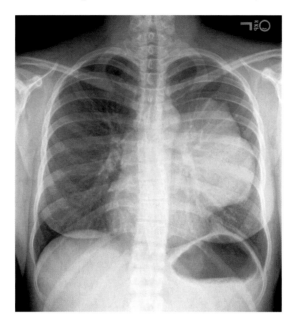

A. Anterior
B. Superior
C. Posterior
D. Middle

13b What is the most likely diagnosis?

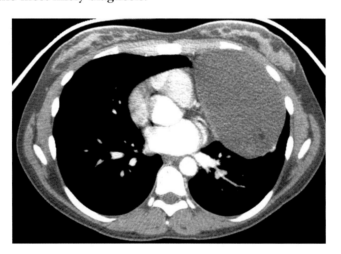

A. Thymoma
B. Teratoma
C. Pericardial cyst
D. Lymphoma

13c What is the most common extragonadal location of germ cell tumors?
A. Retroperitoneum
B. Mediastinum
C. Intraperitoneum
D. Head and neck

14a What is the best recommendation based on the image alone?

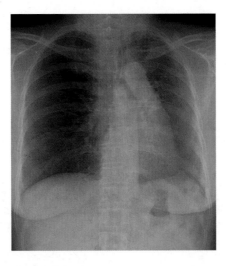

    A. No follow-up
    B. Surveillance radiograph in 6 to 8 weeks
    C. Chest CT
    D. Chest tube placement

14b Which diagnosis best matches the CT findings?

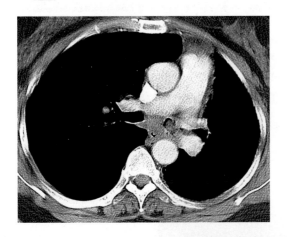
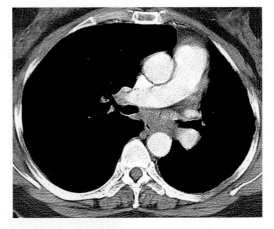
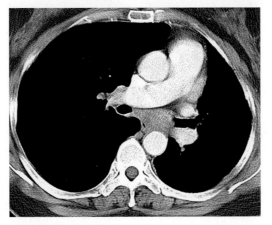

    A. Pulmonary embolism
    B. Endobronchial mass
    C. Aortic aneurysm
    D. Duplication cyst

14c What is the most common tracheal tumor?

    A. Bronchial carcinoid
    B. Adenoid cystic carcinoma
    C. Mucoepidermoid carcinoma
    D. Squamous cell carcinoma

15a What diagnosis is most likely?

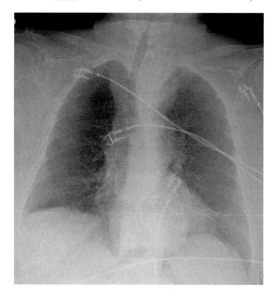 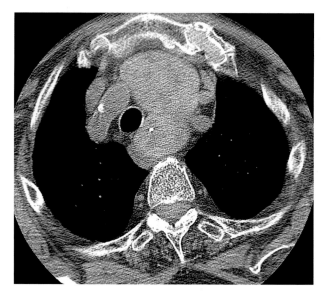

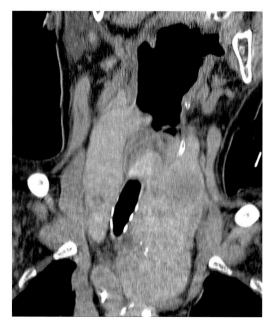

    A. Multinodular goiter
    B. Thymoma
    C. Teratoma
    D. Lymphoma

15b What percentage of intrathoracic goiter lesions are posterior?

    A. 0% to 5%
    B. 20% to 25%
    C. 35% to 40%
    D. 50% to 55%

16   What is the most likely diagnosis in this asymptomatic middle-aged woman?

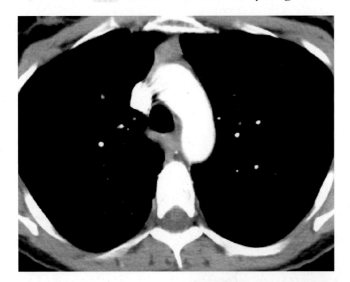

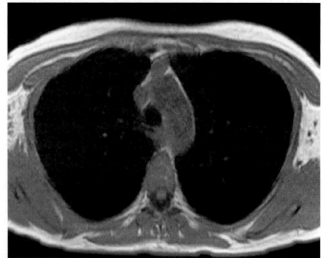

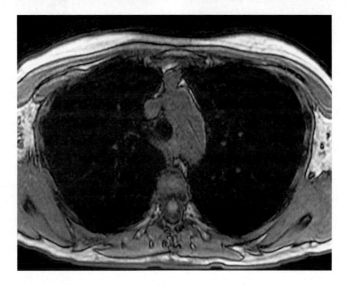

A. Thymic cyst
B. Thymoma
C. Thymic hyperplasia
D. Thymolipoma

17 What is the most likely diagnosis for the anterior mediastinal mass in this patient recently diagnosed with breast cancer? Contrast-enhanced CT (A), precontrast T2-weighted double inversion recovery (B), precontrast T1-weighted fat-saturated (C), and postcontrast T1-weighted fat-saturated subtraction (D) images are provided.

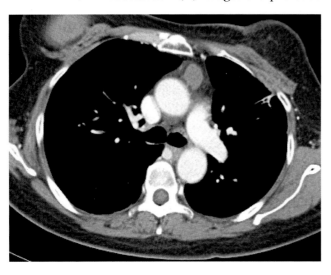
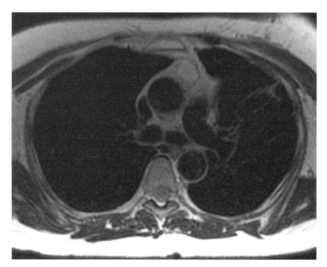
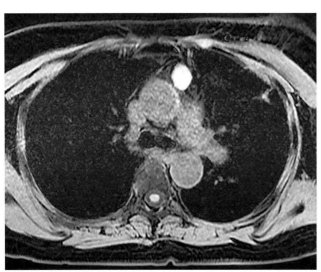
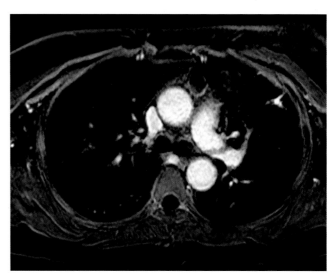

A. Thymic cyst
B. Metastatic breast cancer
C. Lymphoma
D. Germ cell tumor

18a Which systemic condition best explains the findings on the radiograph below?

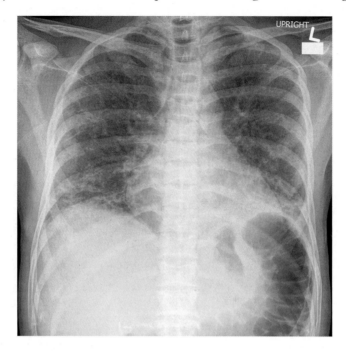

    A. Cystic fibrosis
    B. Systemic lupus erythematosus
    C. Sickle cell disease
    D. Sjogren syndrome

18b What is the most likely etiology of the left paraspinal mass in the CT image below?

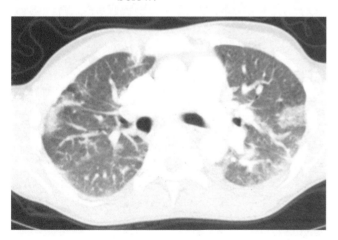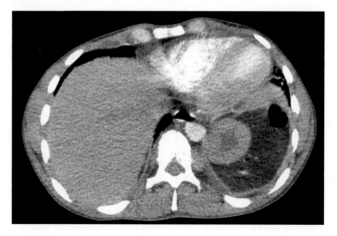

    A. Extramedullary hematopoiesis
    B. Lymphoma
    C. Hematoma
    D. Neurofibroma

19a What is the most likely cause of the mediastinal widening on the chest radiograph?

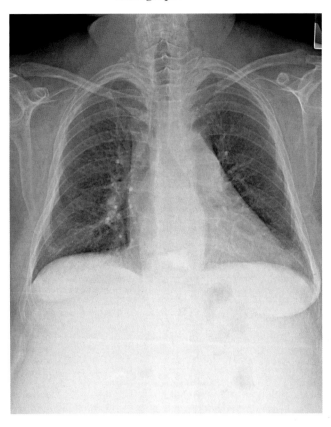

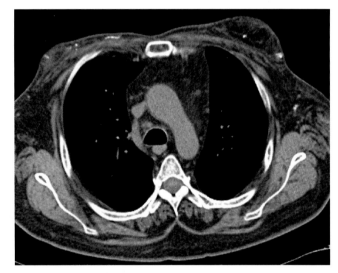

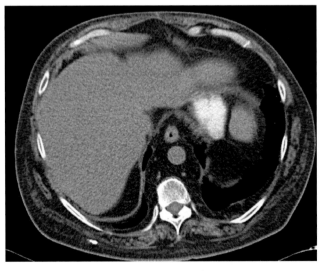

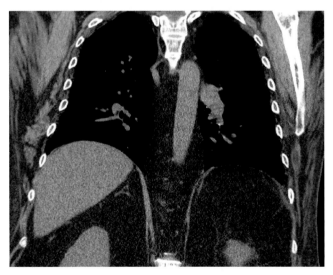

A. Liposarcoma
B. Mediastinal lipomatosis
C. Teratoma
D. Thymolipoma

19b What class of medications is this condition associated with?

A. Steroids
B. Antiemetics
C. Antihistamines
D. Antihypertensives

20a Which mediastinal compartment does the abnormality localize to, per the mediastinal compartmental classification proposed by the International Thymic Malignancy Interest Group (ITMIG)?

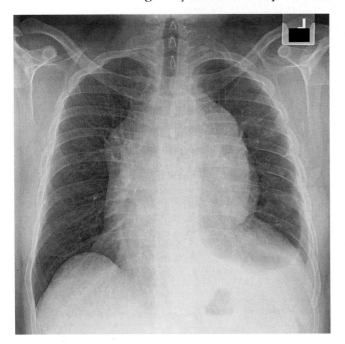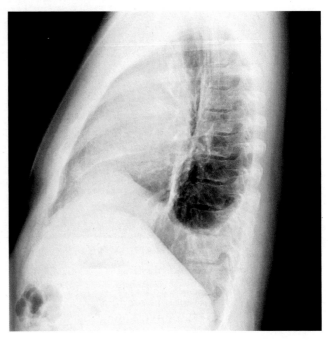

A. Superior
B. Prevascular
C. Visceral
D. Paravertebral

20b Which mediastinal compartment does the abnormality in the below images localize to, per the mediastinal compartmental classification proposed by the International Thymic Malignancy Interest Group (ITMIG)?

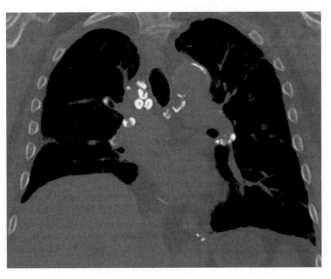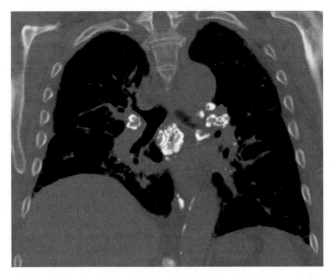

A. Superior
B. Prevascular
C. Visceral
D. Paravertebral

20c What was the most likely occupation of this patient?

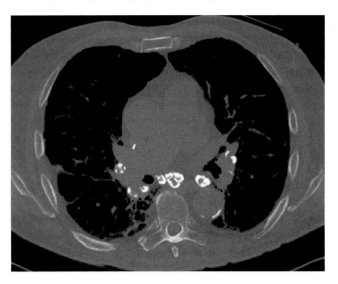

A. Sand blasting
B. Pipe stripping
C. Pigeon breeding
D. Hot tub cleaning

ANSWERS AND EXPLANATIONS

1a **Answer C.**

1b **Answer B.**

1c **Answer A.**   The chest radiograph demonstrates leftward shift of the mediastinum to include the heart and trachea. Lung markings are seen to the periphery bilaterally, excluding pneumothorax as a potential cause of mediastinal shift. Cardiomegaly cannot explain the findings as the heart is not enlarged and would not explain tracheal displacement. Consolidation is absent with diaphragm and mediastinal borders well maintained. Therefore, pulmonary volume loss is the only provided explanation for the radiographic appearance.

CT images reveal left parahilar masslike calcification in addition to an obstructed left pulmonary artery. Chronic pulmonary embolism could cause calcification associated with narrowing of the pulmonary artery, but not extrinsic calcification with occlusion. Also, chronic pulmonary embolism will not cause unilateral volume loss of the lung. Untreated lymphoma is a mediastinal process, which can engulf and obstruct vessels within the mediastinum, but will not cause calcification. Takayasu arteritis can occlude pulmonary vessels and cause calcification, but will not create masslike lesions within the mediastinum or hilum. By elimination, fibrosing mediastinitis can cause each of the findings of hilar masslike calcification, vascular obstruction, and unilateral pulmonary volume loss.

The most common cause of fibrosing mediastinitis in the United States is chronic *Histoplasma capsulatum* infection with alternative infections such as *Mycobacterium* tuberculosis and *Aspergillus* being less common. Radiation-caused mediastinitis is less common and requires a history of prior radiation exposure. Idiopathic fibrosing mediastinitis is a less common cause but should be considered in the setting of mediastinal fibrosis without calcification or with associated alternative sites of fibrosis such as Riedel thyroiditis or retroperitoneal fibrosis.

References: Gurney JW, Conces DJ. Pulmonary histoplasmosis. *Radiology* 1996;199:297–306.

McNeeley MF, Chung JH, Bhalla S, et al. Imaging of granulomatous fibrosing mediastinitis. *AJR Am J Roentgenol* 2012;199:319–327.

2a **Answer B.**

2b **Answer C.**

2c **Answer A.**   Imaging demonstrates a right anterior mediastinal mass, which is infiltrating around the aorta and pulmonary arteries. The superior vena cava is not visualized secondary to complete obstruction. Maximum intensity projection (MIP) and axial CT image both demonstrate contrast filling of large collateral vessels predominantly in the chest wall. While each of these symptoms has been described in the setting of SVC syndrome, head and neck swelling is one of the most common presenting symptoms. Other common presenting symptoms include headache and dyspnea. Stridor and altered mental status can be seen with severe cases of SVC syndrome but are not as common. Nausea has been described with SVC syndrome but is neither characteristic nor specific.

With obstruction of the SVC, multiple collateral venous pathways develop, generally tracking to the abdomen to reach the IVC. In this case, the collaterals are transiting the liver and creating a classic hot quadrate lobe or "hot spot sign." Multiple dense collateral pathways are also seen. While the region of liver is near the gallbladder fossa, it does not demonstrate the expected eggshell calcification of a porcelain gallbladder. Likewise, the stomach wall and spleen are within normal limits on this exam.

Collectively, cancers are by far the most common cause of SVC syndrome, with common cancers including bronchogenic carcinoma, lymphoma (as in this case), and metastatic disease. Iatrogenic causes, fibrosing mediastinitis, and Behcet disease all are potential benign causes of SVC syndrome but are less common etiologies than cancer.

Reference: Sheth S, Ebert MD, Fishman EK. Superior vena cava obstruction evaluation with MDCT. *AJR Am J Roentgenol* 2010;194:336–346.

3a **Answer B.**

3b **Answer C.**

3c **Answer D.** Dividing up the mediastinum into specific compartments (anterior, middle, posterior, and occasionally superior) allows for a narrowing of the differential diagnosis to a manageable number. Here, the lateral chest radiograph best demonstrates an opacity in the retrosternal window. The frontal chest radiograph exhibits the hilum overlay sign, with a rounded border overlying the right hilum but not obscuring the hilar vessels, further confirming the anterior location of the lesion.

Location and internal characteristics on CT can occasionally narrow the differential for an anterior mediastinal mass. Unfortunately, the lesion on the CT provided does not help differentiate the lesion. Its location at the junction of the heart and great vessels, homogeneous density, and projecting to one side of the mediastinum are all characteristic of thymoma, but they are not specific.

Multiple conditions are seen associated with thymoma, the most common being myasthenia gravis with 15% of patients with thymoma having myasthenia gravis and 35% of patients with myasthenia gravis having thymoma. Other common conditions have been grouped into "parathymic syndromes" and include pure red cell aplasia, hypogammaglobulinemia, and disorders of the endocrine system, skin, or connective tissue. Relationships with cardiac disease and renal disease have been published, but the specific conditions listed have not shown any significant association.

References: Rosado-de-Christenson ML, Galobardes J, Moran CA. From the archives of the AFIP thymoma: radiologic-pathologic correlation. *Radiographics* 1992;12:151–168.

Whitten CR, Khan S, Munneke GJ, et al. A diagnostic approach to mediastinal abnormalities. *Radiographics* 2007;27:657–671.

4 **Answer C.** There has been rapid development of a focal rim-enhancing lesion in the anterior mediastinum. Note the new surrounding inflammatory changes as well. Thymoma would be expected to be better defined and homogeneous. Necrosis and internal gas such as in this case would be unusual. Thymic carcinoma and invasive thymoma can have a more aggressive appearance but still would not develop over such a short interval. Normal thymus should not be space occupying such as the lesion demonstrated and would be triangular or bilobed in shape.

Acute mediastinitis is uncommon but most frequently occurs after recent surgery, esophageal perforation, or direct spread from neck infections. Of note, diffuse mediastinitis has a very high mortality (upward of 80% at 30 days). Gas bubbles, such as those seen, can be identified in up to 50% of cases and are an important differentiator for infection versus neoplasm.

Of note, differentiation of normal postmedian sternotomy changes from mediastinal infection or hemorrhage can be difficult in the immediate postoperative period. The normal postoperative appearance can include variable degrees of retrosternal fluid, air, and hematoma but should largely resolve by 2 to 3 weeks.

Reference: Webb WR, Higgins CB. *Thoracic imaging*. Philadelphia, PA: Lippincott Williams & Wilkins, 2010.

5 | **Answer A.**   Alveolar rupture is the most common cause of pneumomediastinum in this setting. This is referred to as the Macklin effect and is characterized by (1) alveolar rupture, (2) air dissection along the bronchovascular bundles (resulting in pulmonary interstitial emphysema), and (3) spread into the mediastinum. This can also occur in other settings such as blunt force trauma, although excluding a direct bronchial or tracheal laceration in that case would be critical. Extension from pneumothorax would be unusual as the parietal pleura would normally prevent gas from entering the mediastinum unless there is a preexisting violation of the pleura such as in the setting of recent thoracic surgery. Tracheal rupture from cuff overinflation is an unusual iatrogenic cause of pneumomediastinum that should be avoidable in most cases due to early identification of the overinflated cuff on chest x-ray and new endotracheal tubes that limit cuff volume and pressure. Esophageal rupture would be unusual without an underlying esophageal abnormality such as esophageal cancer, trauma, foreign body ingestion, or corrosive ingestion. Improper Blakemore tube placement for varices can result in esophageal rupture if the gastric balloon is inflated in the esophagus.

References: Webb WR, Higgins CB. *Thoracic imaging*. Philadelphia, PA: Lippincott Williams & Wilkins, 2010.

Wintermark M, Schnyder P. The Macklin effect: a frequent etiology for pneumomediastinum in severe blunt chest trauma. *Chest* 2001;120(2):543–547.

6 | **Answer C.**   Although this mass appears large and circumferential, the likely diagnosis is that of leiomyoma given the dystrophic areas of calcification (biopsy proven in this case). Metastases only rarely calcify with possible calcification in osteogenic or cartilaginous tumors and some mucinous GI tumors. Liposarcoma metastases are very unlikely to calcify (although they could potentially contain fat elements). Similarly, primary esophageal malignancies, either squamous cell carcinoma or adenocarcinoma, are unlikely to calcify. Untreated lymphoma almost never calcifies.

Leiomyomas are the most common benign tumor of the esophagus. The majority are asymptomatic and smaller than 3 cm in size although some can grow larger. They are most frequently round or mildly lobulated although some grow circumferentially (~10%) as this example demonstrates. They are more frequently seen in men than women (2:1) and less frequently in children. They are generally found in the mid and lower esophagus, and the vast majority are intramural arising from esophageal smooth muscle cells. Unlike the remainder of the gastrointestinal tract, gastrointestinal stromal tumors (GISTs) are less common in the esophagus. GISTs can calcify but have a higher predilection for necrosis or cyst formation within the mass than does leiomyoma, which is generally more homogeneous. Duplication cysts and granular cell tumors are less frequent benign esophageal masses. There is a rare pattern of esophageal leiomyomatosis, which is a more diffuse smooth muscle proliferation giving rise to multiple leiomyomas. This is associated with genetic abnormalities such as Alport syndrome with an increased risk of leiomyomas elsewhere in the body such as the airways.

Reference: Lewis RB, Mehrotra AK, Rodriguez P, et al. From the radiologic pathology archives: esophageal neoplasms: radiologic-pathologic correlation. *Radiographics* 2013;33(4):1083–1108.

7a **Answer B.**

7b **Answer B.** The initial chest radiographs demonstrate a rounded opacity overlying the heart that is difficult to see on the lateral but is localized to the middle mediastinum as a subtle opacity anterior to the spine. The corresponding CT demonstrates tubular structures that enhance more on venous phase imaging than arterial (note the difference in aortic enhancement to distinguish arterial from venous phase imaging). These are large esophageal varices in the setting of cirrhosis. Note, esophageal cancer and lymphadenopathy would not be expected to be tubular as seen here. The esophageal wall is thickened in this case, but that is related to esophagopathy rather than malignancy. Secondary features include splenomegaly and a small nodular liver with a small amount of perihepatic ascites in this case.

Esophageal varices develop as a collateral drainage pathway in the setting of portal hypertension. The collateral pathway is from the portal system into the azygos system. These are the classic "uphill" varices seen in the setting of cirrhosis and portal hypertension. "Downhill" varices can also be seen due to SVC obstruction but are typically noted more superiorly in the upper third of the esophagus. Typical causes of downhill varices include lung cancer, lymphoma, and mediastinal fibrosis.

Reference: Gore RM, Livine MS, eds. *Textbook of gastrointestinal radiology*, 2nd ed. Philadelphia, PA: WB Saunders Co, 2000:454–463, 2082.

8a **Answer A.**

8b **Answer B.** Although distal esophageal ruptures are more common (classically the distal left posterior wall for spontaneous rupture), proximal esophageal ruptures do occur. In the setting of a proximal esophageal rupture, a right effusion is the most common feature of those listed. For distal esophageal rupture, left effusion or hydropneumothorax is more common. On initial radiograph, pneumomediastinum is the most common feature and generally takes at least 1 hour to manifest after initial injury. Pleural effusion and mediastinal widening may take several hours. Etiologies to consider for esophageal perforation include esophagitis, foreign body impaction, trauma, and increasingly iatrogenic causes (such as related to balloon dilatation). Life-threatening mediastinitis, empyema, and lung abscess are complications to consider on follow-up imaging.

References: Wu JT, Mattox KL, Wall MJ Jr. Esophageal perforations: new perspectives and treatment paradigms. *J Trauma* 2007;63(5):1173–1184.

Young CA, Menias CO, Bhalla S, et al. CT features of esophageal emergencies. *Radiographics* 2008;28(6):1541–1553.

9a **Answer B.**

9b **Answer A.**

9c **Answer B.** The CT demonstrates a fluid attenuation lesion abutting the pericardium in the right chest. The location and imaging appearance are typical of a pericardial cyst, and in the majority of patients, no further imaging is warranted. However, in some patients, the appearance may be less typical or there may be a history of malignancy that warrants further evaluation. PET/CT of this area is sometimes difficult due to adjacent myocardial uptake. Additionally, a lack of uptake does not exclude malignancy. Radiographs would not demonstrate anything the CT has not already shown. Echocardiography is an option but can be of limited value due to available echo windows and body habitus. MRI is an excellent method for further evaluation and can demonstrate the fluid nature of the abnormality, even in cases with higher-density proteinaceous fluid. In this example, the high T2-weighted image (note the spinal fluid) confirms fluid within the lesion.

Reference: Jeung MY, Gasser B, Gangi A, et al. Imaging of cystic masses of the mediastinum. *Radiographics* 2002;22(Spec No):S79–S93.

10a **Answer D.**

10b **Answer B.** The cardiac silhouette is markedly enlarged on the frontal radiograph with a typical "water bottle" configuration. On the lateral, there is a vertically oriented density anterior to the heart and posterior to the sternum. This is visible because of vertically oriented low densities on either side. This is termed the "Oreo Cookie" or, less commonly, the sandwich sign, double-lucency sign, or epicardial fat pad sign and reflects pericardial effusion outlined by epicardial fat (anteriorly) and pericardial fat (posteriorly). This is a specific sign for pericardial effusion but is infrequently seen (low sensitivity). Note that there is no relationship with this sign and the double Oreo cookie sign of SLAP tears or the sandwich/hamburger sign of mesenteric lymphoma.

Classic clinical findings for significant effusion and tamponade are the Beck triad of hypotension, muffled heart sounds, and jugular venous distension. Symptomatology is variable and significantly related to acuity. As little as 80 mL of fluid may be symptomatic if acute, but more chronic effusions have been reported as large as 2 L and even 3 L without symptoms. Up to 50 mL is considered physiologic in some patients with 15 to 50 mL generally considered the normal range (some quote a lesser volume of 25 mL as the upper limit of normal).

The causes of pericardial effusion are many, and understanding the clinical context of the patient is critical for determining the cause of effusion. Consider the general differential of infection (in the immunosuppressed, remember tuberculosis), malignancy (especially lung cancer, breast cancer, lymphoma, or melanoma), trauma, radiation therapy, collagen vascular disease (such as lupus), or metabolic disorders (such as uremia).

References: Bogaert J, Francone M. Pericardial disease: value of CT and MR imaging. *Radiology* 2013;267(2):340–356.

Rienmüller R, Gröll R, Lipton MJ. CT and MR imaging of pericardial disease. *Radiol Clin North Am* 2004;42(3):587–601.

Wang ZJ, Reddy GP, Gotway MB, et al. CT and MR imaging of pericardial disease. *Radiographics* 2003;23:S167–S180.

11a **Answer C.**

11b **Answer D.** While only massive circumferential esophageal thickening (>20 cm) can accurately differentiate esophageal carcinoma from other benign esophageal processes like esophagitis, significant thickening with additional imaging characteristics can help exclude certain conditions. The CT shown demonstrates circumferential thickening of the esophagus measuring up to 17 mm (measurement not given) that is soft tissue in density. Esophageal varices will generally contrast fill similar to the other vasculature with a serpentine appearance. A duplication cyst would not create circumferential thickening with central lumen. Barrett esophagus would not cause this degree of thickening.

CT is limited in its staging of esophageal cancer but can be useful in cases of identifying direct invasion, regional lymph node involvement, and distant metastases. If direct invasion of adjacent nonresectable structures is demonstrated, the lesion then meets criteria for a "T4" lesion in the TNM classification. A T4 lesion stages the cancer at III or IV dependent on the presence of distant metastases and excludes treatment with surgery alone.

References: Kim TJ, Kim HY, Lee KW, et al. Multimodality assessment of esophageal cancer: preoperative staging and monitoring of response to therapy. *Radiographics* 2009;29:403–421.

Reinig JW, Stanley JH, Schabel SI. CT Evaluation of thickened esophageal walls. *AJR Am J Roentgenol* 1983;140:931–934.

12a **Answer B.**

12b **Answer C.** On CT, there is a rounded left posterior mediastinal lesion that abuts the adjacent vertebral body as well as the proximal descending aorta. The lesion is homogeneous and slightly lower in attenuation than is the aortic blood pool, suggesting that this could be fluid. Given the location, neurogenic tumors such as neuromas or paragangliomas are possible in addition to foregut duplication cysts or even a pseudoaneurysm. Further imaging is warranted, and MRI would be best suited to identify the exact relationship of the lesion to the adjacent structures and provide information as to its soft tissue or fluid nature.

On MRI, the lesion is homogeneous and of low intensity on T1-weighted sequence and high intensity on T2-weighted sequences. This is consistent with fluid content. Neurogenic tumors can have low T1- and high T2-weighted signal but would be expected to show vivid enhancement after contrast administration, which is not shown. Note that the thin rim of peripheral enhancement shown is typical of wall enhancement in foregut duplication cysts. Furthermore, the lesion does not invaginate into the neuroforamina, which is frequently found in schwannomas. There is no connection to the aorta to suggest pseudoaneurysm. There is a bilobed component more anteriorly to the vertebral body consistent with a middle mediastinal component. These findings are classic for a foregut duplication cyst.

Bronchogenic cysts, esophageal duplication cysts, and neurenteric cysts are all congenital foregut duplication cysts related to abnormality of the budding embryonic foregut. Mediastinal bronchogenic cysts are typically fluid attenuation and located in the middle mediastinum (80%) or less likely posterior mediastinum (17%). As many as 15% to 25% can be extramediastinal such as in the pleura, diaphragm, or lungs. MRI can be a very useful tool for confirmation of the cystic nature of the abnormality, especially for those cases that contain proteinaceous fluid or have had complications such as infection or internal hemorrhage. Treatment options favor surgical removal for larger lesions (especially if symptomatic or in a young patient). There is a theoretical risk of subsequent infection or hemorrhage. Some advise removal for all lesions, and some lesions have been treated percutaneously in high–surgical risk patients. The presence of any mural nodularity would be a reason to suggest removal as the lesion is more likely to be a cystic malignancy.

Reference: McAdams HP, Kirejczyk WM, Rosado-de-Christenson ML, et al. Bronchogenic cyst: imaging features with clinical and histopathologic correlation. *Radiology* 2000;217(2):441–446.

13a **Answer A.**

13b **Answer B.**

13c **Answer B.** The hilum overlay sign indicates location of the lesion either anterior or posterior to the hilum as the hilar structures remain well visualized despite the overlying lesion. Therefore, this case cannot be in the middle mediastinum. The lesion also obscures the left heart border, meaning the large lesion is displacing the lingula, an anterior structure. The lesion is centered below the aortic arch. Altogether, these findings are consistent with an anterior mediastinal mass.

The subsequent CT redemonstrates the large anterior mediastinal mass, which is primarily cystic, but does contain a small portion of fat, making this lesion consistent with a mature teratoma. Approximately 15% of mediastinal mature teratomas do not exhibit fat or calcium on CT. The anterior mediastinum is the most common location of extragonadal germ cell tumors and represents about 1/7 of the total anterior mediastinal masses. Treatment for mediastinal teratoma is complete surgical resection.

References: Moeller KH, Rosado-de-Christenson ML, Templeton PA. Mediastinal mature teratoma: imaging features. *AJR Am J Roentgenol* 1997;169:985–990.

Rosado-de-Christenson ML, Templeton PA, Moran CA. Mediastinal germ cell tumors: radiologic and pathologic correlation. *Radiographics* 1992;12:1013–1030.

14a Answer C.

14b Answer B.

14c Answer D.   Presenting chest radiograph demonstrates leftward shift of the mediastinum with some rotational change in the mediastinal contour. Some may be tempted to diagnose a pneumothorax and recommend chest tube placement, but no direct findings are present to suggest pneumothorax. Without a clear cause "pushing" the mediastinum, the shift is therefore due to left lung volume loss and without comparison needs further workup with CT or potentially bronchoscopy. Some may recognize an abrupt cutoff in the left mainstem bronchus, further supporting the need for timely workup.

The subsequent CT reveals an endobronchial mass obstructing the left mainstem bronchus and projecting beyond the expected bronchial borders. No additional findings are present, such as calcification, that may support a particular tumor type. Statistically, squamous cell carcinoma is the most common adult tracheal tumor, followed by adenoid cystic carcinoma. While this case is in the left mainstem bronchus, it is an adenoid cystic carcinoma (ACC), which is known to extend into or be centered in the mainstem bronchi. Regional adenopathy or distant disease is uncommon, with local recurrence being the primary concern following resection.

Reference: Ngo AH, Walker CM, Chung JH, et al. Tumors and tumorlike conditions of the large airways. *AJR Am J Roentgenol* 2013;201:301–313.

15a Answer A.

15b Answer B.   Extending through the thoracic inlet from the paratracheal thyroid bed, this lesion is consistent with a multinodular goiter with intrathoracic component. On radiograph, the lesion displaces the trachea to the right with widening of the superior mediastinum. Follow-up CT in axial and coronal planes reveals the mildly heterogeneous lesion with small calcifications directly connecting to the thyroid.

The goiter extends lateral and posterior to the trachea on axial image. Up to 25% of intrathoracic goiters are posterior in location and therefore should be included with the differential for a superior posterior mediastinal mass. This lesion is atypical for the fact that it extends along the left trachea, where the vast majority of thyroid goiter, which extends to the posterior mediastinum, descends along the right trachea.

References: Kawashima A, Fishman EK, Kuhlman JE, et al. CT of posterior mediastinal masses. *Radiographics* 1991;11:1045–1067.

Whitten CR, Khan S, Munneke GJ, et al. A diagnostic approach to mediastinal abnormalities. *Radiographics* 2007;27:657–671.

16 **Answer C.** CT demonstrates an indeterminate soft tissue attenuation nodule in the anterior (prevascular) mediastinum. Precontrast in phase (IP) and opposed phase (OP) MRI images demonstrate homogeneous loss of signal on OP images relative to IP images, consistent with microscopic fat. Therefore, the best answer choice is thymic hyperplasia. The signal loss can be quantitated using the chemical shift ratio (CSR) by placing regions of interest on the least suppressing region of the tissue in question as well as the paraspinal muscle on both IP and OP images. The CSR = [OP signal intensity of the thymus/OP signal intensity of the paraspinal muscle]/ [IP signal intensity of the thymus/ IP signal intensity of the paraspinal muscle]. A CSR $\leq$ 0.7 indicates normal thymus or hyperplastic thymus. Another parameter, the signal intensity index (SII), can be calculated using [(IP thymus SI − OP thymus SI)/IP thymus SI] $\times$ 100. A SII $\geq$ 9% indicates normal thymus or hyperplastic thymus.

There are two types of thymic hyperplasia: true hyperplasia and lymphoid hyperplasia. True thymic hyperplasia, an increase in volume of thymic tissue, is associated with recovery from a systemic stressor, such as chemotherapy. Lymphoid thymic hyperplasia, an increase in the number of lymphoid follicles within the thymus, is associated with a variety of conditions, most commonly myasthenia gravis. True hyperplasia and lymphoid hyperplasia cannot be reliably differentiated on imaging.

References: Inaoka T, Takahashi K, Mineta M, et al. Thymic hyperplasia and thymus gland tumors: differentiation with chemical shift MR imaging. *Radiology* 2007;243(3):869–876.

McInnis MC, Flores EJ, Shepard JAO, et al. Pitfalls in the imaging and interpretation of benign thymic lesions: How thymic MRI can help. *Am J Roentgenol* 2016;206(1):W1–W8.

Nishino M, Ashiku S, Kocher O, et al. The thymus: a comprehensive review. *RadioGraphics* 2006;26(2):335–348.

Priola AM, Priola SM, Ciccone G, et al. Differentiation of rebound and lymphoid thymic hyperplasia from anterior mediastinal tumors with dual-echo cchemical-shift MR imaging in adulthood: Reliability of the chemical-shift ratio and signal intensity index. *Radiology* 2015;274(1):238–249.

17 **Answer A.** CT demonstrates a well-circumscribed anterior mediastinal (prevascular) mass that is of higher attenuation than simple fluid (40 Hounsfield units, in this case) and is therefore indeterminate. On MRI, this lesion is homogeneously hyperintense on both precontrast T2-weighted double inversion recovery images and precontrast T1-weighted fat-saturated images. Enhancement is absent on postcontrast T1-weighted fat-saturated subtraction images. These characteristics are consistent with a thymic cyst. Thymic cysts can occasionally demonstrate thin, smooth wall enhancement, but should have no discrete solid or nodular components. Nodular or enhancing components should raise suspicion for a cystic neoplasm. While simple fluid is hypointense on T1-weighted images, proteinaceous or hemorrhagic material within the fluid can result in T1 hyperintensity. In the setting of hemorrhage, a thymic cyst may enlarge and a hematocrit level may be visible. Congenital thymic cysts are typically unilocular. Acquired thymic cysts are associated with mediastinal radiation and surgery and can be either unilocular or multilocular.

References: Ackman J, Wu C. MRI of the thymus. *AJR Am J Roentgenol* 2011;197(1): W15–W20. doi:10.2214/ajr.10.4703

Jeung M, Gasser B, Gangi A, et al. Imaging of cystic masses of the mediastinum. *RadioGraphics* 2002;22(Special Issue):79–93. doi:10.1148

18a **Answer C.**

18b **Answer A.** Sickle cell disease results from a genetic alteration in the hemoglobin molecule, causing it to become more adherent, form into a "sickle" shape, and become less flexible than normal hemoglobin molecules, resulting in microvascular obstruction and hemolysis. Chest radiograph demonstrates streaky bilateral opacities throughout both lungs, with patchy airspace opacities, greatest in both lower lungs. Peripheral, wedge-shaped ground-glass opacities are present on the CT image, consistent with pulmonary infarcts in the setting of acute chest syndrome. Acute chest syndrome is defined as a new opacity on chest radiograph in addition to clinical manifestations such as acute chest pain, fever, hypoxia, and leukocytosis. It can be precipitated by a number of factors including infection and microvascular occlusion. Over time, repeated episodes of acute chest syndrome can result in pulmonary fibrosis and pulmonary hypertension. Pulmonary-related complications are one of the leading causes of mortality in patients with sickle cell disease. The radiograph also demonstrates several extrapulmonary manifestations of sickle cell disease: bone infarcts (sclerotic humeral head and "H"-shaped vertebral bodies), absent spleen (secondary to autoinfarction), and cholecystectomy (due to increased pigment gallstone formation in the setting of hemolysis). The left paraspinal mass in the second CT image is the result of extramedullary hematopoiesis in the setting of anemia. Extramedullary hematopoiesis may present as paraspinal masses but can also form in the intercostal spaces, as well as a variety of organs including the spleen and kidneys. Extramedullary hematopoiesis can be seen in conditions other than sickle cell disease, for example, myelofibrosis and thalassemia.

References: Lonergan G, Cline D, Abbondanzo S, et al. From the archives of AFIP sickle cell anemia. *RadioGraphics* 2001;21(4):971–994.

Madani G, Papadopoulou A, Holloway B, et al. The radiological manifestations of sickle cell disease. *Clin Radiol* 2007;62(6):528–538.

19a **Answer B.**

19b **Answer A.** The chest radiograph demonstrates lateral displacement of both paraspinal lines, enlargement of the cardiac silhouette, and blunting of the left lateral costophrenic sulcus. On CT, these regions correlate with excessive fat in the anterior, middle, and posterior mediastinum, as well as the bilateral extrapleural spaces inferiorly. While there are vessels coursing through the regions of increased fat, no significant soft tissue component is present. These findings are consistent with mediastinal and pleural lipomatosis, the deposition of excessive unencapsulated fat. Mediastinal and pleural lipomatosis is associated with exogenous steroid use, Cushing's, and obesity. As in this case, it can result in the appearance of mediastinal widening, paravertebral masses, and/or pleural effusions on chest radiograph. Patients are usually asymptomatic. Teratoma, liposarcoma, and thymolipoma are typically more focal and would contain soft tissue components.

Reference: Gaerte S, Meyer C, Winer-Muram H, et al. Fat-containing lesions of the chest. *RadioGraphics* 2002;22(Special Issue):61–78.

20a **Answer B.**

20b **Answer C.**

20c **Answer A.** In the first case, the PA radiograph demonstrates an abnormal mediastinal contour, which is widened due to bilateral lobulated opacities with well-defined lateral margins. Because pulmonary vessels are visible through the masses and not silhouetted (hilum overlay sign), the finding cannot be within the visceral (middle) mediastinum. Lateral radiograph demonstrates opacification of the retrosternal window, localizing the mass to the prevascular (anterior) mediastinum. In the second case, coronal CT images demonstrate lymph nodes with peripheral "eggshell" calcifications within the visceral (middle) mediastinum. The differential for calcified lymph nodes is large and can include granulomatous infection, sarcoidosis, silicosis, coal worker's pneumoconiosis, treated lymphoma, calcifying metastases, and amyloidosis. While not specific, peripherally calcified lymph nodes are classically associated with sarcoidosis, silicosis, and coal worker's pneumoconiosis. Sandblasting is associated with exposure to silica dust, making that the correct answer. Pipe stripping is associated with asbestos exposure, while pigeon breeding and hot tub cleaning result in exposure to organic antigens, increasing susceptibility to hypersensitivity pneumonitis.

The conventional mediastinal compartment designations of superior, anterior, middle, and posterior were based on lateral plain radiograph landmarks. In 2017, the International Thymic Malignancy Interest Group (ITMIG) proposed a new classification based on landmarks from CT, now the predominant modality used to diagnose and follow mediastinal pathology. This system divides the mediastinum into prevascular, visceral, and paravertebral compartments based on specific anatomic landmarks visible on CT. The superior and inferior margins of each compartment are the thoracic inlet and diaphragm, respectively. The prevascular compartment is bounded by the sternum anteriorly, the anterior pericardium posteriorly, and the parietal mediastinal pleura laterally. The visceral mediastinum is bounded by the posterior aspect of the prevascular compartment anteriorly and a vertical line 1 cm posterior to the anterior margin of the thoracic vertebral bodies. The paravertebral compartment is bounded by the posterior boundary of the visceral compartment anteriorly and a vertical line against the posterior margin of the chest wall at the lateral aspect of the thoracic vertebral body transverse processes. Division into these groups aids in constructing a differential based on the compartment of origin.

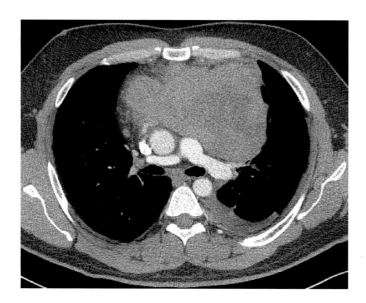
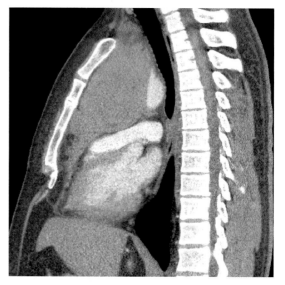

Axial and sagittal CT images from the same patient with the prevascular mass demonstrate a soft tissue mass causing posterior displacement of the aorta and pulmonary artery. The diagnosis of lymphoma was made on biopsy.

References: Carter B, Benveniste M, Madan R. ITMIG classification of mediastinal compartments and multidisciplinary approach to mediastinal masses. *RadioGraphics* 2017;37(2):436–438.

Cox C, Rose C, Lynch D. State of the art: imaging of occupational lung disease. *Radiology* 2014;270(3):681–696.

14 Vascular Disease

Michael Winkler, MD • Mohamed Tarek Seleem Ahmed, MBBCh, MSc

QUESTIONS

1a What is the salient abnormality on this upright PA chest x-ray?

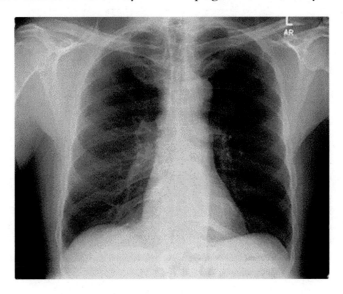

A. Unilateral hyperlucency
B. Unilateral hilar enlargement
C. Unilateral pleural effusion
D. Unilateral pneumothorax

1b Unilateral hyperlucency due to oligemia is referred to as what eponym?

A. Hampton hump
B. Westermark sign
C. Galaxy sign
D. Reverse halo sign

2a In the setting of suspected acute pulmonary embolism in pregnancy, which of the following examinations both is appropriate AND results in the lowest radiation dose to the **fetus**?

A. CTA of the pulmonary arteries
B. V/Q scan
C. CT of the chest without contrast
D. MRA with contrast of the pulmonary arteries

2b In the setting of suspected acute pulmonary embolism in pregnancy, which of the following examinations both is appropriate AND results in the lowest radiation dose to the **mother**?

   A. CTA of the pulmonary arteries

   B. V/Q scan

   C. CT of the chest without contrast

   D. MRA with contrast of the pulmonary arteries

3 The most likely cause of the pulmonary embolus in this case is which of the following?

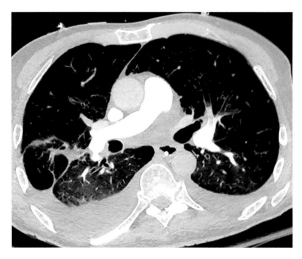 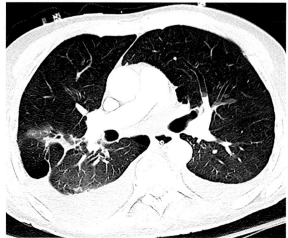

   A. Parturition

   B. Trauma

   C. Arrhythmia

   D. Iatrogenic

4 A patient suffers multiple long bone lower extremity fractures as the result of a high-speed motor vehicle collision. Twenty-four hours after the event, he develops a diffuse rash and acute shortness of breath prompted a CT of the chest. Of the following, which is the most likely cause for the lung abnormality?

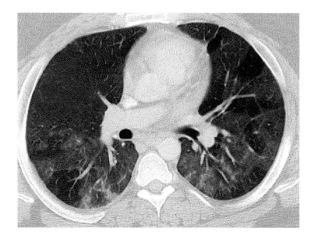

   A. Aspiration

   B. Contusion

   C. Atypical infection

   D. Fat embolism

5 Given the finding present on this radiograph, the most likely diagnosis is which of the following?

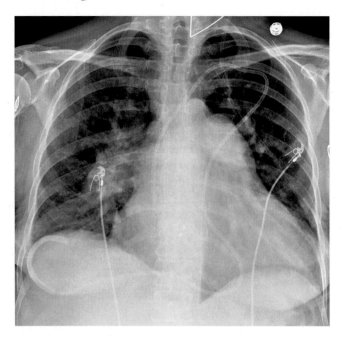

A. Small cell lung cancer
B. Pulmonary hypertension
C. Sarcoidosis
D. Lymphoma

6a The most likely diagnosis, based on the imaging findings, is which of the following?

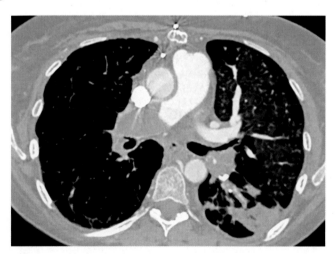

A. Acute pulmonary embolus
B. Pulmonary artery sarcoma
C. Chronic pulmonary embolus
D. Behçet disease

6b The most likely diagnosis, based on the imaging findings, is which of the following?

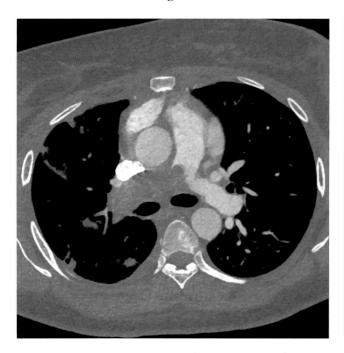 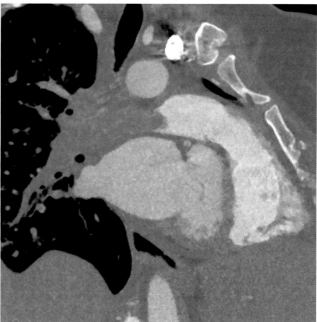

    A. Acute pulmonary embolus
    B. Pulmonary artery sarcoma
    C. Chronic pulmonary embolus
    D. Behçet disease

7 Observe the lesion in the left upper lobe. The radiographic "sign" associated with this lesion is which of the following?

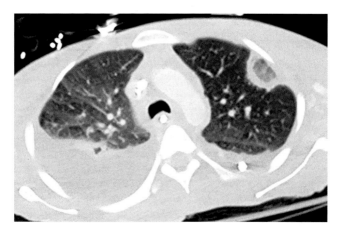

    A. Reversed halo sign
    B. Bull's eye sign
    C. Monod sign
    D. Signet ring sign

8   What is the likely cause of mosaic attenuation seen on this image?

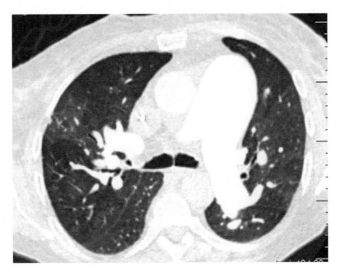

A. Obliterative bronchiolitis
B. Chronic pulmonary embolus
C. Alpha 1 antitrypsin deficiency
D. Asthma

9   Based on these images, which of the following options is the most likely diagnosis?

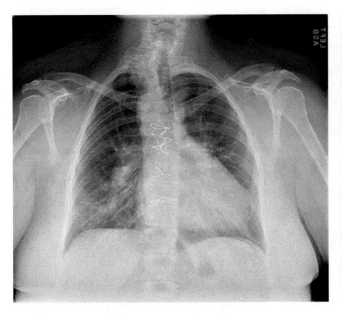
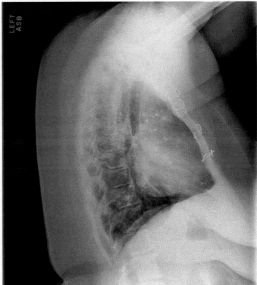

A. Tetralogy of Fallot
B. L-Transposition of the great vessels
C. Chronic pulmonary embolus
D. Pulmonary artery sling

10   In the setting of a young patient with pulmonary hypertension and these CT findings, what is the likely diagnosis?

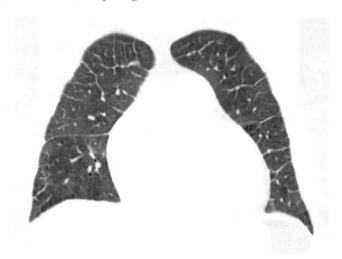

A. Hepatopulmonary syndrome
B. Scleroderma
C. Lymphangitic carcinomatosis
D. Pulmonary veno-occlusive disease (PVOD)

11a   Refer to the exhibits. Which of the following is most likely to be present?

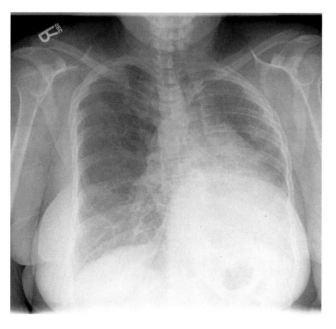 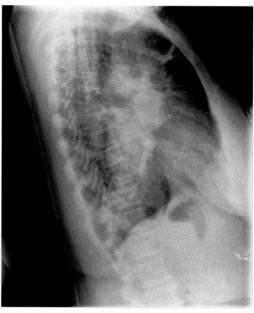

A. Hilar adenopathy
B. Abscesses
C. Mediastinal cysts
D. Hypoplastic left lung

11b The right lung abnormality is most likely due to which of the following?

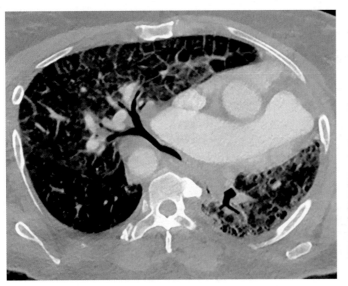 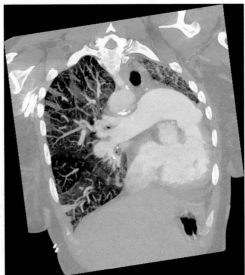

    A. Pneumonia
    B. Aspiration
    C. Edema
    D. Thrombosis

12 What is the source of high density within the nodular opacity demarcated by the arrow?

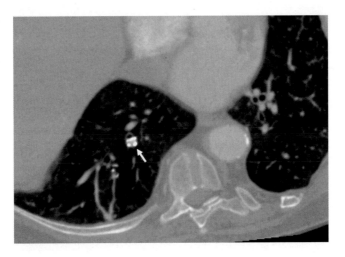

    A. Pulmonary ossification
    B. Dental amalgam
    C. Calcified thrombus
    D. Coil embolus

13   A 14-year-old male presented to the ED with hemoptysis. On examination, his
      SaO$_2$ was 82% and "clubbing" of his fingertips was noted. Given this history
      and the findings present on the image provided, the most likely diagnosis is
      which of the following?

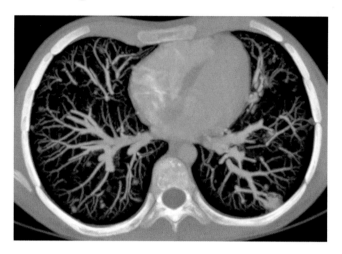

A. Granulomatosis with polyangiitis
B. Hereditary hemorrhagic telangiectasia
C. Blastomycosis
D. Septic emboli

14   Which of the following can be seen in the accompanying image?

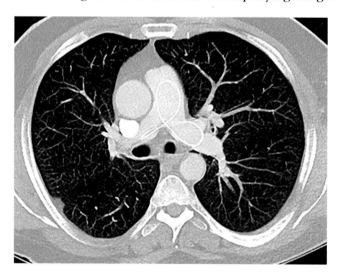

A. Swan-Ganz catheter
B. EKOS catheter
C. Catheter fragment
D. Guidewire

15 What is the cause of the linear high density in the right lower lobe pulmonary artery based on these CT images?

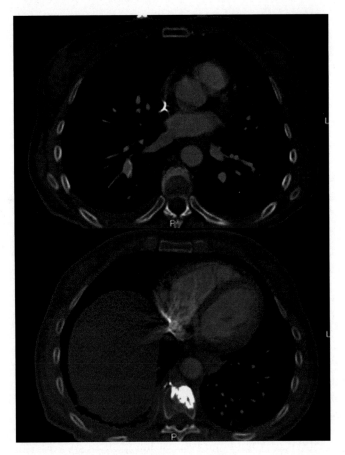

A. Dendriform pulmonary ossification
B. Methyl methacrylate embolization
C. Calcified chronic pulmonary embolus
D. Embolized guidewire

16 What is the most common pulmonary arterial manifestation of Behçet disease involving the lungs?

A. Pulmonary artery aneurysms
B. Pulmonary artery occlusion
C. Pulmonary embolism
D. Pulmonary hemorrhage

17 Which of the following conditions is most likely responsible for these imaging findings?

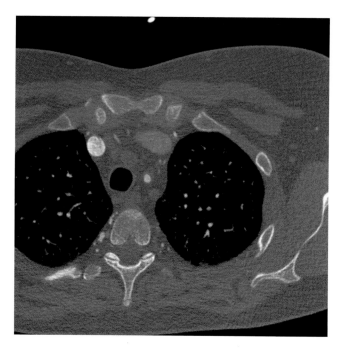

    A. Behçet disease
    B. Granulomatosis with polyangiitis
    C. Takayasu arteritis
    D. Goodpasture syndrome

18 The shunt evident on the image is most likely secondary to which of the following?

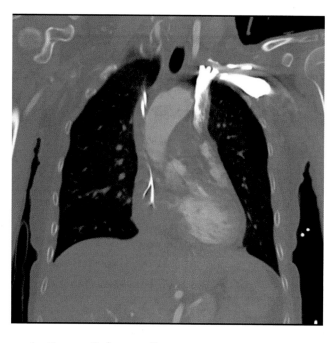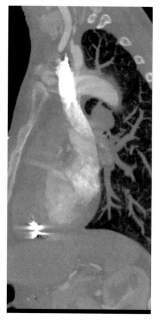

    A. Congenital anomaly
    B. Chronic disease
    C. Traumatic injury
    D. Surgical intervention

19 Note the bronchial artery enlargement present on the image to the left. The cause of enlargement falls into which of the following general categories?

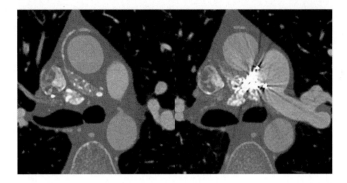

A. Congenital
B. Postsurgical
C. Neoplastic
D. Inflammatory

20 Which of the following is the most likely diagnosis?

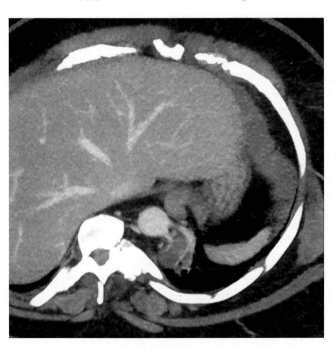
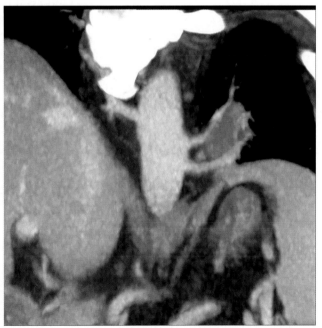

A. Splenic herniation
B. Round atelectasis
C. Lung cancer
D. Pulmonary sequestration

ANSWERS AND EXPLANATIONS

1a **Answer A.**

1b **Answer B.** An obstructive left-sided pulmonary embolism has reduced blood flow to the left lung. As a result of this oligemia, the left lung is hypolucent and the left lung vessels diminutive relative to the right. Together, these findings comprise the "Westermark" sign which, unfortunately, is difficult to perceive prospectively. Additional findings associated with this sign are asymmetrically sized hila and abrupt truncation of the central pulmonary arteries. An anterior pneumothorax or layering effusion can also cause one lung field to appear less dense than the other. However, these causes of asymmetric lung density are only encountered on supine radiographs, and the radiograph presented was acquired with the patient upright.

Reference: Westermark N. On the Roentgen diagnosis of lung embolism. *Acta Radiol* 1938;19:357–372.

2a **Answer A.**

2b **Answer B.** Pulmonary embolism (PE) is both difficult to diagnosis clinically and a leading cause of death for pregnant women. Lower extremity venous Doppler ultrasound is useful in the setting of suspected PE in pregnancy. A positive study initiates the same treatment pathway as PE and therefore can circumvent the use of ionizing radiation for imaging. However, a negative Doppler study has poor predictive value. Pulmonary artery CTA and V/Q scans, while requiring small amounts of ionizing radiation, diagnose PE through direct anatomic visualization rather than by inference.

CTA results in a higher estimated effective radiation dose to the mother than V/Q scanning primarily due to breast exposure, although recent research suggests that the risk of breast cancer is no great after CTA than V/Q. During the perfusion portion of a V/Q scan, technetium macro aggregated albumin circulates throughout the mother's body, including through her uterus, resulting in a relatively higher dose to the fetus. V/Q scans utilization in all settings has fallen over the last two decades because of its inconvenience relative to CTA and because of the impression (among both radiologists and clinicians) that CTA is the superior modality.

While the use of most iodine-based contrast media is thought to be safe, the American College of Radiology recommends that the use of gadolinium-based contrast media be avoided when possible in the setting of pregnancy. A CT without contrast could potentially provide an alternative diagnosis but cannot diagnose PE reliably.

References: Davenport MS, et al. ACR Manual on Contrast Media. American College of Radiology. Available at https://www.acr.org/-/media/ACR/Files/Clinical-Resources/Contrast_Media.pdf. Accessed June 20, 2020.

van der Pol LM, et al. Pregnancy-adapted YEARS algorithm for diagnosis of suspected pulmonary embolism. *N Engl J Med* 2019;380(12):1139–1149.

3 **Answer D.** Note the air column within the left upper lobe pulmonary arteries. There is also a layer of unopacified blood (not thrombus) proximal to the air column which has not mixed with contrast media due to a lack of antegrade flow. Air pulmonary embolism, as seen in this case, is almost always iatrogenic. It can occur as a complication of central line placement, pacemaker implantation, lung biopsy, or even during the power injection of contrast media.

Amniotic fluid and fat embolism, after parturition or trauma, respectively, manifest as ground-glass opacities on CT most commonly. Arrhythmia-related cardiac thrombi are left sided and present with systemic arterial (rather than pulmonary) embolism.

Reference: Malik N, Claus PL, Illman JE, et al. Air embolism: diagnosis and management. *Future Cardiol* 2017;13(4):365–378.

4 **Answer D.** Fat embolism syndrome (FES) is most often the result of traumatic long bone or pelvic fracture. Other causes include orthopedic procedures, liposuction, bone tumor lysis, pancreatitis, and lipid infusion. Clinically FES presents with a classic triad of respiratory distress, cerebral abnormalities, and petechial hemorrhages (rash) 24 to 48 hours after the inciting event. Severe cases carry a high mortality rate upward of 20%. The CT findings of FES are variable but most frequently multifocal bilateral ground-glass opacities that may progress to consolidation. The fat emboli are multiple and microscopic; filling defects within the pulmonary arteries are not generally seen on CT.

Aspiration also manifests as ground glass opacities is common in the setting of trauma. However, the presence of a rash points toward FES. Atypical infection, although possible, would be purely coincidental.

Reference: Malagari K, Economopoulos N, Stoupis C, et al. High-resolution CT findings in mild pulmonary fat embolism. *Chest* 2003;123(4):1196–1201.

5 **Answer B.** Although all of the options listed cause hilar enlargement, the pronounced enlargement of the second "mogul" (the shape of a mound of packed snow) of the left cardiomediastinal border reveals that pulmonary artery hypertension, rather than adenopathy, as the cause of hilar enlargement. Disproportionately small peripheral pulmonary arteries (a phenomena know in the parlance of radiology as "pruning") is another finding evident in this case. The presence of an atrial septal defect occlusion device points to chronic left to right shunting via an atrial septal defect as the etiology of pulmonary hypertension.

Reference: Altschul E, et al. Imaging of pulmonary hypertension: pictorial essay. *Chest* 2019;156(2):211–227.

6a **Answer C.**

6b **Answer B.** Acute pulmonary emboli tend to straddle pulmonary artery bifurcations (aka "saddles"). A branch pulmonary artery that contains an acute embolus will appear to have a central filling defect when viewed in cross section. Acute emboli may be accompanied by signs of pulmonary infarction, such as peripheral consolidation with central sparing and pleural effusion.

In contrast, chronic pulmonary emboli exhibit complete or eccentric filling defects because thrombus eventually adheres to the vessel wall. Other signs of chronic emboli include central pulmonary artery enlargement due to pulmonary hypertension, recanalization of occluded arteries, stenoses, webs, and mosaic attenuation of the lungs due to regions of oligemia. Pulmonary parenchymal signs of chronic pulmonary emboli include peripheral parenchymal bands, wedge-shaped opacities, and linear opacities related to scarring from prior infarcts.

Behçet disease, well known despite its rarity as a cause of pulmonary artery aneurysm, also can manifest with findings that are indistinguishable from acute or chronic pulmonary emboli.

Primary pulmonary artery sarcoma, an even rarer entity, is a mimic of chronic pulmonary embolus. Findings such as unilateral intrapulmonary artery enlargement and occlusion are suggestive of this diagnosis. Statistically, however, these findings are still much more likely to be attributable to chronic pulmonary embolus. Haziness (increased density) of mediastinal fat adjacent to the affected central pulmonary artery is a more specific sign. Direct invasion of adjacent mediastinal structures or a positive CT-PET study are required to make an imaging diagnosis.

References: Castañer E, et al. CT Diagnosis of chronic pulmonary thromboembolism. *Radiographics* 2009;29(1):31–50.

Seyahi E, et al. Pulmonary artery involvement and associated lung disease in Behçet disease: a series of 47 patients. *Medicine (Baltimore)* 2012;91(1):35–48.

Wyler von Ballmoos MZ, et al. Imaging and surgical treatment of primary pulmonary artery sarcoma. *Int J Cardiovasc Imaging* 2019;35(8):1429–1433.

Xi XY, et al. Value of 18F-FDG PET/CT in differentiating malignancy of pulmonary artery from pulmonary thromboembolism: a cohort study and literature review. *Int J Cardiovasc Imaging* 2019;35(7):1395–1403.

7 **Answer A.** The reversed halo sign is characterized by central ground-glass opacity surrounded by a ring of consolidation (i.e., the inverse of the "halo" sign created by a central nodule surrounded by a ring of ground glass). An alternate name for the sign is "atoll," which is the name for a ringed coral reef. Common differential diagnoses include pulmonary infarct, as in this case, and organizing pneumonia. Rare causes include bacterial and fungal pneumonias (e.g., paracoccidioidomycosis, mucormycosis, tuberculosis), sarcoidosis, radiofrequency ablation, or granulomatosis with polyangiitis (aka Wegener's). Monod sign describes a fungus ball in a preexisting pulmonary cavity. "Signet ring" is a sign of bronchiectasis that refers to a dilated airway that is much larger than the accompanying pulmonary artery on axial images. "Bull's-eye" sign refers to the appearance of ulcerated submucosal masses in the gastrointestinal tract seen on fluoroscopic studies.

References: Raju S, Ghosh S, Mehta AC. Chest CT signs in pulmonary disease: a pictorial review. *Chest* 2017;151(6):1356–1374.

Walker C, Mohammed TL, Chung J. Reversed halo sign. *J Thorac Imaging* 2011;26:W80.

Xiang H, et al. Bull's-eye sign: various manifestations in the gastrointestinal tract. *J Med Imaging Radiat Oncol* 2018;62(Suppl 1):60.

8 **Answer B.** In this instance, mosaic attenuation is due to heterogeneous lung perfusion. The constellation of the findings of (1) enlarged central pulmonary arteries, (2) mosaic attenuation of lung tissue, and (3) reduced caliber of peripheral vessels in the regions of relative hypoattenuation are consistent with the diagnosis of chronic pulmonary thromboembolism. Mosaic attenuation caused by heterogeneous respiratory bronchial and alveolar inflation, termed "air trapping," is seen with bronchiolar pathologies, such as obliterative bronchiolitis or asthma. Alpha-1 antitrypsin deficiency presents with destruction of lung parenchymal, which is not present in the image provided.

Reference: Castañer E, Gallardo X, Ballesteros E, et al. CT diagnosis of chronic pulmonary thromboembolism. *Radiographics* 2009;29(1):31–50.

9 **Answer A.** Findings evident on these radiographs include prior sternotomy, right aortic arch, and severe enlargement of the pulmonary artery and its proximal branches, right greater than left. In addition, radiopaque markers overlie the expected position of the pulmonic valve on both PA and lateral images. In this case of surgical correction of tetralogy of Fallot, pulmonary artery enlargement is due to long-standing pulmonary regurgitation. The surgical changes and right aortic arch favor this diagnosis over chronic pulmonary embolus, which also presents with enlarged pulmonary arteries.

In ʟ-transposition, the heart's vascular pedicle will appear to be straightened. The normal convex silhouette of the pulmonary artery along the left mediastinum will be absent. Pulmonary artery sling (aka anomalous origin of the left pulmonary artery) has a CXR finding of widening of the inferior aspect of the right paratracheal stripe.

References: Ammash NM, et al. Pulmonary regurgitation after tetralogy of Fallot repair: clinical features, sequelae, and timing of pulmonary valve replacement. *Congenit Heart Dis* 2007;2(6):386–403.

Castañer E, et al. Congenital and acquired pulmonary artery anomalies in the adult: radiologic overview. *Radiographics* 2006;26(2):349–371.

Castañer E, et al. CT diagnosis of chronic pulmonary thromboembolism. *Radiographics* 2009;29(1):31–50.

Warnes CA. Transposition of the great arteries. *Circulation* 2006;114(24):2699–2709.

10 **Answer D.** In pulmonary veno-occlusive disease (PVOD), a disease of young adults, post capillary vein obliteration leads to pulmonary arterial hypertension. Imaging findings include interlobular septal thickening, poorly defined centrilobular ground-glass nodules, pleural effusions, lymphadenopathy, and pulmonary artery enlargement. Pulmonary capillary hemangiomatosis, although rare, presents similarly. Patients with PVOD are preload dependent and may develop fatal pulmonary edema if treated (as other causes of pulmonary hypertension) with vasodilators. Scleroderma, while associated with pulmonary hypertension, presents with interstitial fibrosis. Lymphangitic carcinomatosis presents with more irregular interlobular septal thickening and is usually accompanied by nodules. Hepatopulmonary syndrome, related to cirrhosis, presents with peripheral pulmonary vessel dilatation or arteriovenous malformations.

Reference: Pena E, Dennie C, Veinot J, et al. Pulmonary hypertension: how the radiologist can help. *Radiographics* 2012;32(1):9–32.

11a **Answer D.**

11b **Answer C.**

Left lung hypoplasia accompanies agenesis of left pulmonary artery. It is easier to note its absence on the lateral CXR (as increased lucency posterior to the trachea). Other findings include distortion of the tracheobronchial tree and severe enlargement of the right pulmonary artery. Direction of right heart output to a single lung results in increase pulmonary arterial pressure and pulmonary edema, which manifests as ground-glass haziness and interlobular septal thickening. Although patients with unilateral pulmonary agenesis are at risk for infection, the diffuse pattern and distribution of these finding is more likely to represent edema than infection or aspiration.

Reference: Govindaraj V, et al. Isolated left-sided pulmonary artery agenesis with left lung hypoplasia: a report of two cases. *J Postgrad Med* 2017;63:262–264.

12 **Answer D.** Two arteriovenous malformations (AVMs) are seen, one coiled and the other yet to be treated (in the most posterior lung with a draining artery and vein). Chronic pulmonary emboli can calcify, but the high density of the coil seen in this image exceeds that cortical bone. Dendriform pulmonary ossification is associated with underlying evidence of aspiration or pulmonary fibrosis in a majority of cases. Dental amalgam will be at least as dense as a coil but located in a bronchus rather than in a vessel.

Reference: Tokunaga K, et al. Can the "pine-needle sign" on computed tomography be used to differentiate pulmonary arteriovenous malformation from its mimics? Analysis based on dynamic contrast-enhanced chest computed tomography in adults. *Eur J Radiol* 2017;95:314–318.

13 **Answer B.** Of the choices provided, only hereditary hemorrhagic telangiectasia (HHT aka Rendu-Osler-Weber) causes clubbing on its own.

Multiple small pulmonary arteriovenous malformations (AVMs), which are the hallmark of this disease, mimic nodules on this maximum intensity image. Both granulomatosis with polyangiitis (aka Wegener's) and blastomycosis manifest as multiple pulmonary nodules with ground-glass halos. In this case however, there is a moderate-sized AVM in the posterior aspect of the left lung. Both an enlarged artery and an enlarged vein connect to this lesion, confirming its nature. The manifestations of septic emboli include cavitating nodules, ground-glass opacities, consolidation, infarcts, effusions, and pneumothorax.

References: Filocamo G, et al. Lung involvement in childhood onset granulomatosis with polyangiitis. *Pediatr Rheumatol Online J* 2017;15:28.

McBride JA, et al. Clinical manifestations and treatment of blastomycosis. *Clin Chest Med* 2017;38(3):435–449.

Nozaki T, et al. Syndromes associated with vascular tumors and malformations: a pictorial review. *Radiographics* 2013;33(1):175–195.

14 **Answer C.** There is a catheter loop in the main pulmonary artery. No catheter portion appears to be exiting the XY plane of the image via the main pulmonary artery. The two ends of the catheter both exit the plane or terminate in the right pulmonary artery. This indicates that the catheter is a fragment rather than a Swan-Ganz. A portion of a port catheter reservoir can be seen just anterior to the left pectoralis muscle. An EKOS catheter additionally would have opaque markers at regular intervals. A guidewire would be much dense and would create beam hardening and streak artifacts.

Reference: Yen HJ, Hwang B, Lee PC, et al. Transcatheter retrieval of different types of central venous catheter fragment: experience in 13 cases. *Angiology* 2006;57(3):347–353.

15 **Answer B.** Methyl methacrylate embolization occurs when cement leaks during vertebroplasty or kyphoplasty into the paravertebral venous plexus. The exact incidence is not well established, but it likely occurs in approximately 5% of cases. Outcomes are also variable with many patients being asymptomatic and others suffering death (although death is very rare). As in this case, MAA cement is often laced with a radio-opacifier, such as barium sulphate, to help proceduralist avoid this complication. The presence of a kyphoplasty on the same image confirms the diagnosis. Chronic pulmonary emboli can calcify but will not be as dense as the heavy metal laced MAA. Dendriform pulmonary ossification can be seen on x-ray and CT but is associated with aspiration or pulmonary fibrosis in a majority of cases.

Reference: Pelton WM, Jacobo K, Candocia FJ, et al. Methylmethacrylate pulmonary emboli: radiographic and computed tomographic findings. *J Thorac Imaging* 2009;24(3):241–247.

16 **Answer A.** Behçet disease is a multisystem large- and small-vessel vasculitis. Patients tend to be young adults of Middle Eastern, Mediterranean, or Far Eastern decent with a strong male predominance. There is a classic triad of symptoms including oral ulcers, genital ulcers, and uveitis. Involvement of additional organ systems is present in approximately one-third of patients. Upward of 85% of cases also involve the venous system, resulting in extrapulmonary venous thrombi. Pulmonary artery aneurysms are the most common pulmonary arterial manifestation in Behçet disease and are frequently accompanied by hemoptysis, which can be life threatening.

Reference: Ceylan N, Bayraktaroglu S, Erturk SM, et al. Pulmonary and vascular manifestations of Behçet disease: imaging findings. *AJR Am J Roentgenol* 2010;194(2): W158–W164.

17 **Answer C.** This image demonstrates circumferential wall thickening with stenosis of the left carotid artery and occlusion of the innominate and left subclavian arteries. Takayasu arteritis and Behçet disease both involve large

vessels. Behçet disease is more likely to involve the abdominal aorta or pulmonary arteries rather than the thoracic aorta or neck great vessels, making Takayasu's the correct answer. Takayasu's affects large- and medium-sized arteries. There is a predilection for women under the age of 40, who constitute more than 90% of cases. Findings include vessel wall thickening, narrowing, occlusion, and, rarely, dilatation. Note also the compensatory enlargement of the intercostal artery. The pristine nature of the facet joints is indicative of the patient's youth. Granulomatosis with polyangiitis (formerly known as Wegener's) is a small-vessel vasculitis. Thoracic manifestations include multiple pulmonary nodules and masses (frequently cavitary), pulmonary hemorrhage, and airway involvement. Goodpasture syndrome manifests in the chest as a pulmonary capillaritis and hemorrhage.

References: Castañer E, Alguersuari A, Gallardo X. When to suspect pulmonary vasculitis: radiologic and clinical clues. *Radiographics* 2010;30(1):33–53.

Ceylan N, Bayraktaroglu S, Erturk SM, et al. Pulmonary and vascular manifestations of Behçet disease: imaging findings. *AJR Am J Roentgenol* 2010;194(2): W158–W164.

18 Answer A. Based on the imaging findings, one can surmise that contrast reaches the heart from a left-sided peripheral venous injection via a persistent left superior vena cava (PLSVC). However, the right heart does not opacify as one would expect. Typically, a PLSVC drains to the coronary sinus and ultimately to the right atrium. Here, a rare drainage of the PLSVC into the left atrial appendage causes right-to-left shunting. This has resulted in opacification of left heart before the right. Under normal hemodynamic conditions, a traumatic fistula will always result in left-to-right shunting. There is no surgical intervention that purposefully cause a left-to-right shunt. A chronic left-to-right shunt can result in cardiomegaly, pulmonary hypertension, and shunt reversal (Eisenmenger's physiology). However, the pulmonary arteries appear normal and cardiomegaly is not seen.

Reference: Tobbia P, Norris LA, Lane T. Persistent left superior vena cava draining into the left atrium. *BMJ Case Rep* 2013;2013. doi: 10.1136/bcr-2013-010167.

19 Answer D. Fibrosing mediastinitis (FM) is an uncommon inflammatory disorder characterized by fibrous tissue proliferation within the mediastinum. It is a fibrosclerotic disorder similar to retroperitoneal fibrosis or Riedel thyroiditis. The process of fibrosis can cause stenosis of any mediastinal vessel or airway. When FM gradually causes pulmonary artery stenosis, enlargement of the bronchial arteries to augment blood flow to the lungs occurs. CT findings include replacement of mediastinal fat by intermediate-density fibrous tissue that compresses and distorts the hila of the lungs. In most instances, enlarged densely calcified lymph nodes are seen. Occasionally, as in this case, pericardial calcification is also seen. Patients with FM may present with a history of prior histoplasmosis or tuberculosis infection.

Reference: Rossi SE, McAdams HP, Rosado-de-Christenson ML, et al. Fibrosing mediastinitis. *Radiographics* 2001;21:737–757.

20 Answer D. Pulmonary sequestration (PS) is a rare congenital malformation. It is usually identified in children and young adults. PS consists of nonfunctioning pulmonary tissue with or without communication with the tracheobronchial tree that receives an anomalous systemic arterial blood supply. It appears as a soft tissue consolidation with or without emphysematous hyperaerated areas. Lung cancer and atelectasis do not have the characteristic systemic supply.

References: Petersen G, et al. Intralobar sequestration in the middle-aged and elderly adult: recognition and radiographic evaluation. *J Thorac Cardiovasc Surg* 2003;126(6):2086–2090.

Walker CM, Wu CC, Gilman MD, et al. The imaging spectrum of bronchopulmonary sequestration. *Curr Probl Diagn Radiol* 2014;43(3):100–114.

QUESTIONS

1 If similar in size, which of the following nodule types would likely have the longest doubling time if malignant?

A. Ground-glass nodule
B. Semisolid nodule
C. Solid nodule
D. Centrally calcified nodule

2 Precontrast T1-weighted image and postcontrast T1-weighted image with Dixon fat saturation obtained for presurgical planning demonstrate this left apical lung lesion, which had been previously biopsied and shown to be a primary adenocarcinoma of the lung. What features of this lesion render it inoperable?

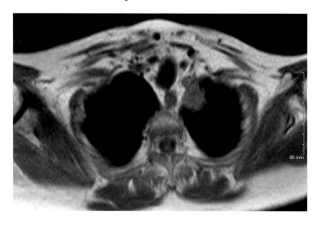 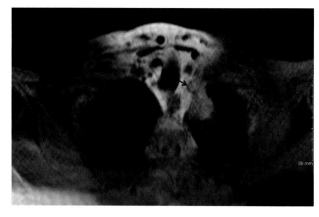

A. Invasion of the brachial plexus
B. Invasion of the left common carotid artery
C. Invasion of the left subclavian artery
D. Invasion of the mediastinal fat

3 Initial radiograph and subsequent CT in a 57-year-old female with chest pain demonstrates this lesion in the left chest. She has no history of trauma. Which of the following diagnoses should be the primary consideration?

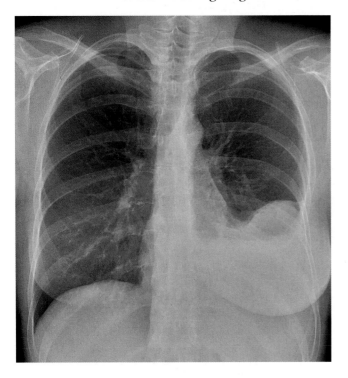

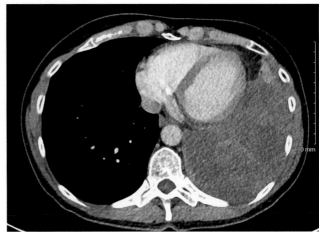

A. Neoplasm
B. Diaphragmatic hernia
C. Empyema
D. Hemothorax

4 Below are CT and FDG-PET images from a 62-year-old female patient. The primary lesion arose from the medial left upper lobe. Based on the provided images, select the most accurate initial staging:

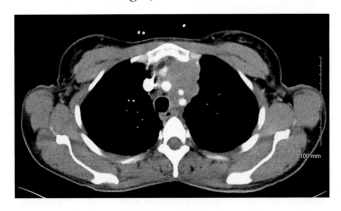

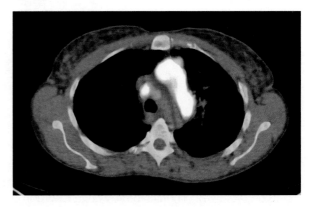

A. T4, N3, M1b, stage IVa
B. T3, N2, M0, stage IIIb
C. T4, N2, M1b, stage IVa
D. T3, N3, M0, stage IIIc

5 A 66-year-old female was treated for pneumonia based on an initial CT (left). On follow-up 3 years later (right), the consolidation in the left lower lobe persists with new development of several nodules such as the one in the right lower lobe. What is the likely diagnosis?

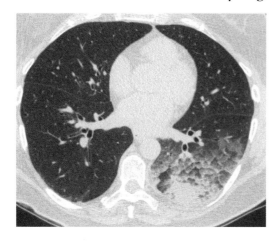 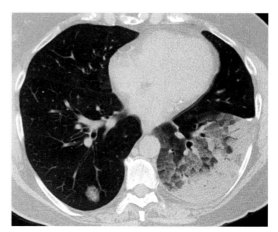

A. Atypical mycobacterial infection
B. Chronic fungal infection
C. Multifocal adenocarcinoma
D. Organizing pneumonia

6 This is an image from a CT scan performed on a 78-year-old female with a long smoking history. The nodule measures 1.5 cm and has persisted for 3 months. No other abnormalities are identified on the chest CT. Assuming that the patient has an acceptable risk profile for surgery, what would be the best evidence-based course for further evaluation and management?

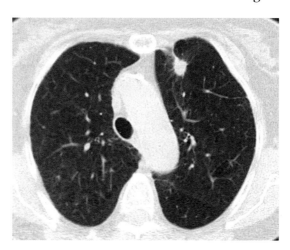

A. Percutaneous transthoracic biopsy
B. Thoracotomy, wedge resection of the nodule, and possible completion lobectomy
C. Preoperative brain MRI
D. Preoperative brain MRI and PET scan

7a With regard to low-dose CT screening for lung cancer, what value should the dose–length product be under for a standard patient?

A. 50 mGy-cm
B. 75 mGy-cm
C. 125 mGy-cm
D. 200 mGy-cm

7b What is the minimum pack-year smoking history recommended for undergoing low-dose CT of the chest for lung cancer screening?

    A. 5 pack-years
    B. 10 pack-years
    C. 15 pack-years
    D. 30 pack-years

8 In this patient with a history of malignancy, what accounts for the lesion marked by the white arrows?

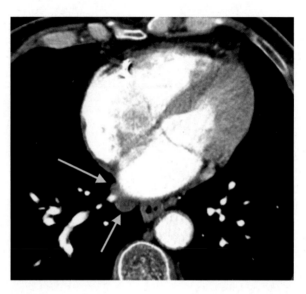

    A. Lymphadenopathy
    B. Metastatic pulmonary nodule
    C. Nonspecific pulmonary nodule
    D. Pericardial fluid

9a An initial staging CT scan on a 61-year-old female patient with iodine-avid thyroid cancer reveals this lesion in the right lower lobe. An FDG-PET/CT scan performed the following week showed only background activity in this lesion and no lesions elsewhere. What is the next best step?

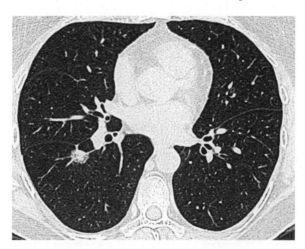

    A. No further follow-up.
    B. Initiate I-131 therapy for metastatic thyroid cancer.
    C. Initiate targeted anti-EGFR therapy for bronchogenic adenocarcinoma.
    D. A 3-month follow-up CT.

9b An outside CT scan from 6 years prior has been obtained, shown below with the new CT for comparison (current on left, 6 years prior on right). What is the likely diagnosis?

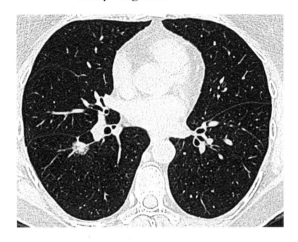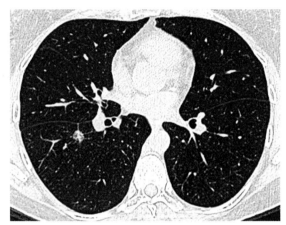

    A. Focal scar
    B. Minimally invasive adenocarcinoma
    C. Thyroid metastasis
    D. Hamartoma

10a What is the most common location of a missed lung cancer on chest radiograph?
    A. Central and upper lobe
    B. Peripheral and lower lobe
    C. Central and lower lobe
    D. Peripheral and upper lobe

10b What type of observer error is the most common in missed lung cancer?
    A. Scanning error
    B. Observer error
    C. Decision-making error
    D. Satisfaction of search error

11a This chest radiograph and CT were obtained from a 45-year-old male complaining of shortness of breath and weight loss. In addition to infectious and inflammatory processes, which of the following malignancies should be considered?

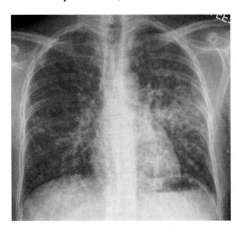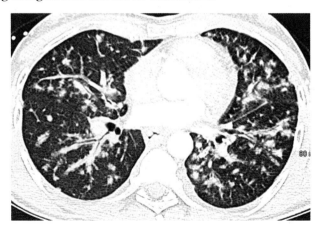

    A. Pulmonary lymphoma
    B. Intraductal papillary mucinous tumor of the pancreas metastasis
    C. Prostate cancer metastasis
    D. Epithelioid hemangioendothelioma

11b During this patient's evaluation, it is discovered that he has HIV infection. What additional diagnoses should be considered?

    A. None

    B. Kaposi sarcoma

    C. Pneumocystis infection

    D. Cryptococcal pneumonia

12a The following frontal radiograph was obtained in a 67-year-old male with chest pain. In the absence of infectious symptoms, which of the following features on the radiograph is the most worrisome for malignancy?

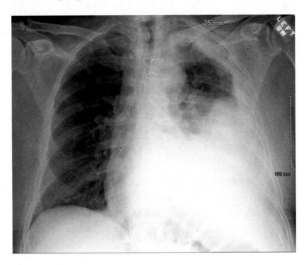

    A. Rib destruction

    B. Mediastinal shift to the right

    C. Large unilateral effusion

    D. Prior CABG

12b A CT scan of this patient was performed. Which of the following is the most LIKELY diagnosis?

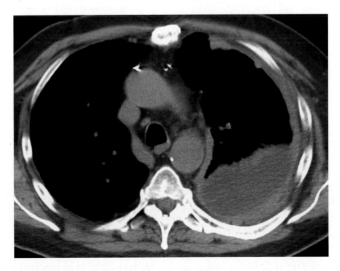

    A. Mesothelioma

    B. Asbestos-related pleural disease

    C. Metastatic adenocarcinoma

    D. Chronic fibrothorax

13 An image from a CT scan performed on a 62-year-old female with chest pain is shown. A percutaneous CT-guided biopsy of this lesion has been requested. What is the most important next step prior to biopsy of this lesion?

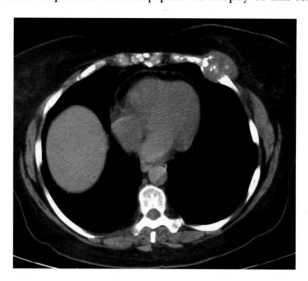

A. Obtain a contrast-enhanced CT, as this may be a highly vascular lesion such as a renal cell carcinoma metastasis.
B. Surgical consultation, as the needle tract will have to be excised.
C. Adrenergic blockage (such as labetalol), as the lesion could be metastatic pheochromocytoma.
D. Anesthesia consultation, as this lesion will be very painful to biopsy.

14a This incidentally discovered nodule measured 12 mm in length. Which of the following is the appropriate action based on the Fleischner Society pulmonary nodule management guidelines?

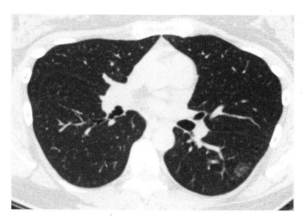

A. Follow-up CT in 3 months.
B. Follow-up CT in 6 to 12 months.
C. Biopsy.
D. No follow-up is required.

14b On follow-up, the nodule is unchanged in size, but has become more solid in density. What is the most appropriate next step?

A. Continued follow-up with CT in 3 months.
B. Continued follow-up with CT in 12 months.
C. Surgical evaluation for possible resection.
D. As the nodule is unchanged in size, no further follow-up is necessary.

15 A 72-year-old female patient with head and neck squamous cell carcinoma had a diagnostic chest CT and PET/CT performed as part of her pretreatment staging. The chest CT demonstrated multiple bilateral pulmonary nodules. Images shown demonstrate two of the larger nodules. The FDG-PET/CT demonstrated increased uptake in the laryngeal primary but did not demonstrate increased uptake in any of the pulmonary nodules. What is the next best step?

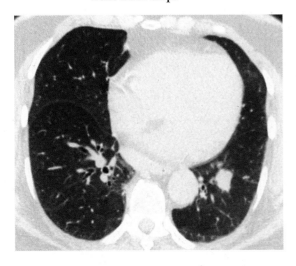 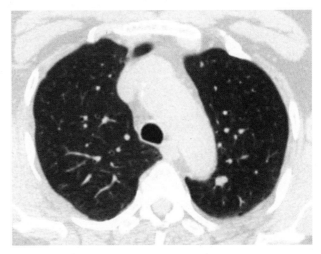

A. No further evaluation, as the lack of PET avidity confirms benignity
B. Repeat PET/CT, as the lack of PET avidity suggests an inadequate study
C. Tissue biopsy, as the nodules are worrisome for metastases
D. Initiation of chemotherapy, as the nodules are definitely metastatic

16a A 76-year-old female presented to her primary physician with chest pain. A PA and lateral chest film was obtained. The PA image is shown. Which of the following findings is present on this radiograph?

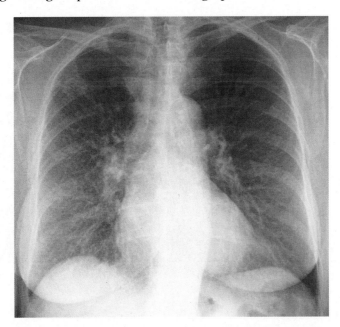

A. Mass lesion projecting behind the right atrium
B. Expansile lesion involving the anterior right second rib
C. Increased interstitial markings only on the right side
D. Diffusely increased interstitial markings, worse on the right

16b A CT was obtained, an image from which is shown. Biopsy demonstrated lymphangitic spread of a previously unsuspected breast cancer. Which of the following findings is most suggestive of lymphangitic spread of cancer on CT imaging?

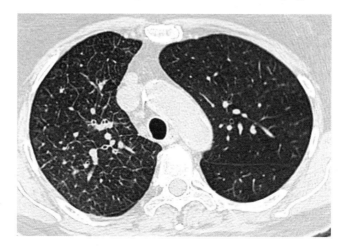

A. Nodular interlobular septal thickening
B. Bronchiectasis
C. Mosaic air trapping
D. Pleural effusion

17 CT image of an 84-year-old man with a significant smoking history and a history of occupational exposure to coal dust. These nodules are unchanged compared to a scan obtained 6 months prior. There is also diffuse partially calcified adenopathy in the mediastinum (not shown). Fused image from an FDG-PET scan demonstrating intense FDG uptake in the larger nodules at the lung bases. There was only mildly increased activity in the partially calcified mediastinal lymph nodes.

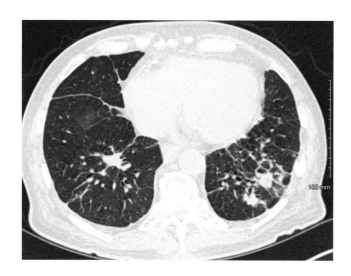

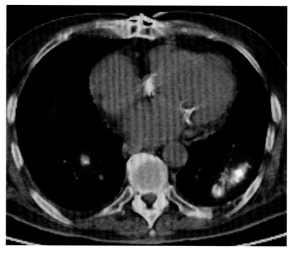

The most likely diagnosis is:
A. Metastatic lung cancer
B. Fungal infection
C. Organizing pneumonia
D. Progressive massive fibrosis

18 The lesion has demonstrated >3 months of stability. Approximately what percentage of this type of lesion will end up being adenocarcinoma on surgical resection?

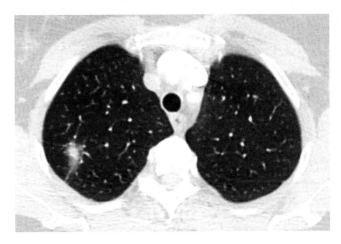

    A. 5%
    B. 25%
    C. 60%
    D. 90%

19a The patient is a 35-year-old nonsmoker. What is the most likely diagnosis?

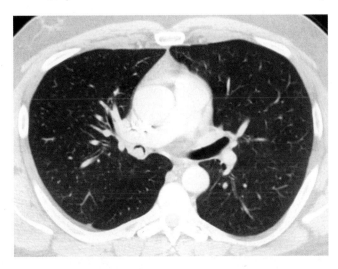

    A. Squamous cell carcinoma
    B. Adenoid cystic carcinoma
    C. Mucoepidermoid carcinoma
    D. Bronchial carcinoid

19b What percentage of bronchial carcinoids cause carcinoid syndrome?
    A. <5%
    B. 10% to 15%
    C. 20% to 25%
    D. More than 30%

20a Portable chest radiograph obtained for suspected pneumonia. What is the best recommendation after initiating antibiotic treatment?

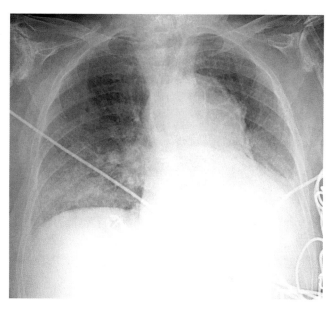

    A. No imaging follow-up
    B. Follow-up chest radiograph in 6 to 8 weeks
    C. Chest computed tomography
    D. Bronchoscopy with transbronchial biopsy

20b Biopsy reveals small cell lung cancer. What criteria would make the cancer "limited stage"?

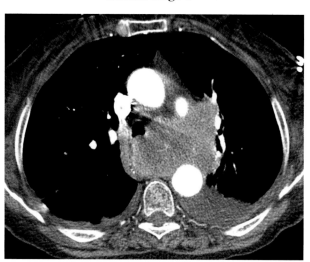 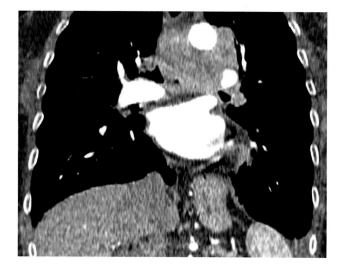

    A. Confined to a single radiation port
    B. Presence of brain metastases
    C. Malignant pleural effusion
    D. Extension beyond a single radiation port

ANSWERS AND EXPLANATIONS

1 **Answer A.** Of the nodule types listed, the ground-glass nodule has the longest potential doubling time. For malignant solid nodules, the doubling time is generally <100 days. Those with a doubling time more than 400 days are usually benign, and stability over 2 years (730 days) is therefore a reliable indicator of benignity for a majority of solid nodules. A doubling time of <20 days is much more likely infectious although this does not hold true for some aggressive malignancies or malignancy in the immunosuppressed. Comparatively, subsolid nodules can demonstrate a doubling time of more than 1,300 days and still be malignant. As such, follow-up of these nodules is generally longer than for the solid nodules, generally now 5 years. Semisolid nodules demonstrate doubling ranges between that of subsolid and solid nodules. A centrally calcified nodule is a benign pattern of calcification. In the remarkably small chance that such a lesion were malignant, such as a cancer that enveloped a calcified nodule, the doubling time would be similar to a solid nodule.

References: MacMahon H, et al. Guidelines for management of incidental pulmonary nodules detected on CT images: From the Fleischner Society 2017. *Radiology* 2017;284(1):228–243.

2 **Answer C.** The precontrast imaging demonstrates an absent flow void within the left subclavian artery seen to the left of the trachea. Postcontrast images demonstrate some enhancement of the thrombus in the left subclavian artery, suggesting tumor thrombus. A normal flow void is seen in the left common carotid artery. The brachial plexus is more superior to the provided images and more anterior to the lesion. There is broad contact with the mediastinal fat, but no clear invasion. Real-time cine sequences may also be helpful in assessing tumor invasion of mediastinal or chest wall structures.

References: Hayes SA, Plodkowski AJ, Ginsberg MS. Imaging of thoracic cavity tumors. *Surg Oncol Clin N Am* 2014;23(4):709–733.

Raptis CA, McWilliams SR, Ratkowski KL et al. Mediastinal and pleural MR imaging: practical approach for daily practice. *Radiographics* 2018;38(1):37–55.

3 **Answer A.** Diaphragmatic hernia would not be a consideration, as no abdominal fat or bowel is appreciated in the lesion. Empyema normally produces significant pleural thickening and has more of a fluid density. Empyema also usually has a slightly contracted appearance and tends to assume a lentiform shape. Hemothorax could be considered, as blood clot can have this density. However, hemothorax will be more heterogeneous in appearance, and the patient has no history or signs of trauma. Thus, the primary concern is neoplasm. As the lung is either completely displaced by or replaced with the tumor, it is difficult to determine if this lesion is of pleural or parenchymal origin.

This lesion proved to be a solitary fibrous tumor of the pleura. These uncommon tumors may exhibit benign or malignant behavior, and the behavior is difficult to predict based on histologic features. Paraneoplastic syndromes occur with a significant minority of these tumors, with hypertrophic pulmonary osteoarthropathy, arthritic symptoms, or refractory hypoglycemia being the most common.

References: Abu Arab W. Solitary fibrous tumours of the pleura. *Eur J Cardiothorac Surg* 2012;41(3):587–597.

Rosado-de-Christenson ML, Abbott GF, McAdams HP, et al. From the archives of the AFIP: localized fibrous tumor of the pleura. *RadioGraphics* 2003;23:759–783.

4 **Answer A.** Based on the provided images, we have a left upper lobe mass with mediastinal invasion and encasement of the great vessels. This is T4. Based on the PET imaging, there is a contralateral right paratracheal lymph node, N3, and there is a rib lesion, M1b. Of course, final staging will be determined by pathology.

Reference: Detterbeck FC, Boffa DJ, Kim AW, et al. The eighth edition lung cancer stage classification. *Chest* 2017;151:193–203.

5 **Answer C.** The initial CT demonstrates significant left lower lobe consolidation and some surrounding ground glass. The appearance is nonspecific and could be related to a lobar pneumonia. However, this case highlights why follow-up is important in many cases, especially those with atypical clinical or radiographic features. The most worrisome cause of chronic consolidation is cancer, and this is a case of multifocal mucinous adenocarcinoma. These lesions can be slow growing, as seen here, and frequently can develop multiple sites of disease over time. These could be aerogenous metastases or metasynchronous primaries, and treatment of these lesions remains controversial. There is some evidence for aggressive treatment including surgical resection especially if the nodal stage is N0 or N1. In addition to surgical resection of the primary cancer, the smaller lesions that are accessible and most aggressive appearing should also be considered for resection. Despite the controversial treatment possibilities, it is clear that those with the more diffuse or multifocal forms of adenocarcinoma have a worse prognosis than do those with an isolated nodule.

References: Gu B, Burt BM, Merritt RE, et al. A dominant adenocarcinoma with multifocal ground glass lesions does not behave as advanced disease. *Ann Thorac Surg* 2013;96(2):411–418.

Liu YY, Chen YM, Huang MH, et al. Prognosis and recurrent patterns in bronchioloalveolar carcinoma. *Chest* 2000;118(4):940–947.

Travis WD, Brambilla E, Noguchi M, et al. International association for the study of lung cancer/American thoracic society/European respiratory society international multidisciplinary classification of lung adenocarcinoma. *J Thorac Oncol* 2011;6(2):244–285.

6 **Answer B.** This is a T1a lesion. We are told that there are no other abnormalities visible on chest CT. In an older patient with a smoking history, it is known that it is more cost-effective and efficient to proceed to surgery, rather than to include the intermediate step of percutaneous biopsy. A spiculated nodule such as this has a >95% chance of being malignant in this patient population. Therefore, answer A is not correct. If the patient was a high surgical risk, and other treatment modalities such as external beam radiation or radiofrequency ablation were being considered, then biopsy would be appropriate.

Preoperative brain MRI is currently recommended in patients with T1b lesions and in all stage II and stage III lesions, but not in patients with T1a N0 disease. Likewise, FDG-PET scans are not currently recommended in this patient population, though they are performed in many centers. Therefore, answers C and D are incorrect.

In patients who are good candidates for potential lobectomy with T1a N0 disease, the sequence of events in answer B corresponds to the current management recommendations. Thoracotomy with wedge resection and immediate evaluation with frozen-section pathology will allow for completion lobectomy in the same setting if proven malignant. Preoperative lymph node sampling, by bronchoscopy or mediastinoscopy, is also not required in this patient population, although lymph node dissection will be performed in conjunction with the lobectomy.

Reference: Ettinger DS, Akerley W, Bepler G, et al.; NCCN non-small cell lung cancer panel members. Non-small cell lung cancer. *J Natl Compr Canc Netw* 2010;8:740–801.

7a **Answer B.**

7b **Answer D.**   The American Association of Physicists in Medicine (AAPM) does recommend that the dose–length product (DLP) be <75 mGy-cm for a lung cancer screening CT. Remember that this is for the AAPM "standard patient," who is 170 cm tall and weighs 70 kg (BMI = 24). As many of your patients will be larger than this, the actual DLP will be frequently higher than this.

The National Lung Screening Trial population, where a screening benefit was shown, ranged in age from 55 to 74. Some recommendations, including the U.S. Preventive Services Task Force, expand the age of recommended screening to 80, based on evidence from other trials. Some groups advocate for extension of the lower age bound to 50, although there are currently no good data to support this. There are currently no data to support lung cancer screening in patients with a lower pack-year history than 30.

Reference: Aberle DR, Adams AM, Berg CD, et al.; National Lung Screening Trial Research Team. Reduced lung-cancer mortality with low-dose computed tomographic screening. *N Engl J Med* 2011;365(5):395–409.

8 **Answer D.**   When the pulmonary veins penetrate the pericardium to join the atrium, a "sleeve" of pericardium surrounds the vein. As such, the right pulmonary venous recess or pericardial "sleeve" recess (of which this is an example) is a normal space within the pericardial sac that can occasionally fill with fluid. Knowing this anatomic space is important to avoid misclassifying it as a malignancy or other abnormality. When seen, there is frequently anterior and posterior fluid surrounding the right inferior pulmonary vein with the posterior component generally slightly larger. Superior and inferior components are possible but less frequently seen unless a larger volume of fluid is present. Features to help distinguish from adenopathy in this space include being well circumscribed, a lack of mass effect, and having fluid/water attenuation. Additionally, adenopathy more frequently appears on one side of the vessel.

Reference: Truong MT, Erasmus JJ, Sabloff BS, et al. Pericardial "sleeve" recess of right inferior pulmonary vein mimicking adenopathy: computed tomography findings. *J Comput Assist Tomogr* 2004;28(3):361–365.

9a **Answer D.**

9b **Answer B.**   Both metastatic and primary neoplasms may elicit sufficient immune response to produce localized fibrosis and scarring, which can produce tethering of the fissure such as this. It is true that thyroid cancer may be negative on FDG-PET, but there are many potential causes for this lesion, and a biopsy proving that this lesion represents metastatic thyroid cancer would be required before initiating therapy. Likewise, while it is true that bronchogenic adenocarcinomas may have this appearance, tissue is required to assess for the appropriate mutation before initiating targeted therapy. Given the semisolid appearance of the lesion, a low-grade adenocarcinoma is the most likely etiology, and comparison with priors if available and obtaining a follow-up CT in 3 months are the next best steps in management.

Many neoplasms may exhibit very slow growth. The FDG activity of this lesion does not actually add any additional information in this case, once the prior CT scan has come to light, as it would be surprising if such a slowly growing lesion had significant metabolic activity and FDG uptake. On the other hand, bronchogenic adenocarcinoma may exhibit very slow growth. In fact, this lesion was resected and was a minimally invasive adenocarcinoma (MIA). MIA is a relatively new pathologic subtype of adenocarcinoma and encompasses the lesions formerly known as bronchioloalveolar cell carcinoma (BAC). These lesions are characteristically slow growing and occur more commonly in nonsmokers than do other types of adenocarcinoma. They are often partly or wholly ground glass in attenuation on CT. For the same reasons, answer C is incorrect. Similarly, although hamartomas can grow, the semisolid nature of this nodule would be extremely atypical for a hamartoma.

It could be argued that, at this growth rate, this lesion would be very unlikely to kill the patient and should therefore be left alone. This can indeed be a reasonable course of action with many patients. There are no good data on the optimal management of these lesions, and the ultimate course of action will be determined by the patient's surgical risk, comorbidities, and the patient's personal preference. As a caveat, the growth rate of such lesions is not necessarily constant. In the absence of good data on the long-term behavior of these lesions, note that in our institution's experience with unresected MIA, roughly 5% will undergo aggressive transformation and become metastatic while they are being monitored.

Reference: Gardiner N, Jogai S, Wallis A. The revised lung adenocarcinoma classification—an imaging guide. *J Thorac Dis* 2014;6:S537–S546.

10a **Answer D.**

10b **Answer C.** In a study spanning from 1993 to 2001, non–small cell lung cancers that proved to be evident and missed on prior chest radiograph were reviewed for lesion location. The majority of missed NSCLC lesions were peripheral (85%) and upper lobe (72%). Specifically, the most common lobe for missed lung cancers was the right upper lobe (45%). The average lesion measured 1.9 cm in diameter. Other important lesion characteristics include density and shape.

The body of literature for missed lung cancers on chest radiograph is sizable, but a few landmark studies are commonly quoted. In particular, Kundel et al. performed several studies examining visual tracking with search patterns of radiologists related to missed lung cancers. They described three different observer errors: scanning, recognition, and decision-making errors. While the scanning error (no visual fixation on the lesion) made up 25% of observer errors and recognition error (visual fixation in the region of the lesion, but not on the lesion specifically) made up 30% of observer errors, decision-making error occurred in 45%, where the radiologist visually fixated on the lesion but incorrectly interpreted it as a normal structure. Satisfaction of search is another observer error where lung cancers are more easily recognized with fewer distracting abnormalities. While important to recognize, satisfaction of search is secondary relative to the aforementioned errors.

References: Shah PK, Austin JH, White CS, et al. Missed non-small cell lung cancer: radiographic findings of potentially resectable lesions evident only in retrospect. *Radiology* 2003;226:235–241.

White CS, Salis AI, Meyer CA. Missed lung cancer on chest radiography and computed tomography: imaging and medicolegal issues. *J Thorac Imaging* 1999;14:63–68.

11a **Answer A.**

11b **Answer B.** The findings are those of extensive, and largely confluent, small nodules extending along the bronchovascular bundles, with some subpleural nodules also noted. This is a perilymphatic pattern and could be seen with lymphangitic spread of any tumor. IPMT of the pancreas, prostate cancer, and epithelioid hemangioendothelioma do not commonly produce lymphangitic spread in the lungs. As well, on the chest radiograph, the pattern is very diffuse, and there is no dominant mass lesion. In cases of lymphangitic spread from extrathoracic metastatic disease, the lymphangitic pattern is usually more focal, and there is often a dominant central mass. Therefore, pulmonary lymphoma is correct. Pulmonary lymphoma may be either primary or secondary, and may manifest with a perilymphatic pattern, or may present as one or more airspace opacities.

While it is true that HIV patients are at increased risk for pulmonary lymphoma, certainly other diagnoses could be considered. One such diagnosis would be Kaposi sarcoma. In fact, this particular case proved to be Kaposi sarcoma rather than lymphoma.

HIV patients are at increased risk for pneumocystis and cryptococcal infection, but they would not be expected to produce the appearances seen here and are therefore incorrect. Pneumocystis typically produces interstitial and ground-glass opacities, and later in the infection, the eponymous cysts may occur. Cryptococcal pneumonia commonly produces nodules, but a diffuse perilymphatic pattern would not be expected.

Reference: Lambert AA, Merlo CA, Kirk GD. Human immunodeficiency virus-associated lung malignancies. *Clin Chest Med* 2013;34:255–272.

12a **Answer C.**

12b **Answer C.**   There is no rib destruction present. Obviously, if rib destruction was present, there is a high likelihood of malignancy. Likewise, there is no mediastinal shift—the trachea lines up nicely over the spinous processes. However, if mediastinal shift were present, this would also be a concerning feature, as malignant effusions often behave in an expansile fashion, and a tension hydrothorax can even occur with a malignant effusion. Prior CABG has no particular association with malignancy, although tobacco use is a shared risk factor for both coronary artery disease and lung cancer. A large unilateral effusion has a very high likelihood of being either a malignant effusion or an empyema, so any large unilateral effusion in a patient without infectious symptoms is very worrisome for malignancy.

This is a classic appearance for mesothelioma, with the characteristic feature being the marked thickening of the mediastinal pleura. However, mesothelioma is a rare tumor, and it is actually more common for a malignant effusion from metastatic adenocarcinoma (most commonly breast or lung) to produce this appearance. Asbestos-related pleural disease reliably does not involve the mediastinal pleura, so this is incorrect. A chronic fibrothorax, from prior hemothorax or empyema, nearly always calcifies, and the involved hemithorax is usually smaller, with mediastinal shift toward the pleural abnormality, so answer D is incorrect.

Reference: Truong MT, Viswanathan C, Godoy MB, et al. Malignant pleural mesothelioma: role of CT, MRI, and PET/CT in staging evaluation and treatment considerations. *Semin Roentgenol* 2013;48:323–334.

13 **Answer B.**   The key to this question is recognizing the presence of calcified matrix within the lesion. Further, the location at a costochondral junction is very typical for this lesion, which is a chondrosarcoma. As chondrosarcomas, like the chondrocytes from which they derive, grow readily in an avascular environment, they may seed the biopsy tract. Management guidelines call for excision of the biopsy tract along with the tumor, so careful planning is required, and answer B is correct. Renal cell carcinoma metastases do not typically contain calcifications, so answer A is not correct. We are given no reason to suspect a metastatic pheochromocytoma, which would require alpha- and beta-adrenergic blockade, so answer C is incorrect. Malignant tumors are not generally painful to biopsy, as they contain no organized nerves. Any pain is usually derived from the needle path through surrounding normal tissues. Answer D is incorrect.

Reference: Souza FF, de Angelo M, O'Regan K, et al. Malignant primary chest wall neoplasms: a pictorial review of imaging findings. *Clin Imaging* 2013;37:8–17.

14a Answer B.

14b Answer C. This is a pure ground-glass nodule, and current guidelines suggest a 6- to 12-month follow-up CT. Earlier recommendations were for an initial 3-month follow-up, but the new guidelines recommend the longer follow-up interval, because "earlier follow-up is unlikely to affect the outcome of these characteristically indolent lesions." Increasing solidity in a ground-glass nodule indicates a high risk for adenocarcinoma and future aggressive behavior, and consideration of biopsy or resection is recommended.

Reference: MacMahon H, Naidich DP, Goo JM, et al. Guidelines for management of incidental pulmonary nodules detected on CT images: from the Fleischner Society 2017. *Radiology* 2017;284(1):228–243.

15 Answer C. Metastases may demonstrate more or less FDG uptake than the primary lesion, as they are often biologically distinct from the primary, with additional mutations. Therefore, answer A is incorrect. It is true that FDG-PET is insensitive to lesions under 8 mm, and this is particularly true in the lungs with the additional consideration of respiratory motion. However, the larger lesion shown in this case exceeds 2 cm in size and should be readily apparent on PET imaging if it takes up FDG. In some cases, depending on the individual clinical situation, a cancer patient who develops new bilateral pulmonary nodules during the course of treatment is assumed to have metastatic disease without tissue proof being obtained. However, this is an initial staging evaluation, and it is never appropriate to make assumptions that alter treatment. Answer C reflects appropriate patient management at initial cancer staging as these are highly worrisome for metastases, but this should be proven by pathology.

In this case, in fact, the larger nodule shown above was percutaneously biopsied, and a smaller contralateral nodule was biopsied thoracoscopically. The pathology of both lesions was typical carcinoid and not metastatic squamous cell carcinoma. Multiple pulmonary carcinoid tumors are not uncommon and may mimic metastatic disease. When they are discovered during evaluation for another malignancy, they often do not have significant impact on the patient's survival or treatment. This patient was able to have curative resection of her head and neck primary.

Reference: Aubry M, Thomas CF, Jett JR, et al. Significance of multiple carcinoid tumors and tumorlets in surgical lung specimens: analysis of 28 patients. *Chest* 2007;131:1635–1643.

16a Answer C.

16b Answer A. The radiograph demonstrates increased interstitial markings only on the right side. There is no evidence of the other answer choices.

Bronchiectasis is not a feature of lymphangitic spread of tumor. Pleural effusions are often present in patients with lymphangitic spread of tumor, but the vast majority of patients with pleural effusions do not, of course, have lymphangitic spread of tumor, so the presence of a pleural effusion is not suggestive of this entity. Mosaic air trapping may occasionally be seen in lymphangitic spread of tumor, because of the thickening of the walls of the small airways, which contain lymphatics. However, other causes of mosaic air trapping are much more common. Nodular or smooth interlobular septal thickening, almost always focal or asymmetric (as in this case), is almost universally present in lymphangitic spread of tumor. Central lymphadenopathy is also often present in lymphangitic spread of tumor and was present in this case (not shown).

Other causes of nodular interlobular septal thickening are few and include sarcoidosis, pneumoconiosis, and pulmonary alveolar septal amyloidosis. These other causes would not likely be as strikingly asymmetric as in this case.

Reference: Honda O, Johkoh T, Ichikado K, et al. Comparison of high resolution CT findings of sarcoidosis, lymphoma, and lymphangitic carcinoma: is there any difference of involved interstitium? *J Comput Assist Tomogr* 1999;23:374–379.

17 **Answer D.**   Metastatic lung cancer is certainly a possible diagnosis, although the presence of irregular nodules and associated architectural distortion, indicating some component of fibrosis, would be unusual. Further, most malignant nodules of this size will demonstrate growth over a 6-month interval. A fungal infection such as blastomycosis could also produce the findings on the current scan, but we would expect both infection and organizing pneumonia to have changed in appearance over a 6-month interval. It is important to recognize that progressive massive fibrosis (PMF) nearly always demonstrates increased FDG avidity. Of course, patients with coal worker's pneumoconiosis and silicosis, who are at risk for developing PMF, also may develop lung cancer. Detecting lung cancer in patients with a large burden of pneumoconiotic nodules can be very difficult. Practically speaking, the best option is serial CT follow-up. Some preliminary data suggest that FDG-PET may be of some benefit in these patients, but there was quite a bit of overlap of the SUV values for malignant lesions and areas of fibrosis.

Reference: Chung SY, Lee JH, Kim TH, et al. 18F-FDG PET imaging of progressive massive fibrosis. *Ann Nucl Med* 2010;24:21. https://doi-org.ezproxy.uky.edu/10.1007/s12149-009-0322-9

18 **Answer C.**   A semisolid nodule is present in the right upper lobe on CT, meaning that some portions of the nodule are definitively ground glass (less dense than pulmonary vasculature) and some portions are definitively solid (obscures the pulmonary vasculature). The best initial recommendation is a 3-month follow-up to exclude an inflammatory or infectious focus. Since this lesion has demonstrated stability over 3 months, it now falls into the category of a persistent semisolid nodule. In a review of lung cancer screening patients with persistent lung nodules measuring from 2 mm up to 45 mm, Henschke et al. found that 32% of solid nodules, 63% of semisolid nodules (partially solid), and 13% of pure ground-glass nodules (nonsolid) ended up being malignant nodules. When subdividing nodules on the basis of malignancy type, all semisolid nodules were found to be adenocarcinoma. Kim et al. found an even higher percentage (75%) of adenocarcinoma in persistent ground-glass nodules measuring 3 cm or less.

References: Henschke CI, Yankelevitz DF, Mirtcheva R, et al. CT screening for lung cancer: frequency and significance of part-solid and nonsolid nodules. *AJR Am J Roentgenol* 2002;178:1053–1057.

Kim HY, Sim YM, Lee KS, et al. Persistent pulmonary nodular ground-glass opacity at thin-section CT: histopathologic comparisons. *Radiology* 2007;245(1):267–275.

19a **Answer D.**

19b **Answer A.**   A nodular filling defect is present in the bronchus intermedius. The most common primary tumor of the bronchi in young adults is carcinoid tumor. Carcinoid tumors can be subdivided into typical and atypical in the spectrum of neuroendocrine tumors along with small cell lung cancer. Carcinoid syndrome is uncommon in bronchial carcinoid (<5%) and generally only in the setting of liver metastases. Approximately 25% of bronchial carcinoids calcify, and evidence of calcification of a nodule with endobronchial component in a young adult is virtually diagnostic. Because it is an endobronchial lesion, patients often present with symptoms related to airway narrowing (cough or wheeze), bleeding (hemoptysis), or obstruction (pneumonia), although approximately a quarter of cases are identified incidentally. Resection of typical carcinoid, as in this case, has an excellent prognosis with a 92% survival rate at 5 years.

References: Jeung M, Gasser B, Gangi A, et al. Bronchial carcinoid tumors of the thorax: spectrum of radiologic findings. *Radiographics* 2002;22:351–365.

Ngo AH, Walker CM, Chung JH, et al. Tumors and tumorlike conditions of the large airways. *AJR Am J Roentgenol* 2013;201:301–313.

20a **Answer C.**

20b **Answer A.** While the portable chest radiograph does demonstrate consolidation in both lung bases, left greater than right, several findings make this more than a typical community-acquired pneumonia. Primarily, a large left mediastinal mass extending into the aortopulmonary window is present. Additionally, there is rightward shift of the trachea from extrinsic compression and leftward cardiac shift due to left lower lobe collapse. No follow-up and follow-up chest radiograph in 6 to 8 weeks after initiation of antibiotic treatment are options for community-acquired pneumonia dependent on patient age. Bronchoscopy is an option here, but the potential for an aortic abnormality as well as guidance for potential biopsy makes CT the best choice before any intervention is performed.

The CT and subsequent biopsy reveal a large middle mediastinal mass from small cell carcinoma. Small cell carcinoma constitutes approximately 15% of all lung cancers, but the overall small cell cancer rate has been decreasing since the 1980s. Highly associated with smoking, small cell carcinoma is the most aggressive of the pulmonary neuroendocrine tumors, and at presentation, more than 60% of patients with small cell carcinoma have metastases. More than 10% will have brain metastases at presentation. Small cell carcinoma can be subdivided into limited stage (LS) and extensive stage (ES), primarily based on disease confined to a single radiation port for limited-stage disease. Debate exists over the importance of contralateral mediastinal or supraclavicular lymph node involvement for determining stage.

Reference: Carter BW, Glisson BS, Truong MT, et al. Small cell lung carcinoma: staging, imaging, and treatment considerations. *Radiographics* 2014;34:1707–1721.

Trauma

James T. Lee, MD • David Nickels, MD, MBA

QUESTIONS

1a A 26-year-old pregnant female post MVC. Which of the following findings are present?

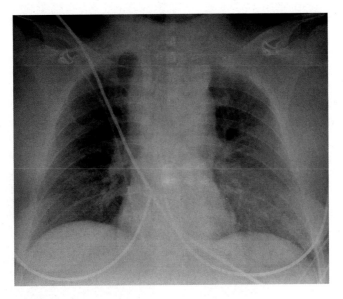

A. Left apical cap
B. Thickened right paratracheal stripe
C. Depression of the left main stem bronchus
D. Widening of the superior mediastinum
E. Indistinctness to the aortic arch
F. All of the above

1b What is the most likely diagnosis?

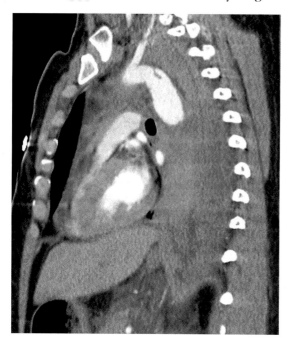

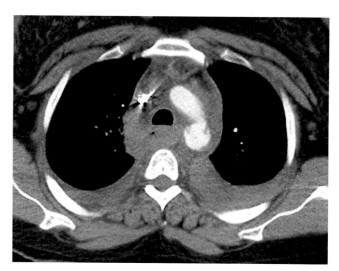

A. Amniotic fluid embolism
B. Traumatic aortic injury
C. Pneumothorax
D. Tension hemothorax

2 A 30-year-old male transferred for evaluation of a cavitary lung mass after motor vehicle collision. What is the most likely diagnosis?

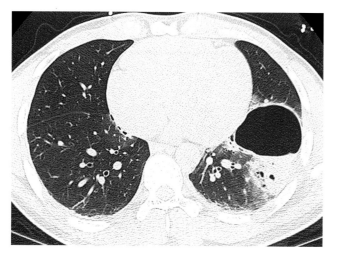

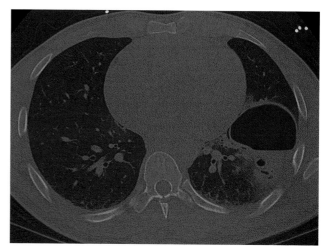

A. Pulmonary laceration
B. Tuberculosis
C. Congenital cystic adenomatoid malformation
D. Cavitary primary neoplasm

3 A 22-year-old female polytrauma patient post exploratory laparotomy, splenectomy, and multiple orthopedic injuries with hypoxemia despite intubation and bilateral chest tube placement. What diagnosis could be considered given the images provided?

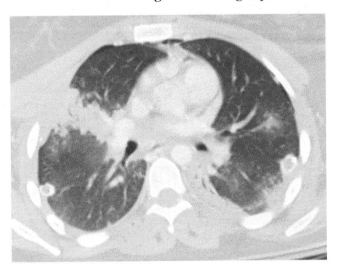

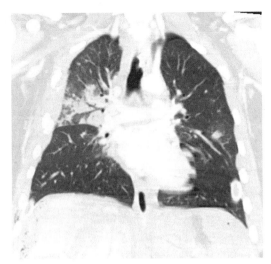

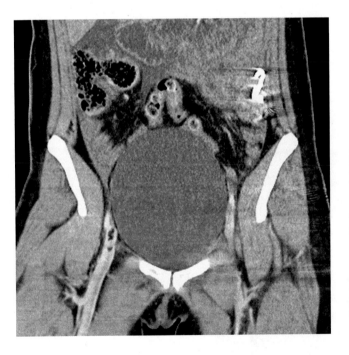

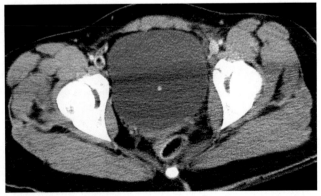

A. Cardiac contusion
B. Abdominal compartment syndrome
C. Tension pneumothorax
D. Fat embolism

4a A 61-year-old post MVC. What radiologic sign is depicted here?

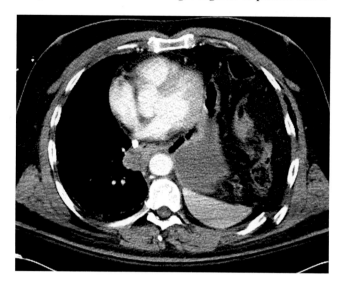

A. Collar sign
B. Dependent viscera sign
C. Bulging fissure sign
D. Cutoff sign

4b What radiologic sign is depicted here?

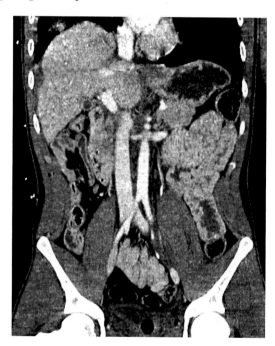

A. Collar sign
B. Dependent viscera sign
C. Bulging fissure sign
D. Cutoff sign

5a What Society of Vascular Surgery grade blunt aortic injury is shown?

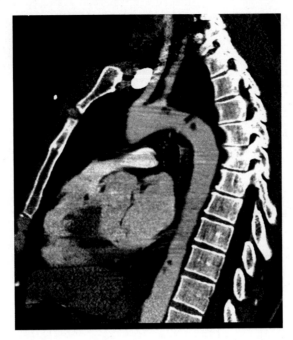

A. Grade 1
B. Grade 2
C. Grade 3
D. Grade 4

5b The patient in question 5A is a 41-year-old male in high-speed MVC with multiple extremity and facial fractures. What is the most appropriate next recommendation?

A. Follow-up CTA of the chest in 2 to 7 days
B. Vascular interventional radiology consult for diagnostic angiogram and possible stent placement
C. Immediate follow-up cardiac gated CTA chest
D. No specific follow-up

6 The salient finding is associated with which of the following?

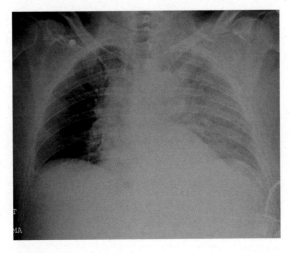

A. Need for prolonged intubation
B. Risk for pneumonia
C. Associated with increased morbidity and mortality
D. All of the above

7   A 36-year-old kicked by a horse. What is the most likely diagnosis?

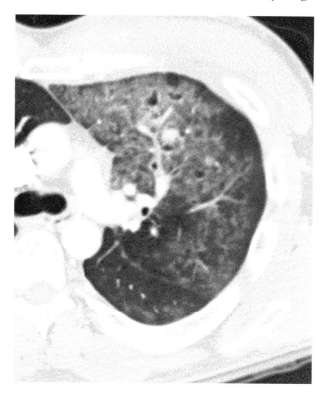

A. Aspiration
B. Pulmonary edema
C. Pulmonary contusion with small lacerations
D. Atypical pneumonia with cyst formation

8a   What is the most important finding in this patient with substernal chest pain?

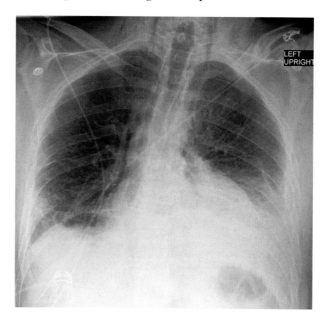

A. Pleural effusion
B. Cardiomegaly
C. Pneumomediastinum
D. Indistinct aortic arch

8b This entity most commonly presents after which of the following?

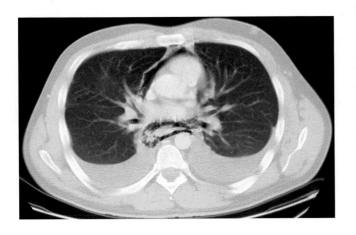

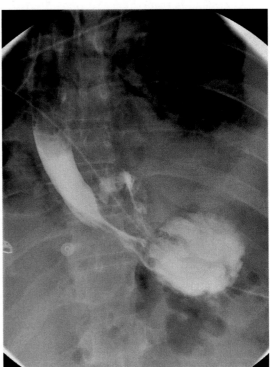

    A. Forceful repetitive vomiting
    B. Blunt trauma
    C. Penetrating trauma
    D. Pressure necrosis secondary to food bolus impaction

9 What pitfall is most likely to interfere with making the diagnosis of a sternal fracture (shown) in the setting of trauma?

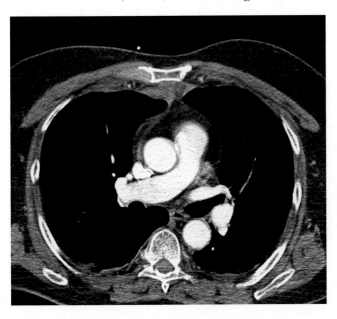

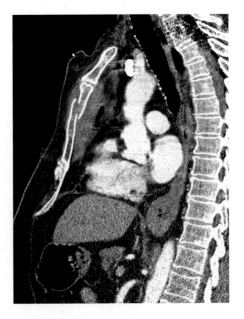

    A. Aortic pulsation artifact
    B. Respiratory motion artifact
    C. Streak artifact
    D. Surrounding soft tissue injury

10a Regarding fractures of the thoracic spinal column, which of the following is true?

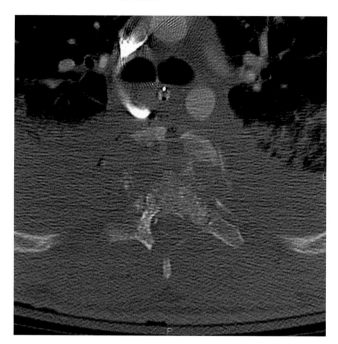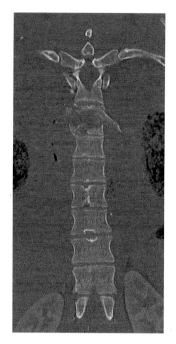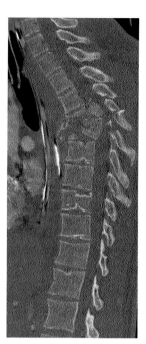

    A. Multiple articulations in the thoracic spinal column gives added load-bearing stability.
    B. Coronal orientation of the thoracic facet joints increases rigidity.
    C. The central canal is most narrow in the thoracic vertebral segments.
    D. All of the above.

10b The fracture shown is best classified as which of the following?
    A. Burst fracture
    B. Compression fracture
    C. Fracture dislocation
    D. Chance fracture

11a What is the diagnosis?

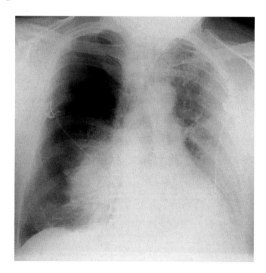

    A. Artifact
    B. Emphysema
    C. Tension pneumothorax
    D. Pulmonary contusion

11b What is the reason a tension pneumothorax can quickly become fatal?

    A. Rapid blood loss
    B. Decreased oxygenation
    C. Decreased arterial blood supply to the brain
    D. Decreased venous blood return to the heart

11c There are several different radiograph techniques that can help to emphasize a small pneumothorax. Which of these techniques requires that the patient be able to follow commands?

    A. Inspiration and expiration views
    B. Upright frontal view
    C. Left lateral decubitus view
    D. Lateral view

12 Persistent pneumothorax after placement of well-positioned and functioning chest tube should raise the concern for what injury?

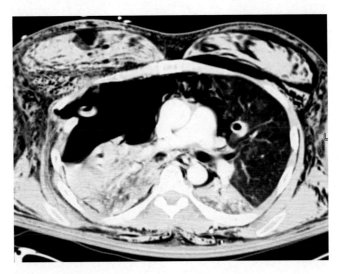

    A. Pulmonary laceration
    B. Tracheal transection
    C. Bronchial tear
    D. Diaphragm injury

13a What is the diagnosis?

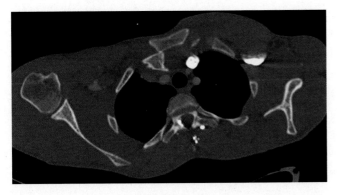 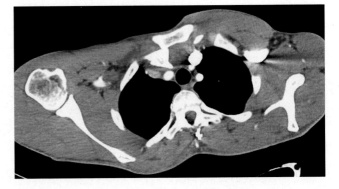

    A. Clavicle fracture
    B. Posterior sternoclavicular dislocation
    C. Manubrial fracture
    D. Sternomanubrial dislocation

13b What vessel injury is associated with a LEFT posterior sternoclavicular dislocation?

    A. Thoracic aorta
    B. Left carotid artery
    C. Left subclavian vein
    D. Superior vena cava

14a What type of acute traumatic aortic injury is present?

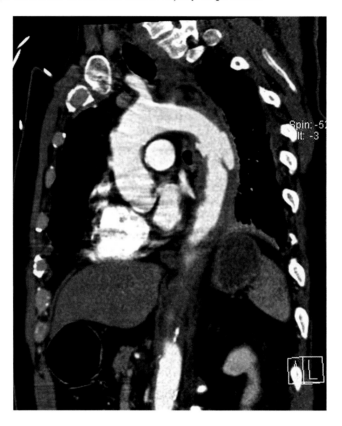

    A. Mural thrombus
    B. Minimal arterial injury
    C. Pseudoaneurysm
    D. Complete transection

14b What grade of injury is present?

    A. Grade 1
    B. Grade 2
    C. Grade 3
    D. Grade 4

14c When a traumatic pseudoaneurysm of the thoracic aorta is present, what layer of the vessel wall remains intact?

    A. Media
    B. Adventitia
    C. Intima

14d Where is the most common site of acute traumatic aortic injury on CT?

    A. At the level of the ligamentum arteriosum (aortic isthmus)
    B. Ascending aorta
    C. Aortic arch
    D. Distal descending thoracic aorta

15 Which of the following is the most likely cause of air adjacent to the trachea and esophagus?

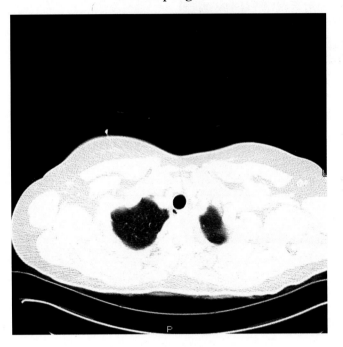 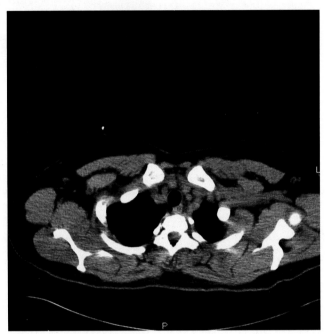

  A. Acute esophageal injury
  B. Soft tissue gas related to rib fracture
  C. Acute tracheal injury
  D. Normal variant

16 The solid white arrows in the given image point to abnormalities in the right subclavian artery. What is the best diagnosis?

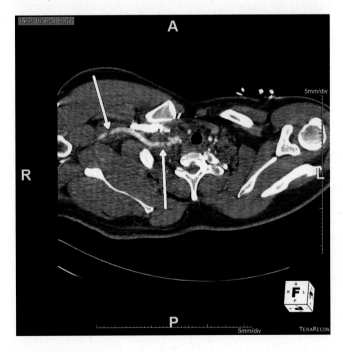

  A. Complete occlusion
  B. Pseudoaneurysm
  C. AV fistula
  D. Intimal flap

17 What is the diagnosis?

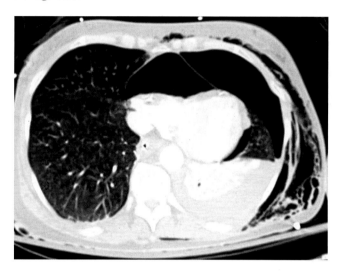

A. Tension pneumopericardium
B. Pulmonary laceration
C. Tension pneumothorax
D. Pericardial effusion

18 What is the diagnosis?

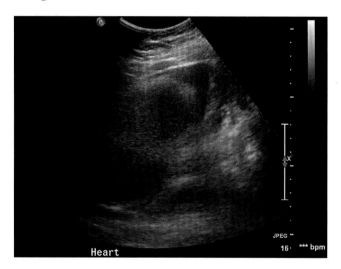

A. Ascites
B. Plural effusion
C. Pericardial effusion
D. Anterior mediastinal hemorrhage

19 What is the most common aspirated foreign body in a trauma patient with maxillofacial injury?

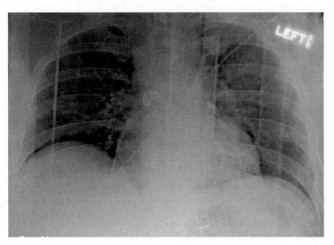 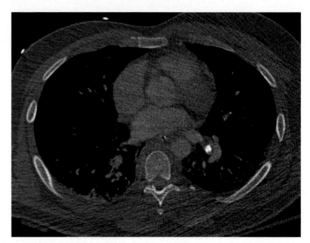

    A. Peanut

    B. Tooth

    C. Food bone (meat/chicken/fish)

    D. Windshield glass

20 Gunshot injury to the left chest. What causes the wide path of pulmonary opacity along the bullet pathway?

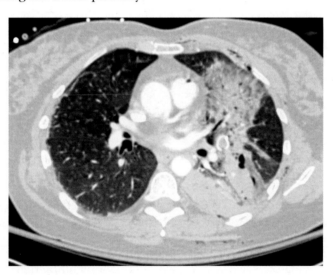

    A. Pulmonary contusion from blast cavity effect

    B. Aspiration

    C. Direct injury from bullet along path

    D. Atelectasis

ANSWERS AND EXPLANATIONS

1a   Answer F.

1b   Answer B.   Although the chest radiograph is a diagnostic examination for many blunt traumatic injuries, it is important to remember that it serves only as a screening examination for acute traumatic aortic injury (ATAI). Many radiographic signs are associated with varying degrees of sensitivity and specificity including widening of the superior mediastinum (>8 cm), enlarged mediastinal to chest width ratio (>0.25), indistinctness of the aortic arch, depression of the left main bronchus, deviation of the trachea to the right, deviation of the nasogastric tube to the right, left apical cap, widening of the paraspinal lines, widening of the right paratracheal stripe, and left hemothorax. Computed tomography angiography (CTA) is the standard for evaluation of suspected traumatic aortic injury. The CT appearance varies with location and associated injuries. Mediastinal hematoma nearly always accompanies ATAI. The most common location for ATAI encountered at imaging is the aortic isthmus. A luminal irregularity is usually seen with surrounding hematoma. Pulmonary contusion and laceration, sternal fractures, and rib fractures are commonly associated injuries.

References: Steenburg SD, Ravenel JG, Ikonomidis JS, et al. Acute traumatic aortic injury: imaging evaluation and management. *Radiology* 2008;248:3.

Woodring JH, Dillon ML. Radiographic manifestations of mediastinal hemorrhage from blunt chest trauma. *Ann Thorac Surg*1984;37:171–178.

2   Answer A.   Pulmonary lacerations occur when a tear of the parenchyma results in a cavity in the lung. The surrounding normal lung pulls away from the laceration resulting in a rounded cavity seen at CT. Lacerations are often accompanied by rib fractures, pneumothorax, hemothorax, and surrounding contusion and may be uni- or multilocular. However, chest wall fracture is not always present. Appearance may also vary depending on contents, for example, air, blood, or both.

Reference: Kaewlai R, Avery LL, Asrani AV, et al. Multidetector CT of blunt thoracic trauma. *Radiographics* 2008;28(6):1555–1570.

3   Answer D.   Fat embolism syndrome should be considered in polytrauma patients with long bone or pelvic injuries and persistent hypoxemia after initial resuscitation. Imaging features of fat embolism syndrome are nonspecific, and common CT findings include areas of consolidation, ground-glass opacities, and small nodules of various sizes. Fat attenuations filling defects in the pulmonary arteries are not typically seen. Imaging given in this case shows fat attenuation clot within the right superficial femoral vein (not typically seen).

Reference: Nucifora G, Hysko F, Vit A, et al. Pulmonary fat embolism: common and unusual computed tomography findings. *J Comput Assist Tomogr* 2007;31(5):806–807.

4a   Answer B.

4b   Answer A.   The dependent viscera sign describes abdominal viscera lying direct on the chest wall, as an intact diaphragm is no longer present to lift the abdominal contents off the posterior chest wall. In the above example for question 4a, the spleen is lying directly on the dependent chest wall, high in the thoracic cavity.

The collar sign describes a collar- or waist-like constriction of abdominal contents as they pass through a tear or defect in the diaphragm. In the above example for question 4b, the liver is constricted by a defect in the right hemidiaphragm. A common pitfall to diagnosis of a diaphragmatic hernia is focal eventration or unilateral paralysis of the diaphragm. The presence of acute traumatic injury (hemothorax, hemoperitoneum, pneumothorax) and the signs described above should aid in the diagnosis of acute diaphragmatic hernias.

References: Cantwell CP. The dependent viscera sign. *Radiology* 2006;238(2):752–753.

Killeen KL, Mirvis SE, Shanmuganathan K. Helical CT of diaphragmatic rupture caused by blunt trauma. *AJR Am J Roentgenol* 1999;173(6):1611–1616.

5a **Answer A**

5b **Answer A.**   The Society for Vascular Surgery adopted a 4-Grade classification scheme: Grade 1, intimal tear only (minimal aortic injury); Grade 2, intramural hematoma or large intimal flap; Grade 3, pseudoaneurysm, or Grade 4, rupture. The associated image demonstrates multifocal intimal injuries. Minimal aortic injury is a newly recognized entity likely owing to improved spatial and temporal resolution of modern multidetector CT. Injury of the aorta is isolated to the intima. Growing data demonstrate that most of minimal aortic injuries resolve or are stable at imaging follow-up. Most experts currently recommend no intervention for minimal aortic injury and would agree that follow-up CTA should be performed to document resolution or stability.

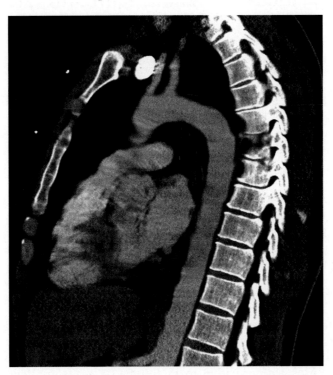

Follow-up CTA in 48 hours (shown) demonstrates complete resolution of the intimal injuries.

References: Azizzadeh A, Keyhani K, Miller CC III, et al. Blunt traumatic aortic injury: initial experience with endovascular repair. *J Vasc Surg* 2009;49(6):1403–1408. doi: 10.1016/j. jvs.2009.02.234.

Steenburg SD, Ravenel JG, Ikonomidis JS, et al. Acute traumatic aortic injury: imaging evaluation and management. *Radiology* 2008;248(3):748–762.

6 **Answer D.** The chest radiograph in this case demonstrates multiple left sided posterior and lateral rib fractures. Flail chest is defined as segmental fractures involving three or more contiguous ribs. The fracture pattern creates a flail segment, which can move paradoxically relative to the remainder of the chest. Flail chest indicates the presence of significant blunt thoracic trauma and is associated with increased morbidity and mortality, prolonged mechanical ventilation, and increased risk of pneumonia. Management depends on each institution's preference and level of expertise. Both surgical and conservative management have been utilized to manage these physiologically complex injuries.

References: Kaewlai R, Avery LL, Asrani AV, et al. Multidetector CT of blunt thoracic trauma. *Radiographics* 2008;28(6):1555–1570.

Tanaka H, Yukioka T, Yamaguti Y, et al. Surgical stabilization of internal pneumatic stabilization? A prospective randomized study of management of severe flail chest patients. *J Trauma* 2002;52(4):727–732; discussion 32.

7 **Answer C.** Imaging appearance of pulmonary contusion consists of patchy airspace opacities or consolidations adjacent to the region of injury without respect to bronchopulmonary distribution. Subpleural sparing or 1 to 2 mm of clear parenchyma beneath the pleural surface is an imaging sign that is often observed. Contusions are frequently not readily visible on conventional radiography.

References: Donnelly LF, Klosterman LA. Subpleural sparing: a CT finding of lung contusion in children. *Radiology* 1997;204(2):385–387.

Kaewlai R, Avery LL, Asrani AV, et al. Multidetector CT of blunt thoracic trauma. *Radiographics* 2008;28(6):1555–1570.

8a **Answer C.**

8b **Answer A.** Boerhaave syndrome is rupture of the esophagus most commonly occurring at the gastroesophageal junction often associated with forceful vomiting. Pneumomediastinum, pneumothorax, and pleural effusions are commonly seen at imaging. Although the fluoroscopic images above demonstrate extravasation of oral contrast, it is important to know that false-negative examinations have been reported to be as high as 20%. Boerhaave's remains a rare cause of esophageal rupture but should be considered among other pathologic entities when the nonspecific imaging findings presented above are encountered.

References: Backer CL, LoCicero J III, Hartz RS, et al. Computed tomography in patients with esophageal perforation. *Chest* 1990;98(5):1078–1080.

Bladergroen MR, Lowe JE, Postlethwait RW. Diagnosis and recommended management of esophageal perforation and rupture. *Ann Thorac Surg* 1986;42(3):235–239.

Ghanem N, Altehoefer C, Springer O, et al. Radiological findings in Boerhaave's syndrome. *Emerg Radiol* 2003;10(1):8–13.

9 **Answer B.** Sternal fractures are relatively uncommon blunt traumatic injuries and occur at a frequency of approximately 5%. Most of the time fractures are associated with anterior mediastinal hematoma, which aids in the detection of these injuries. Unfortunately, many trauma CT scans are degraded by respiratory motion artifact, which serves as a pitfall in diagnosis/misdiagnosis. Conventional radiography can be performed but is of limited utility. It is important to realize sternal fractures are usually accompanied by concomitant injuries (rib fractures, sternoclavicular dislocation, cardiac contusion, pneumothorax, etc.). Management usually depends on concomitant injuries.

Reference: Khoriati AA, Rajakulasingam R, Shah R. Sternal fractures and their management. *J Emerg Trauma Shock* 2013;6(2):113–116.

10a **Answer D.**

10b **Answer C.** Failure of the thoracic spine indicates significant blunt traumatic injury. The thoracic spine is relatively rigid and has approximately four times the axial load-bearing capacity compared to the lumbar spine. Much of the increased strength is attributed to the multiple articulations and connection to the sternum via the ribs. Significant injuries of the thoracic spine are usually catastrophic, and 50% will have neurologic injuries and 5% to 15% will have noncontiguous spinal column fractures. The fracture dislocation patterns of injuries predominate with significant injuries, as shown in the case above.

References: Harris MB, Shi LL, Vacarro AR, et al. Nonsurgical treatment of thoracolumbar spinal fractures. *Instr Course Lect* 2009;58:629–637.

Patel AA, Vaccaro AR. Thoracolumbar spine trauma classification. *J Am Acad Orthop Surg* 2010;18(2):63–71.

11a **Answer C.**

11b **Answer D.**

11c **Answer A.** Tension pneumothorax is caused by large volume of air in the pleural space. Often there is a ball/valve-type mechanism at the site of injury that allows air in but not out. The entire lung on that side eventually collapses under the pressure, and there can also be shift of the mediastinal structures to the contralateral side. This shift can cause vascular compromise, and venous structures being under lower pressure are the first to be affected causing decreased venous return to the heart and eventually reduced cardiac output. On chest radiograph, if a large pneumothorax is present and there is any shift of mediastinal contents to the contralateral side, a tension pneumothorax should be suggested.

For question 11c, answers A, B, and C can be useful in identifying a pneumothorax, but the inspiration and expiration series would require the patient to be able to hold their breath during both inspiratory and expiratory effort. For this reason, lateral decubitus views are a better choice for young pediatric patients if additional imaging is needed beyond an upright frontal view of the chest.

Reference: Pope TL, Harris JH. *Harris & Harris Radiology of Emergency Medicine.* Philadelphia, PA: Lippincott Williams & Wilkins, 2013:522–533.

12 **Answer C.** Persistent pneumothorax after chest tube placement could indicate improper chest tube placement (entire tube or side hole outside of the thoracic cage) or function (clogged or kinked tube). However, if the chest tube is properly positioned, which can be confirmed with imaging, and the chest tube is still functioning (persistent air leak), then air is still entering the plural space. In trauma, a persistent air leak is most likely from a bronchial tear. The larger the injured bronchus, the more brisk the air leak will be. If the chest tube is not able to clear the air faster than it enters the plural space, then a persistent pneumothorax will remain.

Reference: Pope TL, Harris JH. *Harris & Harris Radiology of Emergency Medicine.* Philadelphia, PA: Lippincott Williams & Wilkins, 2013:533.

13a **Answer B.**

13b **Answer C.** A sternoclavicular (SC) dislocation can be difficult to diagnose on radiograph due to overlying structures, but asymmetry of the clavicles should raise concern for this injury. CT is the best modality to diagnose SC dislocation and might demonstrate anterior or posterior position of the medial clavicle in relation to the manubrium. Posterior SC dislocation on the left should raise concern for left subclavian vein injury because of close proximity and impingement by the displaced clavicle.

References: MacDonald PB, Lapointe P. Acromioclavicular and sternoclavicular joint injuries. *Orthop Clin North Am* 2008; 39(4):535–545.

Pope TL, Harris JH. *Harris & Harris Radiology of Emergency Medicine*. Philadelphia, PA: Lippincott Williams & Wilkins, 2013:512.

14a Answer C.

14b Answer C.

14c Answer B.

14d Answer A. Acute traumatic aortic injury (ATAI) includes a wide range of injuries from complete rupture all the way to minimal intimal injuries. Patients with full-thickness tears rarely survive long enough to undergo imaging. A common type of partial-thickness tear is a pseudoaneurysm. In an aortic pseudoaneurysm, the two inner layers (intima and media) are torn, but the outer layer (adventitia) remains intact. The adventitia provides approximately 60% of the tensile strength of the aortic wall.

The most common location of ATAI is at the region of the ligamentum arteriosum, also known as the aortic isthmus. This location accounts for 50% to 71% of ATAI. The reason injuries are common here is because the ligamentum arteriosum acts as a tether point for the otherwise mildly mobile aorta within the thoracic cage.

References: Azizzadeh A, et al. "Blunt traumatic aortic injury: initial experience with endovascular repair." *J Vasc Surg* 2009;49(6): 1303–1408.

Pope TL, Harris JH. *Harris & Harris Radiology of Emergency Medicine*. Philadelphia, PA: Lippincott Williams & Wilkins, 2013:542–564.

Soto JA, Lacey BC. *The requisites: Emergency Radiology*. Mosby Inc., 2009:63–64.

15 Answer D. Tracheal diverticulum or paratracheal air cysts are a normal variant that can be seen along the right posterior aspect of the trachea at the level of the upper mediastinum (as seen in this case). When seen in the setting of trauma, these can be confused for mediastinal gas, but awareness of this normal variant can help the radiologist suggest it instead. Some have speculated that this finding is associated with increased pressures in the trachea and a focal weakness in the wall that allows it to develop over time, but others suggest that it is a congenital anomaly. When a small focus of gas is seen in this location adjacent to the trachea, the radiologist should do a diligent search for other mediastinal gas, but in the absence of other signs of pneumomediastinum, the differential should favor tracheal diverticulum.

Reference: Buterbaugh JE, Erly WK. Paratracheal air cysts: a common finding on CT examinatinos of the cervical spine and neck that may mimic pneumomediastinum in patients with traumatic injuries. *AJNR Am J Neuroradiol* 2008;29(6):1218–1221. doi: 10.3174/ajnr. A1058.

16 Answer D. Vascular injuries at the level of the thoracic inlet are rare but seen more often in penetrating injuries over blunt trauma. The above case involved a patient who was ejected from an MVC and had significant blunt injuries to the right chest. The multiple filling defects seen in the right subclavian artery are most consistent with intimal flap. There is contrast seen past the filling defects, so complete occlusion is not the correct choice. There is no expansion of the lumen; therefore pseudoaneurysm can be ruled out. The contrast is actually higher density in the adjacent vein, so an AV fistula cannot be confidently identified.

Reference: Núñez DB Jr, Torres-León M, Múnera F. Vascular injuries of the neck and thoracic inlet: helican CT-angio-graphic correlation. *RadioGraphics* 2004;24:1087–1100.

17 Answer A.   Tension pneumopericardium is a life-threatening event. Small amounts of air in the pericardial sac can be tolerated without symptoms, but once the amount of air is enough to raise the intrapericardial pressures above 265 mm H_2O, the heart may experience decreased function. Imaging signs include large volume of air in the pericardial sac, flattening of the anterior boarder of the heart, and engorgement of IVC/SVC. Treatment is with emergent needle decompression or pericardial drain placement. Trauma is the most common cause of pneumopericardium.

Reference: Katabathina VS, Restrepo CS, Martinez-Jimenez S, et al. Nonvascular, nontraumatic mediastinal emergencies in adults: a comprehensive review of imaging findings. *RadioGraphics* 2011;31(4):1141–1160.

18 Answer C.   At least one view of the heart should be part of a focused assessment with sonography in trauma (FAST). The heart can be imaged either by a subxiphoid approach or between the ribs just to the left of the sternum. Patient body habitus, lung volume, and current acute injuries might make one location better than the other for viewing the heart. A pericardial effusion in the setting of trauma, especially penetration chest trauma, should raise the concern for cardiac injury. Even a small pericardial effusion might be a sign of bleeding that can enlarge quickly to cause cardiac tamponade.

Reference: Körner M, Krötz MM, Degenhart C, et al. Current role of emergency US in patients with major trauma. *RadioGraphics* 2008 28(1):225–242.

19 Answer B.   While the most common aspirated foreign body in children and adults is food such as a peanut, in the setting of a patient with maxillofacial injury, care should be taken to find any missing teeth to help prevent aspiration of them. Mobile teeth within the oral cavity can be pushed further into the trachea or bronchi during intubation. In the case above, the patient had extensive facial fractures and two missing teeth. One was still in the posterior pharynx, but the second was down in the left lower lobe bronchi as seen on both x-ray and CT.

Reference: Casap N, Alterman M, Leiberman S, et al. Enigma of missing teeth in maxillofacial trauma. *J Oral Maxillofac Surg* 2011;69(5):1421–1429.

20 Answer A.   The actual bullet path causes direct tissue damage and is often referred to as the permanent cavity. The bullet also causes a pressure wave that causes tissue damage from outward stretching and shearing forces. The faster the bullet is traveling, the greater kinetic energy it has, and thus the larger pressure wave it will generate. This additional area of tissue injury is called a blast cavity or temporary cavity. It is important to find the bullet pathway in a patient with gunshot injury so that you can assess for direct damage from the permanent cavity as well as indirect damage from the adjacent blast cavity.

Reference: Patterns of Tissue Injury. Available at: http://library.med.utah.edu/WebPath/TUTORIAL/GUNS/GUNINJ.html

17 Congenital Disease

Anne-Marie G. Sykes, MD

QUESTIONS

1a The vascular anomaly shown is most likely

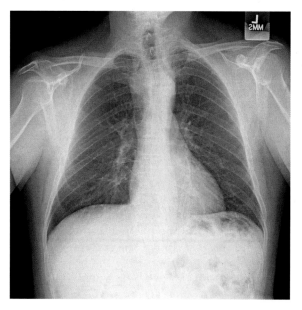

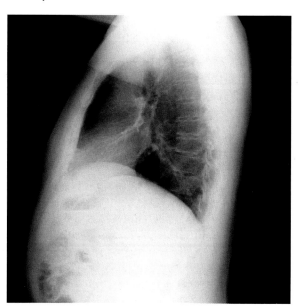

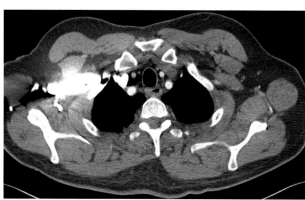

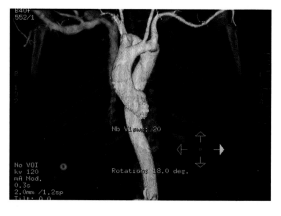

A. Right aortic arch with mirror image branching
B. Double aortic arch
C. Left aortic arch with aberrant right subclavian artery
D. Right aortic arch with aberrant left subclavian artery

1b This anomaly
    A. Is the most common variation of right aortic arch
    B. Is associated with a diverticulum of Kommerell
    C. Is the most common cause of a symptomatic vascular ring
    D. Has a strong association with cyanotic congenital heart disease

2a The radiographic abnormality is localized to the

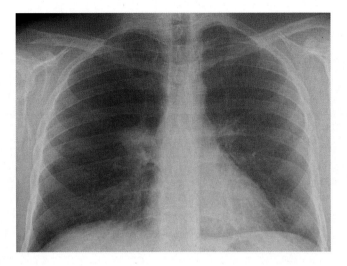

    A. Hilar angle
    B. Right paratracheal stripe
    C. Azygoesophageal line
    D. Chest wall

2b Findings are most consistent with which congenital or developmental anomaly?

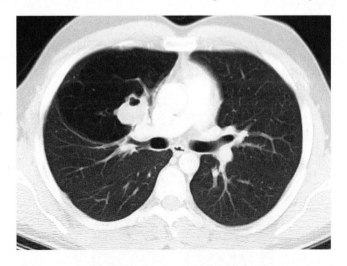

    A. Lobar emphysema
    B. Pulmonary adenomatoid malformation
    C. Bronchial atresia
    D. Swyer-James syndrome

3   What is the characteristic vascular supply and drainage associated with extralobar pulmonary sequestration?

A. Pulmonary arteries and systemic veins
B. Systemic arteries and pulmonary veins
C. Systemic arteries and systemic veins
D. Pulmonary arteries and pulmonary veins

4a   Disease is localized to which pulmonary lobe?

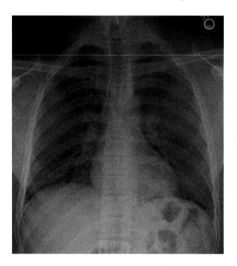 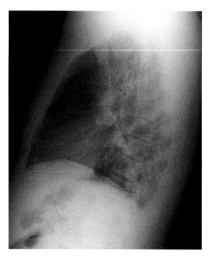

A. Right upper
B. Left upper
C. Right middle
D. Left lower

4b   Which of the following would be most likely in this 28-year-old male with recurrent pneumonias localized to the left lower lobe?

A. Hypogenetic lung syndrome
B. Partial anomalous pulmonary venous return
C. Congenital lobar emphysema
D. Pulmonary sequestration

4c   In this sequestration, the vessel overlying the left hemidiaphragm must:

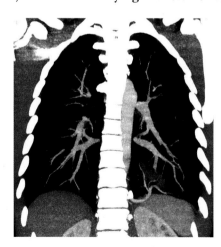

A. Arise from a pulmonary artery
B. Drain into a systemic vein
C. Arise from a systemic artery
D. Drain into a pulmonary vein

5 The vascular anomaly present:

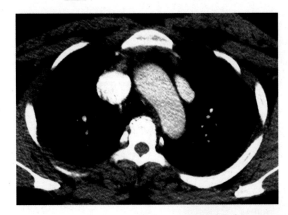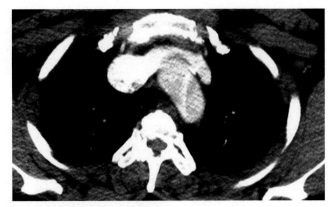

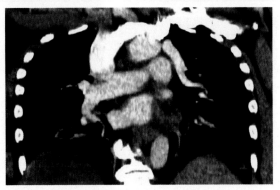

A. Represents a left-to-right shunt
B. Is associated with increased infection
C. Commonly causes dysphagia
D. Most commonly occurs in the left lower lobe

6a Which radiographic shadow is distorted?

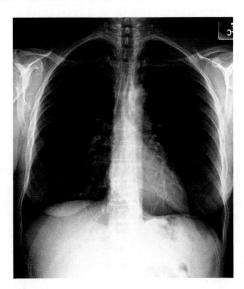

A. Right paratracheal stripe
B. Paraspinal line
C. Azygoesophageal line
D. Anterior junction line

6b What is the most likely cause?

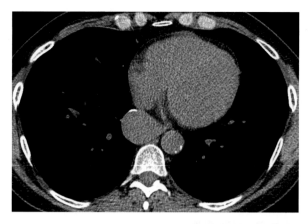 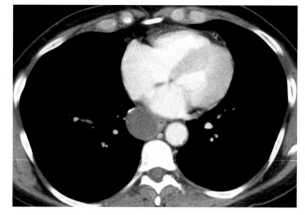

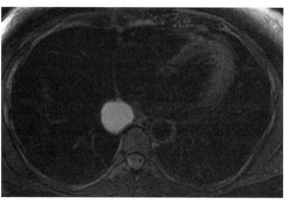

A. Lymphoma
B. Esophageal cancer
C. Foregut duplication cyst
D. Angiosarcoma

7a What imaging pattern is demonstrated on this inspiratory chest CT?

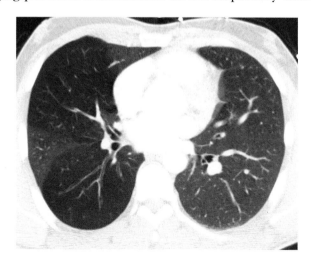

A. Ground-glass opacities
B. Centrilobular nodularity
C. Parahilar nodules
D. Mosaic attenuation

7b What is the most likely cause of the unilateral hyperlucency in this 25-year-old male?

    A. Bronchial atresia
    B. Congenital lobar emphysema
    C. Congenital pulmonary airway malformation
    D. Swyer-James syndrome

7c What is the most common cause of childhood obliterative bronchiolitis (Swyer-James syndrome)?

    A. Human immunodeficiency virus
    B. In utero vascular insult
    C. Toxic fume exposure
    D. Pediatric adenovirus infection

8a The frontal chest x-ray shows an example of what sign?

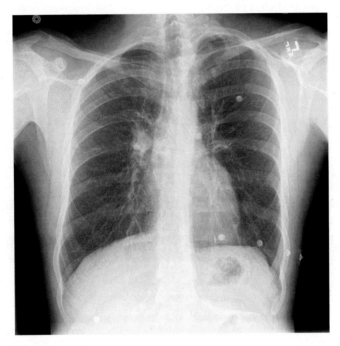

    A. The hilum overlay sign
    B. The positive spine sign
    C. The atoll sign
    D. The S sign of Golden

8b To determine the etiology of the chest x-ray abnormalities, the next best test would be

    A. Pulmonary angiography
    B. Chest CT
    C. Chest MRI
    D. Contrast esophagram

8c Pulmonary arterial venous malformations can be associated with which of the following?

    A. Itchy violet skin lesions, abnormal nails, whitish oral lesions

    B. Recurrent pneumonia, greasy bulky stools, salty skin

    C. Orthodeoxia, polycythemia, cerebral infection

    D. Skin flushing, severe diarrhea, wheezing

8d Treatment of choice for these lesions is

    A. Radiotherapy.

    B. Transcatheter embolization.

    C. Thermal ablation.

    D. None. They are incidental and do not need treatment.

9 What is the most common presentation of the anomaly shown?

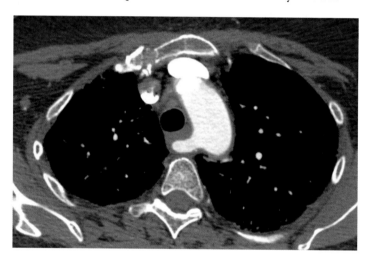

    A. Incidental

    B. Dysphagia lusoria

    C. Aortic dissection

    D. Rib notching

10a What is the diagnosis?

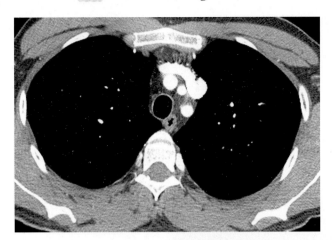 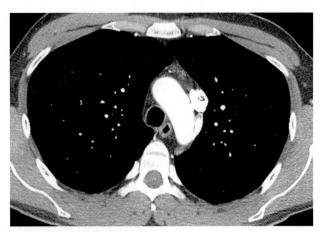

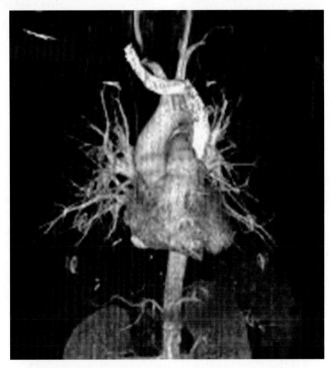

    A. Left-sided superior vena cava
    B. Double aortic arch
    C. Pulmonary sling
    D. Congenital interruption of the inferior vena cava

10b When might this congenital anomaly require surgical correction?

    A. Drainage into the coronary sinus
    B. Drainage into the right atrium
    C. Drainage into the left atrium
    D. Drainage into the hemiazygos vein

11a Localize the radiographic abnormality.

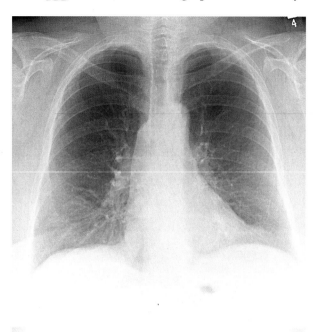
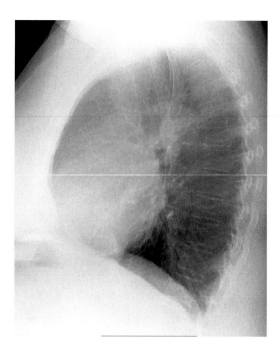

       A. Lungs
       B. Mediastinum
       C. Bones
       D. Chest wall

11b The anomalous vessel on the oblique CT image is a

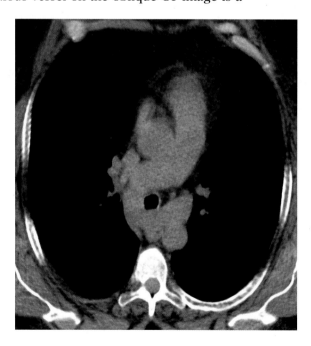

       A. Systemic vein
       B. Systemic artery
       C. Pulmonary vein
       D. Pulmonary artery

11c The anomalous left pulmonary artery courses between the

    A. Esophagus and spine
    B. Esophagus and trachea
    C. Trachea and ascending aorta
    D. Carina and left atrium

12a Which arrow identifies the congenital anomaly?

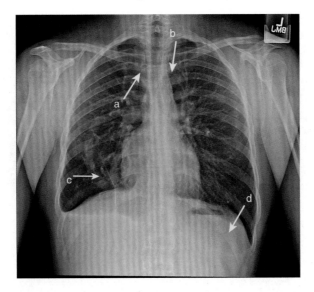

    A. a
    B. b
    C. c
    D. d

12b Which of the following is a feature of scimitar syndrome?

    A. Almost always occurs on the left side.
    B. Is a form of partial anomalous pulmonary venous drainage.
    C. The pulmonary artery on the affected side is usually normal.
    D. Is associated with situs inversus totalis.

13a What chest radiographic finding likely led to obtaining this CT?

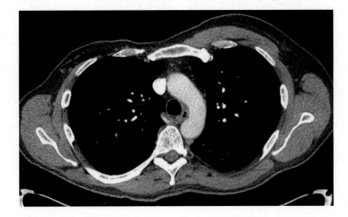

    A. Mediastinal widening
    B. Hyperinflation of one lung
    C. Tracheal narrowing
    D. Unilateral hyperlucency

13b What is the diagnosis?

    A. Poland syndrome
    B. Aortic arch anomaly
    C. Foreign body aspiration
    D. Left chest wall mass

14a What is the diagnosis based on the CT and V/Q scan?

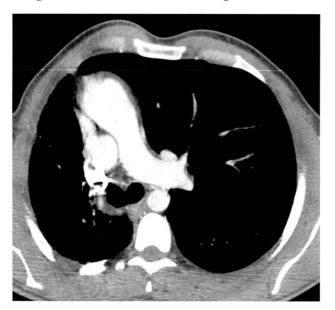

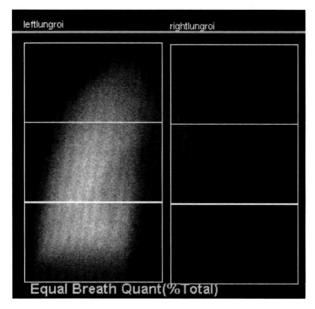

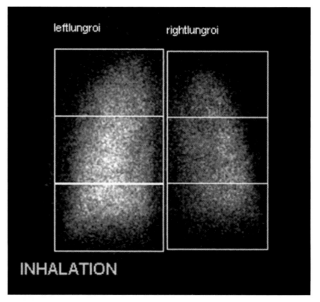

    A. Congenital interruption of the right pulmonary artery
    B. Congenital atresia of the right mainstem bronchus
    C. Congenital absence of the right lung
    D. Congenital interruption of the right pulmonary veins

14b What best describes the usual relationship of the interrupted pulmonary artery to the aorta?

    A. Occurs opposite the side of the aortic arch
    B. Occurs only in the setting of aortic coarctation
    C. Occurs on the same side as the aortic arch
    D. Occurs with a Kommerell diverticulum

15a What congenital anomaly best accounts for the imaging findings?

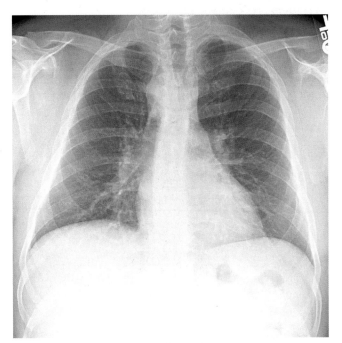
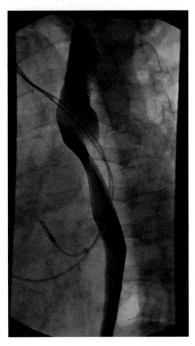

A. Duplicate superior vena cava with left atrial drainage
B. Right-sided aortic arch with mirror image branching
C. Azygos continuation of an interrupted inferior vena cava
D. Right-sided aortic arch with aberrant left subclavian artery

15b What is the most likely presentation for the congenital anomaly shown?

A. Paradoxical emboli
B. Pulmonary artery hypertension
C. Dysphagia lusoria
D. Subclavian steal syndrome

16a The abnormality on the chest is localized to the

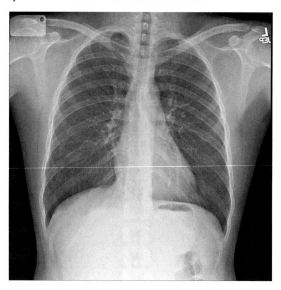

    A. Lung
    B. Mediastinum
    C. Hilum
    D. Diaphragm

16b Which of the following is true of a congenital cystic adenomatoid malformation?

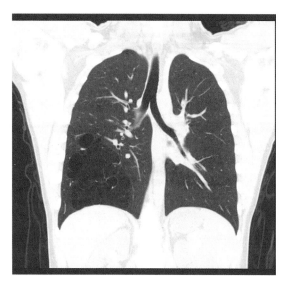
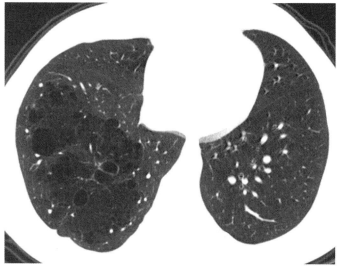

    A. Type 1 CCAM is the most common and has at least 1 dominant cyst larger than 2 cm.
    B. Cannot be diagnosed antenatally.
    C. The vascular supply to CCAMs is usually from systemic arteries.
    D. It has connections to the bronchial tree.

17a The most likely diagnosis is

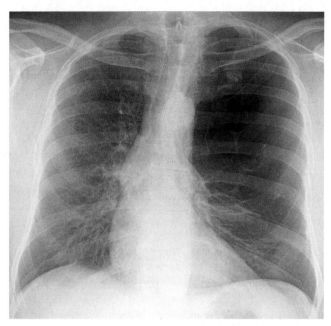

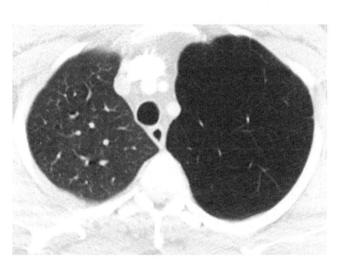
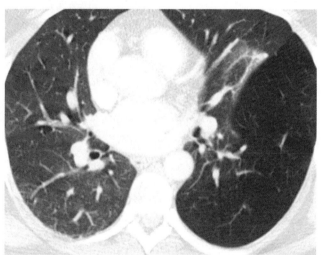

    A. Smoking-related emphysema
    B. Swyer-James-MacLeod syndrome
    C. Congenital lobar emphysema
    D. Left-sided pneumothorax

17b Which of the following is true of a congenital lobar emphysema?

    A. It is usually diagnosed after the age of 1 year.
    B. The most common location is the left upper lobe.
    C. The alveolar walls are abnormal.
    D. It can be effectively treated with chemotherapeutic agents.

ANSWERS AND EXPLANATIONS

1a **Answer B.** The frontal chest radiograph shows an opacity along the left side of the mediastinum in the expected location of the aortic arch; however, there is also a rounded opacity along the right side of the trachea with associated focal impression of the trachea. The lateral chest radiograph shows focal impression along the posterior aspect of the trachea at this level. These findings are suggestive for a double aortic arch. The axial CT image of the upper chest above the aortic arch at the level of the great vessels shows the distinctive branching pattern of the vessels to the head and neck, sometimes referred to as the "four-artery sign." This is because each aortic arch gives rise to a common carotid and subclavian artery. The 3D rendering of the CT angiogram nicely shows both aortic arches.

1b **Answer C.** In a double aortic arch, there are two aortic arches that connect the ascending and descending aortas, encircling the trachea and esophagus (vascular ring), with symptomatology depending on the degree of associated constriction of the trachea and esophagus. The ring associated with the right arch with aberrant left subclavian artery is completed by patent left ductus arteriosus or ligamentum arteriosum and is often relatively loose and therefore less often symptomatic. The right aortic arch with left subclavian artery is a more common anomaly than double aortic arch; however, the double aortic arch is more often symptomatic and makes up most of the cases of symptomatic vascular rings. The diverticulum of Kommerell is a diverticulum at the proximal descending aorta, either right or left configuration, that gives rise to an aberrant subclavian artery. The double aortic arch is rarely associated with congenital heart disease, though when present the most common disorders are tetralogy of Fallot and transposition of the great arteries.

References: Hanneman K, Newman B, Chan F. Congenital variants and anomalies of the aortic arch. *RadioGraphics* 2016;37(1):32–51.

Ramos-Duran L, Nance JW, Schoepf UJ, et al. Developmental aortic arch anomalies in infants and children assessed with CT angiography. *AJR Am J Roentgenol* 2012;198:W466–W474. 10.2214/AJR.11.6982.

2a **Answer A.**

2b **Answer C.** Bronchial atresia often manifests on radiograph as a hilar fullness or branching pulmonary opacity from mucoid impaction. In this case, the noncommunicating airway is nearly completely opacified causing the expected hilar angle, the radiographic right hilar concavity on frontal view at the crossing of the right pulmonary artery and the superior pulmonary vein, to become convex. Lymphadenopathy, hilar mass, and congenital lesions are all considerations and necessitate CT for further evaluation.

The CT image confirms the hilar lesion, which is nonenhancing and of low attenuation and contains a small air component. The associated right upper lobe is hyperexpanded and hyperlucent. Lobar emphysema and Swyer-James syndrome produce varying degrees of hyperlucency and hyperinflation but are not associated with obstructed airway with impaction. Pulmonary adenomatoid malformation generally creates a more bubbly cystic lesion that can look like focal emphysema, again not with the characteristic airway changes.

Occurring most often in the apicoposterior segment of the left upper lobe, the second most common location for bronchial atresia is in the right upper lobe segmental airways. Patients are generally asymptomatic, although some patients may present with recurrent infection. In this latter setting, resection may be required.

Reference: Zylak CJ, et al. Developmental lung anomalies in the adult: radiologic-pathologic correlation. *Radiographics* 2002;22:S25–S43.

3 **Answer C.** Extralobar pulmonary sequestration accounts for approximately 25% of all pulmonary sequestrations with the remaining being intralobar. Nearly all pulmonary sequestrations receive blood supply from the systemic arteries and have variable venous drainage, where the majority of intralobar sequestrations drain to the pulmonary veins and the majority of extralobar sequestrations drain to the systemic veins. Extralobar sequestrations by definition are divided from the normal lung by a pleural investment and most commonly reside between the left lower lobe and hemidiaphragm, although they can occur elsewhere to include the mediastinum, pericardium, diaphragm, and extrathoracic locations. Most commonly identified in infancy, a minority of cases present in adulthood with around 10% of cases incidentally identified in asymptomatic patients. Extralobar sequestrations have a higher rate of associated congenital anomalies compared with intralobar sequestrations, with diaphragmatic hernia being most common. Although these may be asymptomatic, treatment consists of surgical resection.

Reference: Rosado-de-Christenson ML, Frazier AA, Stocker JT, et al. Extralobar sequestration: radiologic-pathologic correlation. *Radiographics* 1993;13:425–441.

4a **Answer D.**

4b **Answer D.**

4c **Answer C.** Positive spine sign on lateral view radiograph supports a lower lobe process, and frontal view correlates with a retrocardiac opacity consistent with a left lower lobe mass-like consolidation. No additional pulmonary parenchymal opacities are present, further confirmed on the follow-up chest CTA.

Recurrent pneumonias isolated to a particular region should raise concern for an underlying lesion or abnormality. In this case, a contrast-filled vessel is seen on coronal MIP CT images extending from the lower mediastinum and diaphragm region to the area of consolidation. In this case, the opacities seen primarily represent mucoid impaction within noncommunicating bronchi. Pulmonary sequestration is defined by systemic arterial supply with rare bronchial connection and variable venous drainage. The affected lung in intralobar sequestration, as seen here, is inseparable from the adjacent normal lung, as opposed to extralobar sequestration, which develops with a pleural boundary separating it from normal lung. Intralobar sequestrations occur most commonly in the left lower lobe. Cases may be discovered incidentally on imaging but can manifest as recurrent infection or massive hemoptysis.

Reference: Zylak CJ, et al. Developmental lung anomalies in the adult: radiologic-pathologic correlation. *Radiographics* 2002;22:S25–S43.

5 **Answer A.** A pulmonary vein is shown draining into the left brachiocephalic vein. By draining a portion of the lung into a systemic vein, the anomaly represents partial anomalous pulmonary venous return (PAPVR). In bypassing the left heart and systemic arterial supply, the oxygenated blood returns to the right heart, increasing the ratio of right heart blood flow consistent with a left-to-right shunt. The majority of PAPVR cases are left upper lobe venous drainage to the left brachiocephalic vein as in this case. Scimitar syndrome is an uncommon variant of PAPVR.

Reference: Rahiah P, Kanne JP. Computed tomography of pulmonary venous variants and anomalies. *J Cardiovasc Comput Tomogr* 2010;4:155–163.

6a   **Answer C.**

6b   **Answer C.** The azygoesophageal recess represents a portion of the right lower lobe, which extends medially, marginated by the posterior margin of the heart, the anterior margin of the spine, and the right lateral margin of the esophagus. Radiographically, this results in a border that runs vertically over the lower thoracic spine and may deviate a little to the left near the esophageal hiatus. Here, the azygoesophageal border deviates to the right, even extending lateral to the right heart border. The right paratracheal stripe is a line along the right trachea in the superior mediastinum. The anterior junction line is also a superior mediastinal shadow. The paraspinal border by definition will not overlie the spinal column as the azygoesophageal border will.

Noncontrast and contrast-enhanced CT images better demonstrate a low-attenuation nonenhancing right paraesophageal lesion in the lower mediastinum. A small amount of peripheral calcification is present along the anterior aspect, and MR reveals a homogeneous high T2 signal within the lesion all consistent with a foregut duplication cyst. Originating from the embryologic primitive foregut, these mediastinal congenital cysts represent anomalies in the divisions of the foregut from the tracheobronchial tree and neural tube and include bronchogenic cyst, esophageal duplication cyst, and neurenteric cyst.

Reference: Zylak CJ, et al. Developmental lung anomalies in the adult: radiologic-pathologic correlation. *Radiographics* 2002;22:S25–S43.

7a   **Answer D.**

7b   **Answer D.**

7c   **Answer D.** CT image provided in lung window at the level of the aortic root demonstrates relative hyperlucency in regions of the right middle lobe and right lower lobe. This is differentiated from patchy ground-glass opacities by the attenuation of vessels in the hyperlucent lung. While air trapping may be associated with the regions of low attenuation, air trapping is typically an expiratory CT finding, where mosaic attenuation is identified on inspiratory imaging. No significant centrilobular nodularity or parahilar nodules are present on the examinations, although normal pulmonary vascular structures may appear as such to the untrained eye.

Each of the pulmonary congenital/developmental abnormalities provided can produce a unilateral hyperlucent lung, but only Swyer-James-(MacLeod) syndrome characteristically produces multifocal hyperlucency. In five out of eight patients with Swyer-James syndrome, Moore et al. found multifocal bilateral regions of mosaic attenuation. Congenital lobar emphysema is a consideration for this appearance, but the combination of involvement of the right lower lobe (uncommon) and multifocal nature (rare) makes this diagnosis unlikely. Bronchial atresia is also focal and results from a noncommunicating bronchus often with mucoid impaction, where this case nicely demonstrates patent bronchi in the right lower lobe. Congenital pulmonary airway malformation produces a mass-like or cystic-appearing lesion rather than mosaic attenuation as shown here.

Swyer-James-(MacLeod) syndrome is the result of postinfectious obliterative bronchiolitis, due to pediatric pneumonia, particularly adenovirus, but can be seen with other infections such as mycoplasma. Toxic fume exposure can cause obliterative bronchiolitis but is not reported as a significant contributor to childhood obliterative bronchiolitis. HIV had been rarely reported as a cause of obliterative bronchiolitis and not a significant contributor to childhood obliterative bronchiolitis. Outside of infection, follicular bronchiolitis would be a more characteristic small airway manifestation of HIV/AIDS. Finally, while in utero vascular insults may be associated with various pulmonary malformations, it is not a cause of Swyer-James syndrome.

References: Colum AJ, Teper AM, Vollmer WM, et al. Risk factors for the development of bronchiolitis obliterans in children with bronchiolitis. *Thorax* 2006;61:503–506.

Moore ADA, Godwin JD, Dietrich PA, et al. Swyer-James Syndrome: CT findings in eight patients. *AJR Am J Roentgenol* 1992;158:1211–1215.

Wasilewska E, Lee EY, Eisenberg RL. Unilateral hyperlucent lung in children. *AJR Am J Roentgenol* 2012;198:W400–W414.

8a **Answer A.** The frontal radiograph shows increased density projecting over the right hilum. The hilum overlay sign is due to an opacity projecting over the hilum on the frontal view, whereby the hilar vessels can be distinguished separately from the opacity. This indicates that the abnormality is not within the hilum itself but is either anterior or posterior to the hilum. The spine sign is due to increased opacity projecting over the lower thoracic spine on the lateral radiograph. Normally, opacity over the upper thoracic spine is greater than the lower thoracic spine. The atoll sign is a sign used in chest CT, also known as the reversed halo sign, describing a central ground-glass opacity with a peripheral rim of consolidation. This was originally described in patients with cryptogenic organizing pneumonia. The S sign of Golden is a finding on the frontal chest x-ray describing central convexity in the right suprahilar region with associated right upper lobe collapse.

8b **Answer B.** In order to determine the etiology of these lesions, a chest CT would be the next best imaging examination, as the most common concern with multiple pulmonary nodules would be malignancy, and chest CT can distinguish between pulmonary parenchymal and vascular abnormalities. In the case of a pulmonary AVM, a chest CT scan, either without or with IV contrast enhancement, would demonstrate a feeding artery and draining vein, characteristic of pulmonary AVM. The chest CT scan in this case showed an intensely enhancing complex pulmonary AVM in the right mid lung posteromedially. An additional very tiny AVM (not shown) was also identified in the right lung apex. Pulmonary AVMs can be seen with hereditary hemorrhagic telangiectasia, also known as Osler-Weber-Rendu syndrome, an autosomal dominant syndrome.

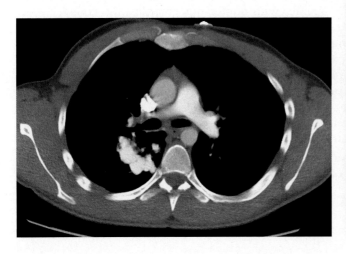

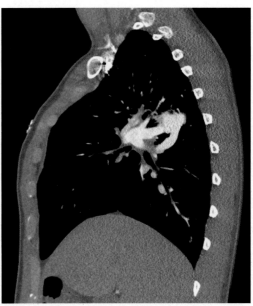

Pulmonary angiography was once considered the "gold standard" for evaluation of pulmonary AVMs; however, for detection, characterization, and follow-up of pulmonary AVMs, chest CT is now predominantly used, particularly as it has superior ability to accurately display complex AVM angioarchitecture.

8c Answer C. A pulmonary AVM is a direct communication between the pulmonary artery and pulmonary vein and therefore is a form of right-to-left shunt, allowing deoxygenated systemic venous blood flow to bypass the lungs, returning to systemic circulation without being oxygenated, resulting in hypoxemia. Pulmonary AVMs are usually more numerous in the lower lungs, and with standing, there is increased blood flow to the lower lungs, accentuating hypoxia in the erect position. The decrease in arterial oxygenation saturation from supine to standing position is known as orthodeoxia.

Chronic hypoxemia triggers increased production of erythropoietin, resulting in polycythemia.

As a right-to-left shunt, thrombi in the pulmonary venous system can be embolized directly into the systemic arterial system, including the arteries supplying the brain, resulting in cerebral infarctions/strokes. Septic emboli can result in brain abscesses.

The combination of itchy violet skin lesions, abnormal nails, and whitish oral lesions can be seen with lichen planus, a rare chronic inflammatory autoimmune skin and mucous membrane disease. Oral and skin lesions seen with pulmonary AVMs are mucocutaneous telangiectases in association with hereditary hemorrhagic telangiectasia and appear as either a central red lesion with dilated capillaries extending out from it or macular circular lesions that can be slightly elevated, which blanch when pressure is applied. They are not itchy.

The combination of recurrent pneumonia, greasy bulky stools, and salty skin is a symptom that is associated with cystic fibrosis, an inherited disorder, which affects cells that produce mucus, sweat, and digestive enzymes, whereby a defective gene causes secretions to become sticky and thick, especially in the lungs and pancreas.

The combination of skin flushing, severe diarrhea, and wheezing can be seen with carcinoid syndrome. Carcinoid tumors are well-differentiated neuroendocrine tumors that most commonly arise in the digestive tract and lungs. Carcinoid tumors can secrete serotonin and other vasoactive substances, which can affect the skin, gastrointestinal tract, and bronchi.

8d Answer B. Transcatheter endovascular embolization is usually the mainstay of treatment for pulmonary AVMs, either with nonferrous embolization coils or with vascular plugs. Vascular plugs are more expensive and take longer to occlude blood flow but allowing for precise deployment near the sac, have a lower risk of device migration, and often only one plug is needed compared to multiple coils. Radiotherapy and thermal ablation have no role. Because of complications associated with pulmonary AVMs (hypoxia, systemic emboli, etc.), the occlusion of pulmonary AVMs with arteries exceeding 2 to 3 mm in diameter is generally recommended. In some cases, surgical excision or even lung transplant may be necessary.

References: Ivanis J, Ding A, Barbon D, et al. *Pulmonary AVM embolization, JOMI preprint.*

Lee EY, Boiselle PM, Cleveland RH. Multidetector CT evaluation of congenital anomalies. *Radiology* 2008;247(3):632–648.

9   **Answer A.** While a left aortic arch with aberrant right subclavian artery can occasionally cause dysphagia, this congenital abnormality is generally identified as an incidental finding on imaging. It is the most common aortic arch anomaly. The aberrant right subclavian artery originates as the last arch branch from the aorta with an occasional dilatation of the aorta at its origin, known as Kommerell diverticulum. There is no direct association of the aberrant right subclavian with aortic dissection or rib notching.

Reference: Yildirim A, Karabulut N, Dogan S, et al. Congenital thoracic arterial anomalies in adults: a CT overview. *Diagn Interv Radiol* 2011;17:352–362.

10a   **Answer A.**

10b   **Answer C.** Despite not seeing the full extent of the anomalous vessel on the provided images, axial CT images demonstrate a contrast-filled structure running vertically along the left lateral aortic arch and connecting to the brachiocephalic veins. The primary differential includes left-sided superior vena cava (the most common superior caval variant) versus partial anomalous pulmonary venous return, but the axial images also reveal an absent right superior vena cava consistent with left-sided SVC. Also, the single projection 3D color reconstruction demonstrates the high density of contrast from the upper extremity intravenous injection, confirming the systemic venous flow toward the heart. The majority of persistent left SVC cases drain into systemic veins, particularly the coronary sinus, or directly into the right atrium, allowing for the normal flow of blood. A small number of cases will drain into the left atrium, which are often associated with other cardiac anomalies and generally require surgical correction.

Reference: Chung JH, Gunn ML, Godwin JD, et al. Congenital thoracic cardiovascular anomalies presenting in adulthood: a pictorial review. *J Cardiovasc Comput Tomogr* 2009;3(1):S35–S46.

11a   **Answer B.**

11b   **Answer D.**

11c   **Answer B.** The radiographs provided are difficult but do demonstrate changes in the normal mediastinal borders. First, a fullness is seen in the region of the azygos arch with a subtle low origin of the right upper lobe bronchus. Second, the lateral radiograph demonstrates a mass-like opacity posterior to the trachea with a well-defined anterior border. Third, the normal arch of the left pulmonary vein over the top of the left mainstem bronchus is absent. No significant findings are present in the lung, bones, or chest wall.

Pulmonary artery sling can mimic a mediastinal mass posterior to the trachea on chest radiographs. CT definitively characterizes this as an anomalous course of the left pulmonary artery originating from the distal right pulmonary artery and coursing between the trachea and esophagus. While the majority of these cases occur with other congenital anomalies identified in infancy, some isolated cases will present incidentally in adulthood as in this patient.

Reference: Castaner E, Gallardo X, Rimola J, et al. Congenital and acquired pulmonary artery anomalies in the adult: radiologic overview. *Radiographics* 2006;26:349–371.

12a   **Answer C.** The abnormality on the chest radiograph is an abnormal tubular structure in the right lower hemithorax that curves medially, with the appearance reminiscent of a Turkish sword (scimitar). Arrow "a" is pointing to the rhomboid fossa of the clavicle, where the costoclavicular (rhomboid) ligament attaches. Arrow "b" is pointing to the superior margin of the manubrium. Arrow "d" is pointing to the normal gastric air bubble.

12b **Answer B.** Scimitar syndrome, also known as hypogenetic lung syndrome or congenital pulmonary venolobar syndrome, almost always occurs on the right side and is an anomaly consisting of partial anomalous venous drainage of the right lung inferiorly (the scimitar vein), most commonly into the IVC, though it can also be into the hepatic veins, portal veins, coronary sinus, or right atrium. There is abnormal development/hypoplasia of the right pulmonary artery and the right lung, which are small. At least some of the vascular supply to the right lung is from systemic arterial vessels. Decreased size of the right lung results in rightward shift of the mediastinal structures, including the heart (cardiac dextroversion). The anomaly is not associated with situs inversus totalis but can be associated with L (left)-isomerism of the bronchial tree, whereby the right bronchial tree is a mirror image of the left side.

References: Hansell DM, Lynch DA, McAdams, HP, et al. Chapter 16: Congenital anomalies. In: *Imaging of diseases of the chest.* 5th ed. 2009. Elsevier Mosby, 2009:1078–1080.

Lee EY, Boiselle PM, Cleveland RH. Multidetector CT evaluation of congenital anomalies. *Radiology* 2008;247(3):632–648.

Paul S. Radiographic appearance of developmental anomalies of the lung. *UptoDate.* August 10, 2017.

13a **Answer D.**

13b **Answer A.** Unilateral hyperlucency on chest radiograph has a differential primarily related to pulmonary pathology such as pneumothorax, foreign body aspiration with hyperinflation, and congenital anomalies. It is important to remember the contribution of the chest wall to the apparent density of the hemithorax. Just as a unilateral mastectomy can create hyperlucency, the congenital absence of the pectoral muscle in Poland syndrome results in a decrease in x-ray attenuation. Similarly, asymmetry on chest CT may cause one to question a contralateral chest wall mass, when in fact the asymmetry is normal pectoral muscle on one side (the left in this case) and absent pectoral muscle on the affected side.

Reference: Mutlu H, et al. A variant of Poland syndrome associated with dextroposition. *J Thorac Imaging* 2007;22:341–342.

14a **Answer A.**

14b **Answer A.** Congenital interruption of the proximal pulmonary artery occurs despite development of the lung and airways. The provided CT demonstrates normal bifurcation of the trachea with a hypoplastic right lung and no associated right pulmonary artery. The subsequent ventilation perfusion scan further demonstrates functional ventilation of the right lung, but an absence of perfusion. Pulmonary vein atresia can occur but would demonstrate a present right pulmonary artery (usually small) with perfusion on ventilation–perfusion scintigraphy.

Interestingly, the interrupted pulmonary artery typically occurs opposite of the aortic arch, meaning that if the left pulmonary artery is interrupted, the patient will also have a right aortic arch. Interruption of the right pulmonary artery, as seen in this case, is more common and occurs with a normal left aortic arch and generally absence of other congenital anomalies. Patients may present incidentally or have associated symptoms from infection, hemorrhage, or general mild dyspnea. Pulmonary arterial hypertension is a common complication.

References: Castaner E, Gallardo X, Rimola J, et al. Congenital and acquired pulmonary artery anomalies in the adult: radiologic overview. *Radiographics* 2006;26:349–371.

Heyneman LE, Nolan RL, Harrison JK, et al. Congenital unilateral pulmonary vein atresia: radiologic findings in three adult patients. *AJR Am J Roentgenol* 2001;177:681–685.

15a **Answer D.**

15b **Answer C.** The frontal chest radiograph demonstrates a right-sided aortic arch producing a well-defined round opacity right of the trachea with absence of the expected arch shadow left of the trachea and superior to the left pulmonary artery. The subsequent image is selected from an esophagram, demonstrating the impression from the right aortic arch and associated focal narrowing due to the vascular ring from an aberrant left subclavian artery connecting to the left pulmonary artery via the ligamentum arteriosum. The vascular ring results in esophageal narrowing, which causes dysphagia lusoria (related to the Greek phrase lusus naturae and translates to "difficulty swallowing in the freak of nature"), although dysphagia lusoria was originally described in the setting of right aberrant subclavian artery. The other provided clinical presentations are not significantly associated with this congenital anomaly.

A right aortic arch with mirror imaging does not produce a retroesophageal vessel and therefore does not contribute directly to dysphagia or esophageal narrowing, but it does have a high association with congenital heart disease. Duplicate SVC would not explain the absence of a normal aortic arch, would not produce a significant right paratracheal shadow, and would not cause focal narrowing of the esophagus at the level of the aortic arch. Azygos continuation of an interrupted IVC could produce dilatation of the azygos arch and increased opacity in the right paratracheal region, but would not explain the absence of the normal aortic arch nor the esophageal narrowing on esophagram.

Reference: Yilirim A, et al. Congenital thoracic arterial anomalies in adults: a CT overview. *Diagn Interv Radiol* 2011;17:352–362.

16a **Answer A.** On the chest radiograph, the vessels in the right lower lung appear abnormal, which represented displaced vascular structures on the CT scan by the demonstrated multicystic lesion. The contours of the mediastinum, hila, and diaphragm are normal.

16b **Answer A.** Congenital cystic adenomatoid malformation (CCAM) is also known as congenital pulmonary airway malformation (CPAM) and is a developmental malformation of the lower respiratory tract. They are hamartomatous lesions that are made up of cystic and adenomatous elements that arise from tracheal, bronchial, bronchiolar, or alveolar tissue. They have connections with the tracheobronchial tree, although the connecting bronchi are usually not normal.

There are several subtypes of congenital cystic adenomatoid malformation (CCAM) that are based on the presumed site of development of the malformation. Type 0 is the rarest form (1% to 3%) and originates from the tracheal or bronchial tissue. The cysts are small (<0.5 cm). This is a diffuse malformation that involves the entire lung. Affected infants die at birth due to severely impaired gas exchange. Type 1 CCAM is bronchial/bronchiolar in origin and is the most common subtype (60% to 70%) consisting of at least one dominant cyst that is larger than 2 cm in size. The cysts are distinct and thin-walled and can be up to 10 cm. Usually, only one lobe of the lung is involved. Type 2 CCAM (15% to 20%) is bronchiolar in origin and consists of numerous small cysts of uniform size measuring <2 cm in diameter (usually 0.5 to 2 cm). These may appear similar to extralobar sequestrations, though the sequestrations have systemic blood supply. Other congenital anomalies are seen in up to 60% of patients with type 2 CCAM. Type 3 (5% to 10%) is bronchiolar/ alveolar in origin. It is made up of microcysts and appears solid when imaged. They are often large and can involve an entire lobe or several lobes. Due to mass effect, these present in utero or at birth. Type 4 CCAM (5% to 10%) is distal acinar in origin and has cysts with a maximum diameter of 7 cm. They may present at birth or in childhood with pneumothorax. This type of CCAM is strongly associated with malignancy, particularly pleuropulmonary blastoma.

CCAMs can be seen with antenatal ultrasound as either solid or cystic intrathoracic masses. They are sometimes associated with polyhydramnios or nonimmune hydrops fetalis, poor prognostic indicators. Some CCAMs may decrease in size on serial antenatal ultrasound examinations and are associated with more favorable prognosis.

Although CCAM and pulmonary sequestration can have a similar appearance on both chest x-ray and CT, the pulmonary sequestration has systemic arterial supply that can be demonstrated on CT. The arterial supply and venous drainage of CCAMs are almost always from the pulmonary circulation.

References: Hansell DM, Lynch DA, McAdams HP, et al. Chapter 16: Congenital anomalies. In: *Imaging of diseases of the chest*. 5th ed. 2009. Elsevier Mosby, 2009:1078–1080.

Lee EY, Boiselle PM, Cleveland RH. Multidetector CT evaluation of congenital anomalies. *Radiology* 2008;247(3):632–648.

Oermann CM. Congenital pulmonary airway (cystic adenomatoid) malformation. *UpToDate*. 2019.

Sfakianaki AK, Copel JA. Congenital cystic lesions of the lung: congenital cystic adenomatoid malformation and bronchopulmonary sequestration. *Rev Obstet Gynecol* 2012;5(2):85–93.

17a **Answer C.** The chest x-ray and CT show apparent emphysematous changes involving one hemithorax and only one lobe (the left lower lobe), with associated overexpansion of the hemithorax. There is some compressive atelectasis of the adjacent left upper lobe/lingula.

Congenital lobar emphysema (CLE), also known as congenital lobar overinflation, is thought to be due to deficiency/dysplasia/immaturity of bronchial cartilage with resultant check-valve mechanism, leading to diminished flow of air on expiration and progressive hyperexpansion of one or more lobes of the lung. Adjacent lobe(s) may show some compressive atelectasis, as in this case.

In smoking-related emphysema, the changes usually consist of centrilobular emphysematous change, wherein the appearance predominately consists of scattered cystic-appearing lucencies. The primary lesion is produced by dilation and destruction of respiratory bronchioles within a single acinus that become confluent within the lobule. The changes are usually bilateral and upper lung predominant.

Swyer-James-MacLeod syndrome is a form of constrictive bronchiolitis and pulmonary vascular hypoplasia resulting from a viral injury to the developing lung (before the age of 8). It is a cause of hyperlucent hemithorax, but unlike in this case, the hemithorax is decreased in size. The pulmonary vessels on the affected side are also small.

The chest x-ray and CT scan show vessels within the areas of hyperlucency, ruling out a pneumothorax.

17b **Answer B.** Most cases of CLE are diagnosed within the first 6 months of life due to respiratory distress from mass effect on adjacent structures. The abnormality in congenital lobar emphysema is in the bronchial cartilage. The alveoli are overdistended but otherwise normal. A polyalveolar form of CLE has been described, which is clinically identical, but pathologically distinct, consisting of an increased number of nondistended alveoli.

Most cases of CLE involve the left upper lobe, followed by right upper lobe and then right middle lobe. The lower lobes are infrequently affected. The reason for this is unknown.

Congenital lobar emphysema is not a neoplastic condition; therefore, treatment with chemotherapeutic agents is not indicated. Surgical resection of the affected lobe is usually undertaken for infants <2 months of age and patients of any age who are significantly symptomatic.

References: Hansell DM, Lynch DA, McAdams HP, et al. Chapter 16: Congenital anomalies. In: *Imaging of diseases of the chest*. 5th ed. 2009. Elsevier Mosby, 2009:1078–1080.

Lee EY, Boiselle PM, Cleveland RH. Multidetector CT evaluation of congenital anomalies. *Radiology* 2008;247(3):632–648.

Lynch DA, Austin JH, Hogg JC, et al. CT-definable subtypes of chronic obstructive pulmonary disease: a statement of the Fleischner Society. *Radiology* 2015;277(1):192–205.

Wasilewska E, Lee EY, Eisenberg RL. Unilateral hyperlucent lung in children. *AJR Am J Roentgenol* 2012;198:W400–W414.

18 Postoperative Thorax

Jeremiah T. Martin, MBBch, MSCRD, FRSCI

QUESTIONS

1 A 45-year-old lady has fever and leukocytosis 5 days after a right upper lobectomy. Part of her workup includes the CT scan shown. Findings are most consistent with

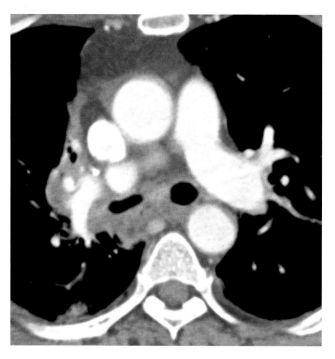 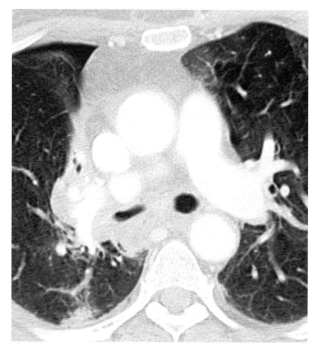

    A. Bronchopleural fistula
    B. Empyema
    C. Lobar torsion
    D. Pneumonia

2   A 78-year-old man underwent pneumonectomy for a central squamous cell carcinoma. Six months postoperatively, his follow-up chest CT is shown demonstrating a significant volume of pleural fluid and diffuse pleural thickening. This pleural fluid most likely represents

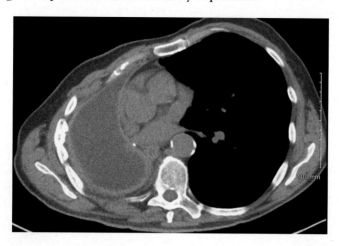

A. Purulent fluid
B. Serous fluid
C. Chylothorax
D. Hemothorax

3   A 24-year-old patient presents for outpatient follow-up after pneumonectomy. Her postoperative course was complicated by bronchial stump dehiscence necessitating reexploration, drainage, and creation of an Eloesser flap. The CT scan below demonstrates an abnormality in the right pleural space, which represents

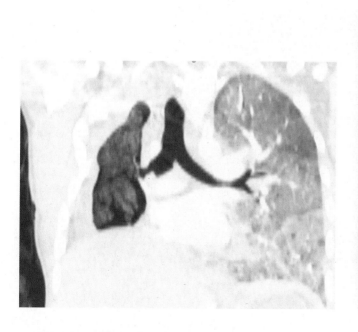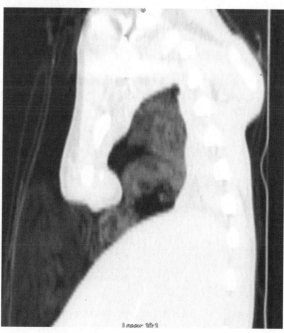

A. *Aspergillus* infection
B. Retained dressing material
C. Muscle flap
D. Blood clot

4   Five years after pneumonectomy, a 62-year-old lady complains of weight loss, worsening wheeze, dysphagia, and acid reflux. Her symptoms, barium swallow, and chest CT (oblique maximum intensity projection images, MIP) are most suggestive of

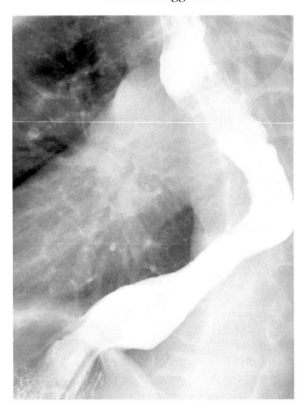

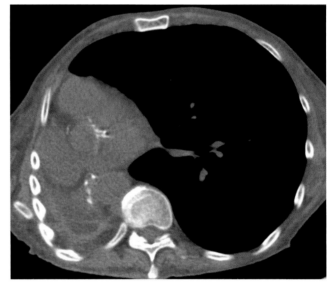

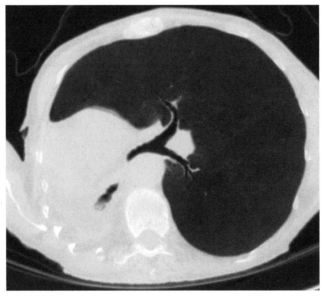

A. Achalasia with aspiration
B. Nutcracker esophagus
C. Postpneumonectomy syndrome
D. Hiatal hernia

5 A tracheal stent has been placed for benign tracheobronchomalacia (TBM) in a patient with COPD. What is the most significant and likely long-term complication of tracheal stent placement in this case?

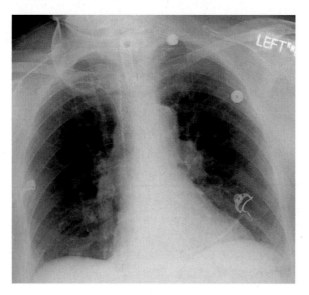

   A. Stent migration
   B. Malposition of tracheostomy
   C. Mucous plug formation
   D. Granulation tissue

6 A 66-year-old lady underwent definitive radiation for a central lung tumor. A long-segment stricture has been treated with an esophageal stent as seen in the x-ray. In the following days, what complication is most likely to occur?

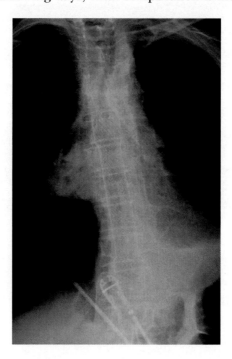

   A. Stent migration
   B. Stent erosion
   C. Stent collapse
   D. Stent occlusion

7   These CT scout films are taken 1 year apart (initial on the left, follow-up on the right) and most likely represent which surgical procedure?

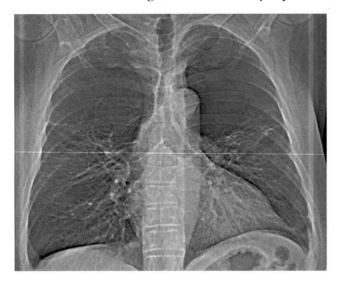 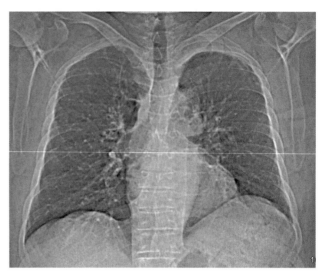

A. Bilateral lung transplant
B. Lung volume reduction surgery
C. Diaphragm plication
D. Pleurodesis

8   A 51-year-old patient returns after surgical treatment for esophageal cancer. He complains of reflux. His CT scan is shown, and findings are suggestive of a(n):

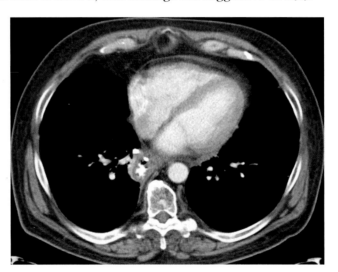

A. Hiatal hernia
B. Normal postoperative appearance
C. Anastomotic stricture
D. Ventral hernia

9 A 39-year-old patient underwent a CT scan in the emergency room for chest pain. He has a recent history of thoracotomy for hiatal hernia. Representative images from the IV contrast CT are shown. Regarding the left hemidiaphragm, the finding most likely represents

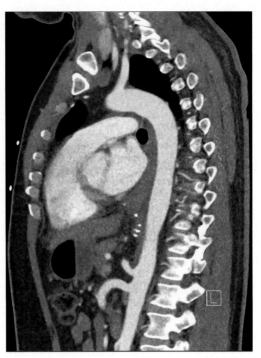

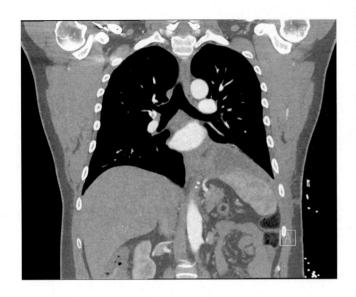

A. Postthoracotomy atelectasis
B. Normal postoperative appearance
C. Failure of hiatal hernia repair
D. Diaphragm paralysis

10 A patient presents with pleuritic chest pain 6 months after a thoracoscopic procedure. CT scan is shown and most likely represents

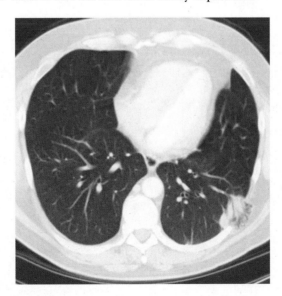

A. Seroma at the surgical site
B. Intercostal lung hernia
C. Osteosarcoma
D. Empyema necessitans

11 This film was obtained in a 58-year-old gentleman who presented to the emergency room with worsening dyspnea. He underwent CABG 1 month previously. Thoracentesis yielded a turbid fluid with resolution of symptoms. The most likely etiology in this case is

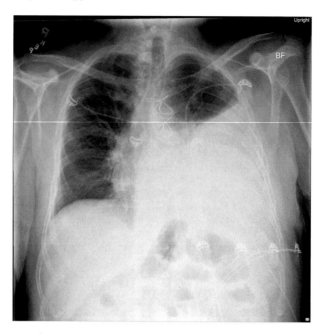

A. Retained hemothorax after IMA harvest
B. Chylothorax
C. Empyema
D. CHF exacerbation with pleural effusion

12 What do these images most likely represent?

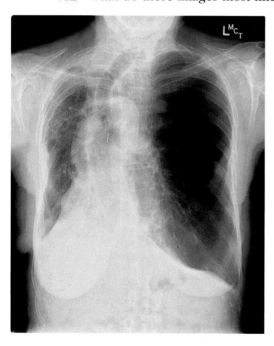
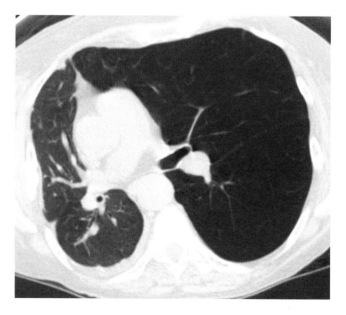

A. Normal right lung, unilateral bullous disease on the left
B. Normal left lung, status post lobectomy on the right
C. Transplanted right lung, hyperinflated native left lung
D. Transplanted left lung, atrophied native right lung

13 A patient who underwent routine CABG 1 month ago presents with new and worsening chest pain. Imaging shown demonstrates

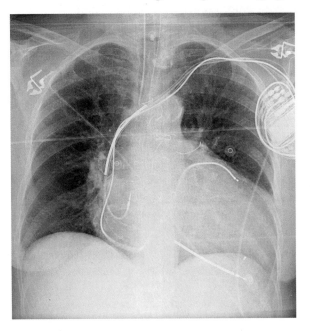
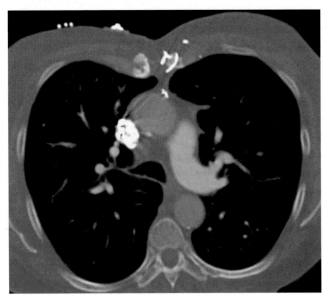

   A. Aortic dissection
   B. Pulmonary embolus
   C. Sternal dehiscence
   D. SVC thrombosis

14 Three months after pacemaker placement, a patient presents with shortness of breath, worse with exertion and leaning forward. Her chest x-ray is shown. Her shortness of breath is most likely due to

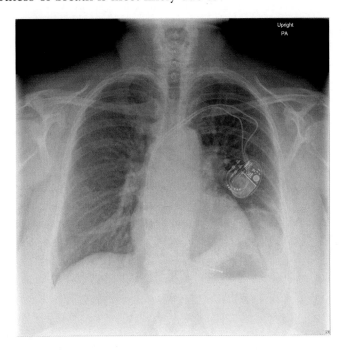

   A. Hiatal hernia
   B. Worsening CHF
   C. Left hemidiaphragm paralysis
   D. Malpositioned pacemaker

15   This x-ray was obtained on the morning after a 64-year-old gentleman underwent a thoracoscopic wedge and talc pleurodesis for secondary spontaneous pneumothorax. He has a history of emphysema with bullae. There are several concerning findings on this film; however, the one most likely correlated with prolonged air leak and potential need for reintervention is

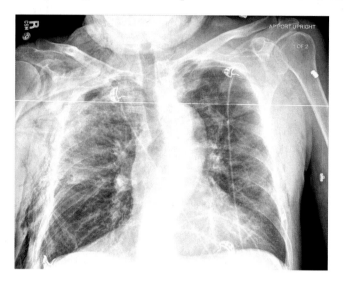

A. Subcutaneous emphysema
B. Chest tube position
C. Partial pneumothorax
D. Diffuse opacity of right upper lung

ANSWERS AND EXPLANATIONS

1 **Answer C.**   Contrast chest CT demonstrates both narrowing of the middle lobe pulmonary artery and bronchial obstruction consistent with a partial torsion. In patients with complete fissures, the middle lobe may have a narrow pedicle, which can rotate partially or completely. During upper or lower lobectomy, intraoperative manipulation of the middle lobe may occasionally cause it to become reinflated in a rotated or torsed configuration. This usually presents with venous congestion of the lobe and signs of inflammation/infection, most commonly 5 to 10 days after the primary procedure. Chest x-ray may demonstrate progressive middle lobe opacity; however, a high index of suspicion is required for correct diagnosis. Contrast CT can confirm the diagnosis with either absence/obstruction of venous and/or arterial flow or focal rotation of hilar structures and associated consolidation/collapse. Delayed diagnosis results in necrosis of the affected lobe necessitating resection. Overall incidence is <0.1% of all pulmonary resections.

Reference: Cable DG, et al. Lobar torsion after pulmonary resection: presentation and outcome. *J Thorac Cardiovasc Surg* 2001;122(6):1091–1093.

2 **Answer B.**   After pneumonectomy, the empty pleural space is gradually obliterated by a sequence of normal changes. Initially, the pleural space fills with fluid with expected complete obliteration and opacification of the chest within 4 weeks of surgery. Skeletal changes include contraction of the intercostal spaces, which may be associated with scoliosis in some patients. Hemidiaphragm elevation and mediastinal repositioning allow almost complete obliteration of the pleural space at 6 months. The remaining lung enlarges and commonly herniates anterior to the heart. The heart is displaced to the side of the pneumonectomy. In an asymptomatic patient, fluid within the pleural space is to be expected and, as this is a sterile collection, should not be manipulated. In contrast, a drop in the pleural fluid volume on successive postoperative chest x-rays should raise suspicion for a bronchopleural fistula.

References: Bazwinsky-Wutschke I, et al. Anatomical changes after pneumonectomy. *Ann Anat* 2011;193(2):168–172.

Smulders SA, et al. Cardiac function and position more than 5 years after pneumonectomy. *Ann Thorac Surg* 2007;83(6):1986–1992.

3 **Answer B.**   An Eloesser flap is used as an intermediate step in the management of a postpneumonectomy bronchopleural fistula. Bronchial stump breakdown is associated with contamination of the pleural space and occurs in upwards of 5% of cases, more commonly on the right. The left-sided bronchial stump is naturally reinforced due to its location beneath the aortic arch. Empyema after pneumonectomy is a challenging problem due to the difficulty of clearing infection in such a large cavity. Open thoracotomy allows for daily dressing changes to promote granulation tissue formation, healing by secondary intention, and preparation of the wound bed for additional attempts at closure. In general, ribs are removed allowing for myocutaneous flap to be sewn to the diaphragm, creating a chronic open cavity. The opacity in this patient's film represents packed dressing material.

References: Miller JI Jr. The history of surgery of empyema, thoracoplasty, Eloesser flap, and muscle flap transposition. *Chest Surg Clin N Am* 2000;10(1):45–53.

Thourani VH, et al. Twenty-six years of experience with the modified Eloesser flap. *Ann Thorac Surg* 2003;76(2):401–406.

4   **Answer C.**   Postpneumonectomy syndrome occurs infrequently in long-term survivors after pneumonectomy and is caused by extreme mediastinal shift after pneumonectomy. The CT scan demonstrates complete rotation of the heart into the right chest and compression of the airway and, in this case esophagus, over the aorta and vertebral column. The most common symptom is progressive central airway obstruction with wheezing. Esophageal obstruction presents with dysphagia as in this case. Mediastinal repositioning is helpful in many of these patients and is generally accomplished with the placement of a Silastic implant in the pneumonectomy bed.

Reference: Avgerinos DV, Meisner J, Harris L. Minimally invasive repair of post-pneumonectomy syndrome. *Thorac Cardiovasc Surg* 2009;57(1):60–62.

5   **Answer D.**   TBM is seen in adults with COPD and results in dynamic airway collapse. Patients who are appropriate risk for surgery should undergo a posterior stabilization of the membranous trachea (tracheoplasty); however, many patients require palliation with a stent. Although stents provide excellent immediate relief (>75%) and may facilitate wean from a ventilator, they are associated with significant long-term complications. All of the listed complications can occur; however, the most significant and likely to occur in the long term is the formation of granulation tissue, which can obstruct the stent and prohibit its removal. The stent shown is a self-expanding metallic stent. Silicone stents are also available and preferred by some surgeons.

Reference: Wright CD. *Optimal management of malacic airway syndromes. Difficult decisions in thoracic surgery.* London, UK: Springer, 2011:363–366.

6   **Answer A.**   Self-expanding esophageal stents are used for both benign and malignant indications. They provide excellent palliation and relief of obstructive symptoms and can restore near-normal ability to swallow for many patients. Unlike the airway, the esophagus in most patients is motile, and peristalsis continues to occur. Various design elements have been introduced to minimize migration; however, distal migration remains the most common early problem with esophageal stents. This can easily be detected on daily x-rays and is more likely to occur when the stent is placed for nonmalignant reasons including perforations and leaks. Endoscopy is required to replace, retrieve, or reposition the stent. Small esophageal leaks and injuries can be treated conservatively with stenting: a recent review demonstrated a 76% clinical success rate in carefully selected patients, which can obviate the need to perform an extensive surgery. However, of the above complications, migration is the most common.

Reference: van Boeckel PG, et al. Fully covered self-expandable metal stents (SEMS), partially covered SEMS and self-expandable plastic stents for the treatment of benign esophageal ruptures and anastomotic leaks. *BMC Gastroenterol* 2012;12(1):19.

7   **Answer B.**   Although transplant would result in replacement of the diseased parenchyma, this patient still has some evidence of bullae in the right medial lung, and there are no sternal wires that should be seen with a transverse sternotomy (clamshell) as is typically performed for bilateral transplantation. LVRS is a good option for patients such as this who have end-stage lung disease, characterized by nonhomogeneous emphysema and preserved exercise tolerance. The National Emphysema Treatment Trial (NETT) found no advantage to LVRS versus medical therapy in terms of survival in patients with homogeneous emphysema (emphysema distributed diffusely in the craniocaudal plane). However, the risk ratio of death was 0.47 in the surgically treated group with nonhomogeneous emphysema such as this patient (upper lung predominant emphysema). In essence, removal of the hyperinflated, nonperfused, apical segments allows for expansion and recruitment of functionally collapsed basilar segments and can be an effective bridge to transplant in select patients.

Reference: Fishman A, et al. A randomized trial comparing lung-volume-reduction surgery with medical therapy for severe emphysema. *N Engl J Med* 2003;348(21):2059–2073.

8 **Answer B.**   Surgery for esophageal cancer generally consists of esophagectomy and reconstruction with a gastric conduit. The stomach is stapled parallel to the greater curvature to separate this gastric tube from the GE junction and tumor, and the conduit is then passed along the esophageal bed to anastomose with the proximal esophagus. The anastomosis may be performed in the neck or in the chest (commonly referred to as Ivor Lewis). This CT scan demonstrates a contrast-filled gastric tube in the esophageal bed, which is appropriately sized, with no evidence of rotation or hernia. Chest CT is not ideal for evaluation of any anastomotic stricture, which is better visualized with barium swallow or esophagoscopy.

Reference: Rubesin SE, Williams NN. Postoperative esophagus. In: Gore RM, Levine MS (eds.). *Textbook of gastrointestinal radiology*. Philadelphia, PA: W.B. Saunders, 2000:449–461.

9 **Answer B.**   Thoracotomy for hiatal hernia is oftentimes a procedure of last resort and in the current era may be performed by general thoracic surgeons in the treatment of multiply failed or recurrent hiatal hernia. Interpretation of these images can be challenging, and reconstructions are helpful to understand landmarks. In this case, the patient continues to enjoy a successful repair, and the pain was due to intercostal neuralgia after thoracotomy. Nevertheless, left-sided pain will commonly result in an exhaustive workup. The transthoracic fundoplication is often referred to by its eponym, the Belsey fundoplication. This operation is useful in providing the surgeon access to new tissue planes—it is less constrained by the need to lengthen the esophagus as the diaphragmatic hiatus is completely mobilized and resutured to the esophagogastric junction. Careful review of the sagittal views in this case demonstrates suture material at the GE junction, with no stomach above the line of the diaphragm. Differential diagnosis should of course include diaphragm paralysis and volume loss, which are known postthoracotomy complications.

Reference: Pennathur A, et al. Chapter 17: Transthoracic fundoplication: belsey fundoplication. In: Khatri VP (ed.). *Atlas of advanced operative surgery*. Elsevier, 2019:134–139.

10 **Answer B.**   The image demonstrates herniation of a portion of the lung parenchyma with opacification suggestive of strangulation. Lung hernias are an uncommon complication of thoracic surgery and may be entirely asymptomatic, present as a bulge that moves with respiration, or be associated with pleurisy or signs of infection. Counterintuitively, they may be more likely to occur due to modern minimally invasive techniques as the thoracic ports are not closed with pericostal suture in the same way that a thoracotomy is closed. Management of the majority of cases is purely observational; however, a case of strangulated parenchyma as shown may require revision, resection of involved lung, and patch repair of the defect.

The abnormality shown is not fluid density, and therefore, a seroma is incorrect. Additionally, there is abnormality of opacified lung, not a chest wall mass, making osteosarcoma incorrect. Empyema necessitans refers to a pleural infection that erodes through the parietal pleura and into the chest wall, especially in the setting of tuberculosis empyema.

Reference: Bhamidipati CM, et al. Lung hernia following robotic-assisted mitral valve repair. *J Cardiac Surg* 2012;27(4):460–463.

11 Answer B.   Unilateral effusion after CABG is not uncommon. The internal mammary artery graft is a key component of surgical coronary revascularization. It is mobilized from the chest wall along its length, which creates the potential for left-sided postoperative issues. Accumulation of shed blood in the left pleural space will result in a left effusion, which may require thoracentesis: this occurs 1 to 2 weeks after surgery when the shed blood completes hemolysis and fluid accumulates in the hyperosmolar environment. Less commonly, injury to the thoracic duct or phrenic nerve during harvest in the thoracic inlet can lead to left-sided issues. This patient was found to have a chylothorax as evidenced by the turbid fluid on thoracentesis. This responded to drainage, NPO, and octreotide and did not require further surgical intervention. A CHF exacerbation is also a common cause for post-CABG effusions, but this would generally be bilateral.

Reference: Kilic D, et al. Octreotide for treating chylothorax after cardiac surgery. *Tex Heart Inst J* 2005;32(3):437.

12 Answer C.   Hyperinflation of the native lung may be seen in COPD patients who receive a single-lung transplant. Mediastinal shift is unlikely after lobectomy, and the different appearance of the parenchyma in both lung fields suggests the presence of a transplant. Unilateral constrictive bronchiolitis such as from prior infection (Swyer-James) is a consideration but considerably less likely given the severity of the abnormality present.

Due to loss of elasticity and destruction of alveoli in the COPD lung, Laplace law explains the overinflation that occurs from decreased surface tension in the native alveoli versus the transplanted lung. Progressive hyperinflation of the remaining native emphysematous lung can compromise function of the transplanted lung, and some of these patients must undergo a staged sequential transplant as a result. As such, bilateral lung transplant is favored for COPD. Single-lung transplantation is reserved for non-COPD patients or for the occasional older COPD patient who would benefit from transplant but would be less likely to be allocated a double graft based on lung allocation score.

Reference: Motoyama H, et al. Quantitative evaluation of native lung hyperinflation after single lung transplantation for emphysema using three-dimensional computed tomography volumetry. *Transplant Proc* 2014;46(3):941–943.

13 Answer C.   Sternal dehiscence is a feared complication after cardiac surgery. Routine closure of the sternotomy is performed with sternal wires, and alternative devices are also available such as metallic plates. On chest x-ray, notice the fracture of multiple sternal wires, which are displaced to opposite sides. On CT, the patient appears to have a broken sternal wire with separation of the sternal edges. Fractured sternal wires in isolation are frequently seen as an incidental finding. It is the lateral displacement that is worrisome for dehiscence.

Dehiscence is strongly associated with both diabetes and morbid obesity. One study of this issue in US patients demonstrated a rate of dehiscence of almost 7% in morbidly obese patients (BMI > 30) compared with 1.6% in nonobese patients. The occurrence of dehiscence was associated with infection and mediastinitis in 96% of patients and carried a 40% mortality. Management generally requires débridement, delayed wound closure, and myocutaneous flap interposition in many cases.

Reference: Molina JE, Lew RS, Hyland KJ. Postoperative sternal dehiscence in obese patients: incidence and prevention. *Ann Thorac Surg* 2004;78(3):912–917.

14 Answer C.   Hemidiaphragm paralysis will present with worsening dyspnea and is exacerbated by patient positioning. Although many cases are unexplained, the course of the phrenic nerve makes it vulnerable to injury during many thoracic surgical procedures. Although very unusual, this case involved percutaneous access of the subclavian vein and either hematoma or instrumentation in the vicinity of the medial thoracic inlet resulted in compromise of the left phrenic nerve. Acute denervation of the diaphragm does not immediately result in elevation. However, as the muscle stretches over time, the radiographic appearance and symptoms become more prominent. In cases of nerve injury rather than transection, recovery may occur in several months. Symptoms are due mostly to paradoxical motion, which limits the ability of the patient to generate negative intrathoracic pressure for inspiration. This is best visualized under diaphragm fluoroscopy ("sniff test"). Plication provides significant relief and may be performed via transabdominal or transthoracic approaches.

Reference: Zwischenberger BA, et al. Laparoscopic robot-assisted diaphragm plication. *Ann Thorac Surg* 2016;101(1):369–371.

15 **Answer C.** Partial pneumothorax in this case is of concern as it represents failure of pleural apposition. Pleurodesis with/without wedge resection is performed to minimize recurrence risk for patients with spontaneous pneumothorax. The goal is to fuse the visceral and parietal pleura, such that if a future source of air leak develops (ruptured bleb), the lung cannot collapse. Pleurodesis may be achieved by mechanical abrasion, or chemical means that include talc and doxycycline. Talc can result in an intense inflammatory reaction in the pleura, which can appear as a diffuse opacity. This patient has radiographic signs of a persistent air leak with subcutaneous emphysema extending along the chest wall, into the neck, and outlining the pectoralis musculature. Subcutaneous emphysema, although alarming for staff and patient, is rarely of clinical significance and usually self-limiting. In this case, however, the persistent pneumothorax places the patient at significant risk for persistent bronchopleural fistula and failure of pleurodesis. The chest tube appears appropriately positioned after surgery. However if applying or increasing suction to the chest tube does not resolve the pneumothorax, an additional chest tube may be needed to facilitate lung expansion. Severe air leaks may require a reoperation.

Reference: Jeon HW, et al. Air leakage on the postoperative day: powerful factor of postoperative recurrence after thoracoscopic bullectomy. *J Thorac Dis* 2016;8(1):93.

Note: Page numbers followed by *f* indicate figures.